THERAPEUTIC
REVOLUTIONS

Other books by Martin Halliwell

Romantic Science and the Experience of Self (1999)

Modernism and Morality (2001)

republished as *Transatlantic Modernism* (2006)

Critical Humanisms: Humanist/Anti-Humanist Dialogues (2003)

(with Andy Mousley)

Images of Idiocy: The Idiot Figure in Modern Fiction and Film (2004)

The Constant Dialogue: Reinhold Niebuhr and American Intellectual Culture (2005)

American Culture in the 1950s (2007)

American Thought and Culture in the 21st Century (2008)

(edited with Catherine Morley)

Beyond and Before: Progressive Rock since the 1960s (2011)

(with Paul Hegarty)

William James and the Transatlantic Conversation (forthcoming)

(edited with Joel Rasmussen)

THERAPEUTIC REVOLUTIONS

Medicine, Psychiatry, and American Culture, 1945–1970

MARTIN HALLIWELL

RUTGERS UNIVERSITY PRESS

New Brunswick, New Jersey, and London

First paperback edition, 2014

Library of Congress Cataloging-in-Publication Data

Halliwell, Martin.

Therapeutic revolutions : medicine, psychiatry, and American culture, 1945–1970 / Martin Halliwell.

p.   cm.

Includes bibliographical references and index.

ISBN 978–0–8135–6064–9 (hardcover : alk. paper) — ISBN 978–0–8135–6065–6 (pbk. : alk. paper) — ISBN 978–0–8135–6066–3 (e-book)

I. Title.

[DNLM: 1. Mental Disorders—history—United States.   2. History, 20th Century—United States.   3. Mental Disorders—therapy—United States.   4. Psychiatry—history—United States.   5. Social Conditions—United States.   6. Therapeutics—history—United States. WM 11 AA1]

362.19689—dc23

2012023503

A British Cataloging-in-Publication record for this book is available from the British Library.

Visit our website: http://rutgerspress.rutgers.edu

Manufactured in the United States of America

Contents

Illustrations

Preface

The cultural history of mental illness in the United States since World War II is marked by both progress and stasis. This doubling is perhaps best illustrated by a brief opening discussion of the anti stigma campaigns of 1999—a year that witnessed the first annual report on mental health by the US surgeon general and, on 7 June, a White House Conference on Mental Health. The opening speaker, First Lady Hillary Rodham Clinton, argued that such a conference could not have happened a decade earlier, let alone in the 1960s or 1970s; she thanked the vice president's wife, Tipper Gore, for her energetic work in the field of healthcare, and called for a national anti-stigma campaign to dispel some of the deeply ingrained myths that continued to inform contemporary conceptions of mental illness.[1]

The White House initiative was an extension of the "Open the Doors" campaign of three years earlier, when the World Psychiatric Association had begun a global program against stigma and discrimination, providing a transnational framework for Tipper Gore and the American Psychiatric Association to argue strongly for parity legislation for the treatment of physical and mental illness. This liberal agenda also chimed with Secretary of Health and Human Services Donna E. Shalala's claim that "mental health is absolutely essential to achieving prosperity."[2] Rather than reinforcing the hegemony of the pharmaceutical industry, Shalala argued in 1999 for the need to combine "safe and potent medications" with "psychosocial interventions" to "allow us to effectively treat most mental disorders" and to educate professionals, mental health sufferers, and the public alike. This agenda was also evident in a spring 2001 conference sponsored by the Substance Abuse and Mental Health Services Administration and a campaign by the World Health Organization in the same year. These initiatives were part of a wave of activity at the turn of the millennium, of which the White House Conference was the most public face.[3]

Despite the historical importance of the 1999 White House Conference, government agendas do not always—and perhaps rarely—map neatly onto social realities. In September 1993 the *New York Times* proclaimed that President Bill Clinton's health security proposal was "Alive on Arrival," only to backtrack a year later, and President Barack Obama has had to deal with as many thorny political and public issues in the move toward national health insurance as Presidents Harry S. Truman, Lyndon B. Johnson, and Clinton before him.[4] The post–World War II story of American medicine is associated closely with presidential attempts to offer a model of responsible governance for healthcare; however, the oscillation between idealism and realism, dreams and pragmatism is woven into the fabric of American life, often creating a "boomerang" effect, as Theda Skocpol has called it. The fierce debates over the 2010 Affordable Care Act (sometimes pejoratively referred to as Obamacare) make clear that this boomerang effect is particularly pertinent for healthcare because medical policy is full of proactive and reactive decisions, plans that work and plans that don't, debates that are hard (or impossible) to win, and budgets that cannot be balanced. Skocpol noted in the mid-1990s that many Americans have grown skeptical about the promises of the federal government and sense that "government institutions are less likely than ever to produce effective and democratically inclusive solutions to pressing national problems."[5] Even in the mid-1940s there was a backlash to President Truman's earnest attempt to reform the healthcare system, a failure that troubled him throughout his administration. Although there have been great medical reforms and breakthroughs since then, the same rhythms of proposition and resistance to healthcare reform are still embedded in American political and civic life, leading Michael F. Hogan, Chairman of President George W. Bush's New Freedom Commission on Mental Health, to assert in 2003 that the "mental health care system is a patchwork relic—the result of disjointed reforms and policies."[6]

The surgeon general's first report on mental health makes salutary reading, not least because the debates about mental health, social stigma, and therapy had not moved very far since the mid-1960s, when Hillary Clinton was a student at Wellesley College. Although the report was able to draw on relatively sophisticated medical nomenclature, it circled around a set of debates similar to those of the years following World War II. In the 1963 book *Stigma,* for example, the sociologist Erving Goffman argued that, on the one hand, medical categories are far too rigid but, on the other hand, they can easily elide disparate conditions. Rather than examining illness, disease, and disability solely through a medical lens, Goffman took his readers beyond public policy and institutional regulation to investigate the sociological implications of stigma and what it means to be unwell in America. He argued that stigma needs to be placed within a broader sociocultural framework to understand the mechanisms that mark sick and disabled individuals as different from members of the dominant group, and that subjects them to surveillance (in most instances) or institutionalization (for severe cases).[7] As we will see in the first two sections of this book, even though the twin emphasis of Presidents Truman and Dwight D. Eisenhower on biomedical knowledge and better hospital care reinforced the joint responsibility of government and medicine, it did little to uncouple medical conditions from their moral status in the postwar period.

We might want to align Goffman's account of widespread misconceptions about mental illness with fears of the outsider during the Cold War, but a third of a century later, Rosalynn Carter, the former First Lady, was arguing that comparable forms of stigma were still evident. Published a year before the 1999 White House conference, Carter's *Helping Someone with Mental Illness* stemmed from three decades of efforts to inject funds into mental health, on which she had begun working during Jimmy Carter's campaign for governor of Georgia in 1970, and which later influenced the President's Commission on Mental Health, established by President Carter in

February 1977. In her 1998 book, Rosalynn Carter illustrates the ongoing hostility toward and stigma of mental illness by citing the case of Missouri Senator Thomas Eagleton, who was forced to withdraw as Democratic vice presidential nominee in 1972 when it became known that he had been voluntarily hospitalized for "nervous exhaustion."[8] The Democratic presidential nominee, George McGovern, initially said he would back Eagleton "1000 percent," only to renege on his promise when news of his running mate's hospitalization became public. Carter does not offer a parallel example from the late 1990s, but Tipper Gore's anti-stigma campaign and testimonies from prominent figures like the actor Rod Steiger about long-standing depression are evidence of continuing concerns over the public understanding of mental illness. As a consequence, the subtitle of Goffman's book, *Notes on the Management of Spoiled Identity*, not only reflects broader discourses in the early 1960s concerning the "injuries" or "damage" that mental illness can exact on the individual, but it also provides a broader historical context for the 1999 report of the surgeon general, David Satcher.

Satcher began the report by claiming that the physical health of the nation "has never been better," but when it came to mental illness "the mind remain[s] shrouded in fear and misunderstanding," only a little more informed, in fact, than in 1963, when the Health Information Foundation concluded that "our knowledge of this terribly difficult problem remains at best scanty."[9] Entitled *Health Progress in the United States: 1900–1960*, that earlier report focused on hospitalized cases of mental illness, but Satcher estimated that at the turn of the century, mental illness accounted for about 15 percent of "the overall burden of disease"—slightly more than diseases such as cancer and, in terms of years lost to premature death, substantially greater than respiratory conditions, alcohol and drug use, and infectious diseases.[10] Perhaps for this reason, Satcher contended that research into physical and mental health has never been granted equal priority.

The surgeon general argued that the "destructive split" between mental and physical health could be remedied only by new research into the causes and treatment of mental illness that would reposition it at the center of healthcare. He realized that the barriers to understanding were both educational and institutional, and as much financial as medical, especially as at the time forty-four million (or one in six) Americans lacked health insurance. For strategic reasons Satcher did not call for massive financial investment, but rather "the willingness of each of us to educate ourselves [and] confront the attitudes, fear, and misunderstanding that remain as barriers before us." Moreover, because brain disease can lead to both mental disorders (of thought, behavior, mood) and somatic disorders (of movement, touch, balance), and because it varies depending on genetics and environment, he argued that health and illness should be seen "as points along a continuum," in which "neither state exists in pure isolation from the other."[11] Thus, Satcher sought to replace the mind-body binary model with a holistic understanding of illness as affecting the whole person.

As the third section of this book explores, holistic discourses came to prominence in the United States in the mid-1960s. Holism was influenced by a wave of European émigrés who worked in the social sciences and were well versed in existential ideas, but it was also shaped by progressive forms of homegrown psychiatric practice that steered away from the normative medical categories that were common in the 1950s. More recently, Anne Harrington has argued that the mind-body split has been a weakness in modern medicine, leading to therapeutic shortcomings and what she calls "existential deficiency," while Charles Rosenberg characterizes the holistic model as a reaction "against the categorical claims of the mechanistic reductionist style of medical explanation."[12] However, although holistic methods assess how illness is embodied within the full range of an individual's experience, Rosenberg reminds us that "holism challenges precise definition" and can often lead to woolly thinking rather than sharp analysis.[13] These rival models of dualism and holism have deep roots in European and North American history but are particularly pertinent for considering health in the period covered by this book: from World War II to the end of the 1960s.

Across the three sections of this work, I pursue these ideas through a study of the twenty-five years between 1945 and the dawn of the 1970s, developing Goffman's sense that a broad sociocultural framework is necessary to do justice to the ways in which medical ideas and practice have an impact on a wide spectrum of experience. Rather than seeing medicine as a circumscribed profession, Goffman realized that the abstract terms "health" and "illness" need to be positioned within broader historical, social, and cultural contexts. Without these reference points, we are left with a specialized scientific and diagnostic language that ignores both the intersections between medicine and culture and the complex social interactions that shape perceptions of illness. It is these issues that my account of the therapeutic revolutions of the postwar period tackles, by combining discussions of subjects that range from national politics, public reports, and healthcare debates with the ways in which culture and the media provide channels for exploring, shaping, and challenging preconceptions about health and illness. Although my primary focus is mental health, I try to capture the spirit of the surgeon general's 1999 report by arguing that mental and physical health need to be brought together holistically, yet without sacrificing precision.

Acknowledgments

I am extremely grateful for the generous support I have been given in all its many forms over the last six years. First, I would like to thank the University of Leicester, the Wellcome Trust, and the British Association for American Studies for providing the financial resources that has made possible my frequent visits to libraries and archives. I am also indebted to the Rothermere American Institute at the University of Oxford, where I was Senior Research Fellow in 2007 (when this project was in its infancy) and Associate Fellow 2008–2013, and I would like to acknowledge the support of the previous and current directors of the institute, Paul Giles and Nigel Bowles.

I have presented papers relating to this project at a range of conferences and symposia, and I am lucky to have received very helpful feedback on each occasion. Among these were papers at the University of Oxford, University of Exeter, University of Nottingham, University of East Anglia, University of London, University of Manchester, Trinity College Dublin, and University of Cambridge, and a keynote lecture sponsored by the Eccles Centre at the British Library and presented at the 2012 European Association for American Studies Conference, "The Health of the Nation," at Ege University, in Izmir, Turkey. I would particularly like to thank the following friends and colleagues for their help and encouragement throughout this project: Erica Arthur, Robert Burgess, James Campbell, Julie Coleman, Tom Coogan, Sue Currell, Philip Davies, Alex Dunst, Nick Everett, Andrew Fearnley, Jacqueline Foertsch, Richard Foulkes, Corinne Fowler, Holly Furneaux, Jo Gill, Sarah Graham, Paul Hegarty, Michael Hoar, John Horne, Michelle Houston, Joel Isaac, Andrew Johnstone, Rob Jones, Emma Kimberley, Richard King, Sarah Knight, Peter Kuryla, George Lewis, Daniel Matlin, Catherine Morley, Andy Mousley, Michael O'Brien, Joel Rasmussen, Mark Rawlinson, Annette Saddik, Emma Staniland, Douglas Tallack, Robin Vandome, and Alex Waddan. I am deeply grateful, as always, to Laraine for being there through the many ups and downs of this project—and to my cousin Kathryn who is no longer here, but who will always be with me. I also pay tribute to the life of my grandmother, Ida Halliwell (1914–2011), who was knowledgeable on so many subjects and with whom I shared a birthday.

I would like to thank the librarians and archivists who have assisted me at the Archives of the History of American Psychology at Akron University; the Lister Hill Library at the University of Alabama at Birmingham; the Helen McLean Library at the Chicago Institute for Psychoanalysis; the Duke University Medical Center Library; the Woodruff Health Sciences Center Library at Emory University; the Library of Congress; the Menninger Historic Psychiatry Collection at the Kansas Historical

Society, Topeka; the National Library of Medicine; the Abraham A. Brill Library of the New York Psychoanalytic Society; the Fondren Library and Texas Medical Center Library at Rice University; Lane Medical Library at Stanford University; the Film and Television Archive and the Louise M. Darling Biomedical Library, both at the University of California, Los Angeles; the Jean and Alexander Heard Library at Vanderbilt University; the Center for Film and Theater Research at the Wisconsin Historical Society, Madison; the Vere Harmsworth Library at the Rothermere American Institute, University of Oxford; and the Wellcome Trust Library, London. I would like to extend my thanks to Peter Mickulas at Rutgers University Press for being such a supportive commissioning editor, and to the Wisconsin Center for Film and Theater Research and the Herb Block Foundation for generously granting me permission to include some fantastic illustrations. All figures are courtesy of the Wisconsin Center for Film and Theater Research, except figures 5.1 and 6.1, which are courtesy of the Herb Block Foundation.

Sections of the first part of this book have been published in shorter forms in the following publications: the *Journal of Literary and Cultural Disability 3*, no. 2 (2009); the *Journal of American Studies 44*, no. 2 (2010); *The Edinburgh Companion to Twentieth-Century British and American War Literature,* edited by Adam Piette and Mark Rawlinson (Edinburgh University Press, 2012); and the British Library pamphlet "Therapeutic Communities and Community Health Care in 1960s America" (2013).

THERAPEUTIC
REVOLUTIONS

Introduction

THE THERAPEUTIC REVOLUTIONS
OF POSTWAR AMERICA

In this book I want to test two contradictory arguments that raise searching questions about the historical conceptions of illness, health, and medical knowledge. The first argument is that social understanding of health, particularly mental health, has developed considerably since the 1960s—thanks to more specific nomenclature, greater sensitivity to stigma, and better access to public healthcare facilities—and that moral and medical categories are now rarely confused. The second argument is that, despite the healthcare proposals of a number of postwar American presidents, the medical and public understanding of illness—especially mental illness—has not advanced significantly since the middle of the twentieth century, with debates about stigma in the 1990s focused on a cluster of issues similar to those that the sociologist Erving Goffman was tackling in the 1960s.

To explore these two positions I examine discourses of illness, health, and therapy as they evolved in the twenty-five years following World War II, through intersecting perspectives that bring the histories of medicine, psychiatry, and psychology together with different strains of intellectual and cultural history. The central focus in the book is on mental health, but I want to examine its historical evolution with respect to physical illness, cognitive disorders, and disability in order to map broader patterns in American thought and culture. My scope is national, but I zoom in on particular issues, medical conditions, and regional examples to show that the story of postwar American healthcare is a multilayered narrative that involves issues of patient care, institutional provision, and medication; relationships among doctors, patients, and communities; and theories, images, and stories of selfhood. In order to untangle these issues and better understand the cultural politics of therapy, I discuss a range of medical accounts and social-scientific studies published between 1945 and 1970, alongside an analysis of how illness is represented in postwar film, fiction, poetry, television, and journalism.

In this book I take "illness" to mean a single diagnosable condition or a number of related factors (biological, psychological, physiological, or social) that unsettle an individual's balance, in contrast to the World Health Organization's definition of health as "a state of complete, physical, mental, and social well-being."[1] Illness is thus used as a descriptive rather than a normative category, sometimes objectively visible but always subjectively felt.[2] As such, illness rests on the fulcrum between the public world of policy and medical treatment and the private world of cognition, emotion, and somatic response. In order to explore this fulcrum, I discuss a range of historical examples, analyzing individual experiences through case studies, clinical records, and a variety of narratives. At heart, the book does not conceive of medicine as a sealed sphere of activity and inquiry; rather, it adopts a panoramic quarter-century perspective on the medical humanities in order to tell a national story of illness as a central facet of American life.

In the following chapters, I show how certain social and medical realities that arose in the 1940s drove the postwar reconceptualization of illness in two opposing directions, characterized by successive historical phases. The first direction looked outward to scientific institutions and biomedical expertise for dealing with illness and was emphasized throughout the Eisenhower administration; the second put the therapeutic needs of individuals and groups above psychiatric and medical controls and was most visible during the 1960s. The rise of a normative model of health in the 1950s and the emphasis on statistics, technology, and the laboratory were key elements in the first phase. In contrast, the second phase featured links to broader ideas of holism, community, and pluralism; was more sensitive to the subjective experience of illness; and had more faith in the patient's self-knowledge and resilience. It is tempting to describe these two phases as conservative (1950s) and liberal (1960s), with the first phase's dogmatic faith in scientific and medical authorities challenged by the more inclusive humanistic understandings of health and illness in the second phase. But, as the following chapters discuss, the ideological implications are more complex than this binary split suggests, with different ideas and practices, thinkers and reformers, and private and state institutions competing to be heard above the many voices of therapy.

The title of this book, *Therapeutic Revolutions*, self-consciously echoes two volumes published in 1979, but with two crucial differences: the first in terms of my historical focus and the second in respect to the revolution itself. The first of the 1979 volumes, *The Therapeutic Revolution: Essays in the Social History of American Medicine*, edited by Morris Vogel and Charles Rosenberg, locates the upheaval in medical and therapeutic practices within the nineteenth century as "the gradual triumph of a critical spirit over ancient obscurantism." The second book, Leon Chertok and Raymond de Saussure's *The Therapeutic Revolution, from Mesmer to Freud* (originally published in French in 1973), focuses on the "psychoanalytic revolution" of the early twentieth century—when Freudian thought, like Einstein's 1905 theory of relativity, turned conventional wisdom on its head.[3] This second study proposes that the late nineteenth century and the early twentieth witnessed the growth of clinical psychology, psychiatry, and psychoanalysis as independent fields of inquiry represented by professional associations. However, I propose here that the most significant therapeutic revolution in the United States occurred after World War II and had a more complex trajectory than Chertok and de Saussure credit. This was partly due to the increased public awareness of medical and psychological ideas and practices via a range of popular media, and partly due to the writings of a wave of European émigré thinkers who helped to revolutionize how medical and social-scientific knowledge was understood and applied. Freud was the obvious intellectual resource for postwar thinkers and writers, but the various and conflicting ways in which Freudian ideas were deployed—from the conservative belief that an individual cannot transcend his or her instincts to a radical sexual philosophy tinged with anarchism—reveals an ideologically complex terrain in which "revolution" is a deeply contested term.

Nevertheless, medical institutional change was slow to come about. Charles Rosenberg points outs that "the inertia of traditional practice" in Europe and the United States "was powerful indeed," with physicians and clinicians seeking "to ensure the greatest possible degree of continuity with old ideas."[4] Rosenberg looks back to the mid-nineteenth century, when the normative concept of health began to replace the idea of health as a "natural state" and started to be defined in terms of population norms and within the framework of laboratory science.[5] This moment also saw the formation of what was to quickly become the official voice of medicine, the American Medical Association, which was established in 1847 and promoted in its 1884 "Code of Medical Ethics" a strict medical training in "anatomy, physiology, pathology and organic chemistry."[6] Forced to compete with a variety of nonprofessional practices and quackery that flourished throughout the nineteenth century, the association focused in the early years of the twentieth century on facilitating the development of better training schools and the improving of medical standards. But, although laboratory research and specialized knowledge became increasingly important for the medical profession, questions about the limits of empirical science persisted. This led to a range of experiments with medication and therapeutic techniques at the turn of the century that, as Chertok and de Saussure discuss, "far from being restricted in its effects to the field of medicine, came to exert an influence in every area of contemporary culture."[7]

However, I would argue that neither of these periods (the second half of the nineteenth century and the early twentieth century) represented a full-scale revolution in the therapeutics of everyday life—at least not in the United States. This is not to say, however, that significant cultural developments did not occur, many of which reached beyond Freud. Although Freud was skeptical about the United States and traveled there only once, a number of American thinkers in the 1890s and 1900s (including Silas Weir Mitchell, William James, G. Stanley Hall, and George Santayana) offered a series of medical and behaviorist insights that resonated with Freudian ideas but also ranged widely across the sciences and humanities, drawing in other elements of European and American thought. This transatlantic mode was extended further after World War II by the wave of émigré thinkers who arrived in the 1930s and 1940s—among them Theodor Adorno, Max Horkheimer, Erik Erikson, Otto Rank, Bruno Bettelheim, Erich Fromm, Herbert Marcuse, and Frederick Perls— and who applied a combination of clinical, existential, and social ideas to their new environment. These émigrés were not alone, though, as the influential Menninger family from Topeka, Kansas; the psychiatrist Harry Stack Sullivan; the sociologist David Riesman; and the self-styled radical Paul Goodman provided fresh approaches to human motivation and behavior. The influence of Freudian psychoanalysis cannot be denied, but American therapeutic currents are more complicated than simply tracing a Freudian lineage, from his only visit to the United States, in 1909, to the advertising work of his nephew Edward Bernays in the 1920s and 1930s; and from Hollywood's and Broadway's love affairs with psychoanalysis in the late 1940s to Woody Allen's films of the 1970s.[8]

In making a claim for the importance of the postwar years in this therapeutic revolution, the 1930s and early 1940s can be seen as a central point. James Capshew points out that the number of American psychologists grew tenfold, from three hundred to three thousand between 1919 and 1939, and World War II brought another increase. In addition, the number of newly professionalized clinical psychologists and members of the American Psychiatric Association (APA) grew rapidly after the war, with many registered psychiatrists geared to treating combat fatigue and other war-related conditions.[9] The publication of the *Diagnostic and Statistical Manual of Mental Disorders* in 1952 was a concerted effort on behalf of the APA to codify the various and often confusing symptoms linked to the experience of war, thereby substantially revising the War Department Technical Bulletin, Medical 203, issued in 1943. Beyond the front line, psychologists and psychoanalysts were engaged in their own methodological battles: analysts started to argue between themselves, and psychologists, intent on emphasizing the supremacy of science, placed greater emphasis on statistical methods, practical application, and scientific instrumentation.[10] Still, despite the supreme confidence that many had in science and medicine, the number of cases of combat fatigue during World War II indicated that the nation, which seemed purposeful and prosperous on the surface, underneath suffered from uncertainty and anxiety. This was emphasized after the war when veterans, some diagnosed as ill or permanently disabled, struggled to reintegrate into civilian society while facing deep-seated structural problems in their working and domestic lives. And not just personal and family health were at stake. The ideological cauldron of the Cold War into which medicine and psychiatry were thrown and another hot war in Korea, where experiments with consciousness-altering drugs and "thought reform" were widespread, revealed a world in which medical hopes were compromised by the difficulty of distinguishing beneficial from harmful therapy.

Trends did not change sharply in the late 1940s and 1950s, despite the fact that the membership of the APA grew rapidly in the first half of the 1950s.[11] Indeed, in a national symposium on healthcare held in New York City in October 1961, the pragmatist philosopher Sidney Hook reflected on the preceding years and, while bemoaning what he saw as a "genteel timidity" within the medical profession when it came to alternatives, praised versions of socialized medicine and comparative medical practices in other countries.[12] This timidity and the frustrating bureaucracy that accompanied proposals for healthcare reform (what Hook called "the inertia, the inefficiency, the mechanical administration of rules") are part of the broad narrative of this book.[13] It is clear that the health of the nation was closely linked to the health of its citizens, particularly at a time when the scope and nature of democracy was being debated on both sides of the Atlantic.[14] But I also contend that a number of postwar events—coupled with a wave of new research linking social psychology, psychoanalysis, and cultural production—brought about a revolution in medical thought, practice, and representation. There were precursors. Margaret Mead and Karen Horney, for example, worked on the boundaries between psychology, psychoanalysis, sociology, and anthropology in the 1930s in order to emphasize the influence of culture on identity formation; and Theodora Abel, Nathan Ackerman, Erik Erikson, and Paul Goodman, among others, extended this mode of study after the war to focus on children, adolescents, families, and communities. Fieldwork, statistical analysis, and personality tests were important for understanding modal identity structures, but the spread of psychiatric and psychoanalytical ideas across the cultural sphere led Philip Rieff to announce the "triumph of the therapeutic" in his 1966 book of that name, as therapy had begun to take the place of religion at the heart of daily life.[15]

Inflecting these issues, the title of this book plays on those two earlier volumes to suggest that what took place was not just one therapeutic revolution but two: the first reinforcing medical and political authority from above, in the name of helping individuals feel secure and content; and the second challenging the authority of the medical profession and the philosophical model of human nature on which it rested. As I discussed above, this might appear to offer us a neat transition from the conservative 1950s to the liberal 1960s, but the phasing of these revolutions was not that simple. I propose, instead, that the two impulses are best seen as intersecting cyclical revolutions that, taken together, reveal a deep ambivalence toward health issues in American life. The revolutionary dimension of these two impulses is most visible in the mid- to late 1960s, when a normative model of health gave way to radical reappraisals of medical categories and clinical practices in the guise of the human potential and free clinic movements, and more radical groups—such as the American Association for the Abolition of Involuntary Mental Hospitalization, founded in 1970 by Thomas Szasz, George Alexander, and Erving Goffman—sought to abolish imposed psychiatric interventions.

My intention here is not to argue that this second revolution happened overnight, or that it was a unified vanguard. For example, elements of what later became a dominant therapeutic discourse can be identified in 1951 in the collaborative book *Gestalt Therapy*, which begins: "We believe that the Gestalt outlook is the original, undistorted, natural approach to life . . . the average person, having been raised in an atmosphere full of splits, has lost his Wholeness, his Integrity."[16] This holistic understanding was elaborated in the 1950s and 1960s by two of the book's authors, Paul Goodman and Frederick Perls, and therefore runs through the period. It is linked to an important narrative thread of this book, which explores how a range of postwar social experiences—among them demobilization; work-related stress; patient care; and anxieties about parenthood, adolescence, and sexual identity—gave way to full-scale reassessment of medical normativity in the 1960s, although these progressive currents were held in check by the persistence of more conservative ideas and institutional constraints. I am not arguing that the progressive revolution of the 1960s was either complete or enduring: the cost of national healthcare was approaching $75 billion when Richard Nixon entered the White House in 1969, and many of the health and welfare issues Nixon faced as president were similar to those that had been at stake when he became Eisenhower's vice president in 1953.[17] As the discussion of the 1990s anti-stigma campaigns in the preface indicates, normative categories persisted into and beyond the 1970s, revealing both continuity and disjunction during the postwar period and suggesting that to do justice to the contours of medical and social change, we need to keep both progressive and realist perspectives in mind.

Postwar Medical Humanities

In essence, this book presents a two-layered cultural history of US medical humanities after World War II. The first layer is the nexus of ideas and practices that encompass medicine, psychiatry, psychology, psychoanalysis, and related therapeutic discourses; and the second layer links medicine to a number of ancillary services, modes of enquiry, and cultural production.[18] I favor the term "medical humanities" over "health sciences" to describe this broad field because it bridges science, medicine, and the arts. Indeed, in 1913 the Harvard philosopher Hugo Münsterberg argued in his influential study *Psychology and Industrial Efficiency* that medicine had never been a sealed profession in the United States. Münsterberg's primary focus was the extent to which experimental psychology could be practised in industry. However, he highlighted tensions between broad ideas and "the exactitude" of "anatomical, physiological, and pathological examination" that became pertinent for the post–World War II medical scene at a time when laboratory experimentation grated against practical application, health reform jostled with biomedical theories of pathology, and humanistic understanding strained to deal with the impact of technology and pharmaceuticals.[19]

Tracing the tensions between ideas, practices, and institutions is central to the cultural history of medicine, but so too is understanding how medical science functions to "act materially and actually" on bodies and minds, to adopt the language of French theorist Monique Wittig.[20] Consequently, this book aims to balance an account of the positive advances of postwar medicine with recurrent theoretical, ethical, and social problems of the period. The twenty-five years after World War II were an important battleground for such optimistic and skeptical perspectives on medicine. Following John Burnham's 1982 essay "American Medicine's Golden Age: What Happened to It," Bert Hansen has argued that the triumphant seventy-year story of medicine—from "Pasteur to Polio," as Hansen dubs it—was followed by a shift in the late 1950s and 1960s, in which "cracks of hesitation and skepticism" emerged following a spate of articles on and representations of incompetent medical practice.[21] However seductive the "golden age of medicine" model might be, since 1968 the temptation has been to lean just as far the other way and treat medical authority as an ideological state apparatus that subjugates the patient to powerful technology and the scientific gaze. Although this anti-authoritarian approach is an important corrective to the confident march of medical science (as celebrated in a January 1950 issue of *Life* magazine) or the promise that science could be an "endless frontier" (as reflected in the title of Vannevar Bush's famous 1945 report to President Franklin D. Roosevelt), it has an equally problematic tendency toward oversimplification by replacing triumphalism with cynicism.[22]

In fact, neither the medical profession nor illness itself can be treated as either stable or monolithic; the historical relationship between medical ideas and practices is a complex acting out of multiple human transactions between doctors, analysts, patients, nurses, welfare workers, and counselors—often across lines of race, class, region, and gender. This terrain is complicated further when we consider the numerous cultural channels for medical knowledge and healthcare, which extends the discussion of therapy into the public realm. A scholarly article from August 1950 suggested that physicians were beginning to have a "keener awareness of the connections between disease and environment in all its manifestations," which led a number of well-known figures to contribute not only to high-end journals such as the *American Journal of Psychiatry*, the *Journal of the American Medical Association*, and the *Bulletin of the History of Medicine*, but also to mass-market magazines like *Life*, *Look*, *McCall's*, *Collier's*, *Harper's*, and the *Ladies' Home Journal* (the latter had eight million readers by the early 1960s), in an attempt to increase public awareness of health issues.[23] Such attempts to bridge the gap between professional and public knowledge are closely linked to the ways in which medical ideas and practices crisscross in the cultural sphere. What emerges from attempts to map this complex field of knowledge, opinions, stories, and images is a strong sense that the metanarrative of medical authority is not as secure as it first looks—particularly not in the 1960s, when alternative voices challenged the hegemony of professional medicine.

Following the trajectory of Hansen's study on mass media images of medical progress, stories and images in the public eye are particularly important to this book. As one study from 1961 noted, at times the postwar media distorted, exaggerated, or simplified postwar health issues; but at other times it helped to disseminate information about public health or even found ways of critiquing medical authority. On occasion, there was a cultural lag in public information—a number of psychiatric studies published in the early 1960s relied on decade-old data; and *I Never Promised You a Rose Garden*, the widely read story of psychiatric treatment that was published in 1964, drew on personal experiences from the late 1940s. But other new medical ideas were quickly addressed, such as the experimental use of cortisone, the so-called wonder drug, which was critiqued in the mid-1950s in a topical *New Yorker* article and in the Twentieth Century–Fox film *Bigger than Life* (see chapter 5).

The flow of information between medical and cultural spheres was not always smooth. In 1954 the sociologist Earl Koos claimed that "medical science has until recently been somewhat neglectful of social factors in illness," partly because "the magic of the microscope, the X ray, and the test tube often so impress and overwhelm the layman . . . that he sees himself as having little or no part in the processes associated with health and healing."[24] This assertion was true to a degree, but it does not account for the range of postwar filmmakers, writers, and artists who dealt seriously with medical and clinical subject matter. An alternative focus would recognize the many ways in which public knowledge of health and illness was inflected by cultural practitioners working at a remove from official channels of medicine and government. For this reason, the exploration of ideas and practices in the cultural sphere are of equal importance in this book to changes within the health professions and medical practice.

Therapeutic Revolutions narrows the historical frame of reference to the postwar period by drawing on early accounts by Erich Fromm, Philip Rieff, Paul Ricoeur, Donald Meyer, Paul Robinson, and Richard H. King; more recent studies, such as Ellen Herman's *The Romance of American Psychology* (1995), James Capshew's *Psychologists on the March* (1999) and Eva Moskowitz's *In Therapy We Trust* (2001); the resurgence of interest in postwar psychiatry, psychoanalysis, and psychology seen in Mathew Thomson's *Psychological Subjects* (2006), Linda Sargent Wood's *A More Perfect Union* (2010), and Michael Staub's *Madness Is Civilization* (2011); and new institutional histories, ranging from Gerald Grob's *From Asylum to Community* (1991) to Karen Kruse Thomas's important study of health care and race, *Deluxe Jim Crow* (2011).[25] But I also broaden the debate by considering a range of cultural texts (primarily film, fiction, poetry, journalism, and television) in which ideas of health and illness were reshaped through the representation of interaction between patients, doctors, and analysts. This breadth allows me to develop Chertok and de Saussure's claim that therapy began to "exert an influence in every area of contemporary culture," but with the important difference that I argue the American therapeutic revolution actually occurred a half-century later than they propose.

The years between 1945 and 1970 are crucial for framing therapeutic culture as a broad category with multiple nodal points. Tracing the postwar trajectory of medicine and psychiatry helps to explain why the two accounts of how far healthcare has developed since the 1960s that I outlined at the start of this introduction—what we can call "the progressive account," in which medical understanding has advanced considerably, and "the realist account," in which ignorance and misperceptions still fuel understanding—are not actually contradictory but emphasize the push and pull of medical development. Despite postwar advances in specialist knowledge and increasingly sophisticated nomenclature, the relationship between medical ideas, long-held beliefs, and ingrained prejudices remained complex. So, although the primary focus of this book is on the historical routes that medicine and psychiatry took between the end of World War II and the beginning of the 1970s, I argue that this should not be separated from a careful analysis of the broader evolution and representations of health and illness. The discussion will take into account many aspects of social, political, and cultural thought and practice—from scientific and medical studies to psychiatric and psychoanalytic approaches; from public policy and sociological debates to cultural representations and mediations in literature, film, and visual culture; from occupational and physical therapy to self-help manuals and alternative therapies. This layered approach is vital for exploring the intersections and interactions between medicine and everyday life.

Two Cultures

There are two other important frames of reference for charting the cultural shift in the quarter-century following World War II and positioning medicine in a middle ground between the arts and sciences. The first of these is the two-cultures debate, which dominated discussions of the arts and sciences in the United States and United Kingdom in the postwar years. The phrase "two cultures" was given currency in 1959 by the British physicist and novelist C. P. Snow, who pitted literary intellectuals and natural scientists against each other.[26] He argued that each group was suspicious of the other's motives and found it hard, if not impossible, to see the other's point of view. Snow's context was distinctly British in raising questions of labor, class, and education and in returning to the Victorian debate between Matthew Arnold and Thomas Huxley about the relative merits of a classical education versus a scientific one. But Snow's view had a broader reach during the Cold War, when science and technology were priorities for research funding. He claimed that whereas literary culture often held the high moral ground in dealing with the complex human condition, some writers had shown themselves to be morally (and politically) suspect for dallying with extreme ideologies in the 1930s, and he asserted that science was actually a deeply ethical activity in which scientists were responsible for the welfare of humanity. Rather than bracketing off moral issues, Snow's two-cultures argument wrestled ethics back into science. By emphasizing the scientist's ethical responsibility, Snow offered a perspective on ethics that differed from Goffman's idea of medical and moral categories blurring in unhelpful or harmful ways.

Unsurprisingly, Snow's one-sided argument received hostile responses, most famously from the literary critic F. R. Leavis, who argued that Snow's relative claims about the arts and sciences were specious. Leavis thought that Snow had adopted a lowbrow position, and the more exacting New York intellectual Lionel Trilling agreed, arguing that Snow's argument was depoliticized and overgeneralizing.[27] Another American critic who sought a more balanced approach was Archibald MacLeish; in his Christmas Day 1960 *New York Times* feature article, "To Face the Real Crisis," MacLeish argued that poetry (often considered the highest of the literary arts) was being eroded by technocratic impulses, and with it was disappearing the ability to imagine a life any different from the present. MacLeish had been claiming for years that the looming Cold War crisis was not of "a laboratory" or "a launching pad" but had been brought about by "the revolution of knowledge" that had given rise to a "new scientific man."[28] Given Snow's thesis that science at its best is a moral pursuit, MacLeish might be dismissed as a disgruntled man of letters unhappy with the "new, precise, objective, dispassionate observation of the world" that had undermined human understanding and removed the capacity to "feel." But MacLeish's perspective chimed with other views. For example, Lewis Mumford gave a speech at a disarmament vigil in Washington, D.C., in November 1957, only weeks after the launch of the Soviet satellite *Sputnik 1*, in which he argued that the "bright side of science and invention has a dark face," pushing the nation toward "ultimately inhuman and morally repulsive objectives." And, earlier that year, in a piece for the *New York Times*, the poet Paul Engle depicted poetry as a form of expression vital to human health: "Poetry is the only one of the arts which comes literally from inside the body . . . poetry is boned with ideas, nerved and blooded with emotions, all held together by the delicate, tough skin of words."[29]

What we can discern from this intellectual posturing is that it was difficult, especially at the peak of Cold War anticommunism in the late 1940s and early 1950s, to think outside a binary paradigm. The best one could hope for was balance, but very few critics were able to map out a middle space that would draw together elements from the arts and sciences without becoming skewed by one or other pole. Perhaps the mathematician Jacob Bronowski came closest in his 1951 book *The Common Sense of Science,* where he argued that science should be seen as part of a broader culture and not a specialist sphere of activity: "We have fallen into the habit of opposing the artistic to the scientific temper; we even identify them with a creative and critical approach."[30] For Bronowski, the trap was an artificial division between "thinkers" and "feelers," in which artists are seen as uncritical and scientists appear to be intent on destroying culture with unspiritual materialism. The emphasis on physical science and technology during the Cold War was one reason for the perceived divide, but Bronowski affirmed that "science and the arts today are not as discordant as many people think"; the real issue is "the lack of a broad and general language in our culture" that could provide a multidimensional perspective to link personal and social activities.[31]

As Daniel Cordle points out, there are at least three problems with the two-cultures model: first, science is undeniably part of culture; second, "there are overlaps between literary and scientific modes of knowing"; and third, the debate "encourages the unthinking acceptance of stereotypical definitions of literature and science."[32] Even though binary oppositions were hard to avoid during the Cold War, I would suggest that medicine and psychiatry inhabited a unique space in postwar life. Seen by some as a specialist sphere of knowledge akin to the natural sciences, medicine was viewed by others as a human-centered project more akin to the arts: a healing art in which health and illness are concrete terms that affect all human beings, regardless of gender, race, or nationality. In this way, the medical humanities grew in the postwar years in that space between the poles of science and the arts, partly shaped by changes in the medical profession, but partly free from institutional concerns. This middle space was rarely comfortable, with institutional and healing pressures often in conflict with each other. However, in his 1965 book *Freud and Philosophy* (translated into English in 1970), the French philosopher Paul Ricoeur felt able to assert that seemingly divergent "scientific-epistemological" and "artistic-hermeneutic" modes of enquiry are more closely interrelated than often acknowledged.[33] Such a perceived separation was true of the two-cultures debate, but its advocates tended to ignore the emerging trends that dominated the intellectual scene during the 1960s, particularly those given weight by émigré thinkers. Many German émigrés thought that American life was far preferable to the "damaged life" they had experienced in the war-torn Central Europe of the 1930s (to cite the subtitle of Adorno's 1951 book of aphoristic fragments, *Minima Moralia*), but they worried that mass culture might distract individuals from being aware of the material forces that shape their lives and might blind them to the power relationships embedded in medicine and psychiatry.

The second broad frame of reference for understanding postwar cultural shifts is closely linked to the first in that the "one universal language" that Bronowski called for in 1951, in order to unite "art and science, and layman and scientist," was actually the problem rather than the solution.[34] Universalism was certainly a strong characteristic of scientific discourse circulating in the 1940s, especially as regards "human nature," which was thought to be largely free from history, nationality, and ethnicity. One example of this trend is a 1957 science primer by J.A.V. Butler, *Science and Human Life*, the premise of which is that "we now have a fairly complete and adequate scientific picture of life in general and man in particular."[35] Butler was skeptical about whether such a scientific picture "could arrive at solutions of all human problems," but he cherished the power of science "to change the human outlook so radically."[36] The postwar emphasis on humanism also helps to explain why universalism was so dominant, but a number of events in the 1950s—the rise of civil rights activism, the emergence of "third world" countries from the grip of colonialism, generational rifts, and the audibility of public voices outside the privileged spaces of the Northeast—raised questions about the universalistic model by focusing on power relations. Beneath the social organization promoted by the Eisenhower administration lay more complex patterns of response, linking isolated or disaffected individuals to community structures that could better support their health needs. This paradigm shift is explored by Richard King in his 2004 book *Race, Culture, and the Intellectuals, 1940–1970*, which charts the gradual drift from universalism that dominated public discourses in the 1940s toward the particularism and identity politics of the 1960s.[37]

In truth, though, both universalism and particularism punctuated the postwar period. Grand humanist statements became less tenable during the mid-1960s with the Vietnam War abroad and race riots at home, but the fear that particularism in academic circles would lead to logic chopping, specialization, and an inability to clearly see across a wide social field led some, such as Abraham Maslow, to call for a "humanistic revolution" in 1968, and the architect and designer R. Buckminster Fuller to recommend, four years earlier, that we forsake "specialization" and "powerful generalization" in order to become "comprehensionalists."[38] The growth of holistic practices and homeopathic medicine also illustrate a non-institutional countertrend, emphasized by Buckminster Fuller's speech at the Fifteenth Conference on Mental Health Programs in Chicago, in which he encouraged psychologists and program directors to exercise "a general kind of know-how" both within and beyond their professions and creatively apply their training to "very complex problems."[39]

Fragmentation, Organization, Reorganization

These tensions between universalism and particularism and between specialization and holism inform the three historical phases that structure this book. This tripartite structure suggests a dialectic in which irrational forces that came to the fore during the wars of the 1940s and early 1950s met their opposite in the rational emphasis on organization in the mid-1950s. According to this dialectical model, the combination of these two orientations gave rise to a more flexible culture of reorganization in the 1960s, in which health and illness were conceived in more holistic, imaginative, and enabling ways. But, rather than a neat sequence or a natural evolution, the therapeutic revolutions of the postwar period contained traces of each other as discourses of authority and liberation intertwined.

Part 1 of this book, "Fragmentation: 1945–1953," deals with the impact of World War II, particularly the wounding, demobilization, and rehabilitation of soldiers (chapter 1), the mounting interest in psychiatry and clinical psychology within professional and cultural spheres (chapter 2), and the ways in which the Cold War and the Korean War threatened identity in very profound and far-reaching ways as medicine and psychiatry seemed to increasingly become the apparatus of the state (chapter 3). I argue that American cultural practices in the late 1940s and the 1950s helped to explore the injuries and damage of war, at times with more insight than some medical accounts—particularly in relation to mental health, for which metaphors of "fragmentation" and "disorganization" were often deployed in clinical circles.

Parts 2 and 3, "Organization: 1953–1961" and "Reorganization: 1961–1970," explore the therapeutic revolutions of the 1950s and 1960s. At the level of politics, these parts of the book offer a stark contrast between, on the one hand, the emphasis on organized business (chapter 4), nuclear families (chapter 5), and personal identity (chapter 6) during the Eisenhower years and, on the other hand, the more urgent health reforms of Presidents John F. Kennedy and Lyndon Johnson and emerging social movements that brought new voices to public attention. These 1960s trends are examined in part 3 with reference to institutional critiques and new health research into race and urban conditions (chapter 7), humanistic and existential currents (chapter 8), and countercultural thought and practice (chapter 9). In this way, we can contrast the Cold War consensus, which tended to rigidify categories into neatly aligned oppositions, with the dynamism of President Kennedy's promise to get the nation moving again and the grass-roots activism that mobilized the energies of the young and social groups for whom medical services often proved inadequate.

As this discussion will illustrate, the emphasis on medical progress and scientific authority during the Cold War concerned many thinkers working in various parts of the humanities, social sciences, and related health professions. Some of them were troubled by the restrictions of the scientific model; others were disturbed by the ideological directions of domestic and foreign policy; and still others worried about the limitations of medical knowledge and inadequate patient care. Reacting to the image of the medical man as a Cold War laboratory scientist, these thinkers, like others, were coming to realize that, in order to better understand the causes of illness and to provide better medical facilities, health workers needed to collaborate more closely with each other and to take heed of the progressive social goals outlined by President Kennedy in February 1963—goals that will be discussed further in chapter 7. We should not exaggerate the speed of transition, though, nor forget that public perceptions of illness often lag behind changes in medical nomenclature and practice. Neither should we ignore broader social parameters (including race, poverty, age, gender, and sexual identity) that have an impact on conceptions of health. We will see examples of dynamic conceptions of health—those of Sullivan, Goffman, Erikson,

Marcuse, Fromm, Maslow, and Rogers—but the realities of many illnesses did not change as much as champions of the therapeutic revolution of the 1960s believed.

Although the historical phases of this book's three parts are fairly orderly—from World War II to the Korean War (part 1), the Eisenhower years (part 2), and the Kennedy and Johnson administrations (part 3)—the transitions are more multifaceted, at times demanding backward and forward glances. Most notably, the transition from the normative model of social organization to the emergence of community-based practices can be glimpsed in the late 1950s—certainly by 1960, which the World Health Organization dubbed "Mental Health Year"—but a full-scale shift took a few years longer to evolve, culminating at the federal level in the amendment of the Social Security Act of 1965 (ushering in Medicaid and Medicare) and the passing of the Developmental Disabilities Services and Facilities Construction Act in 1970. Signed into law by President Nixon but conceived by the Kennedy administration, this act acknowledged that public provision for those with developmental disabilities was at best patchy and at worst nonexistent. The signing of the act, the launch of the anti-psychiatry association (the American Association for the Abolition of Involuntary Mental Hospitalization), countercultural research initiatives, and the curbing of federal welfare spending are the main reasons why this book ends in 1970. But I want to resist countering one heroic narrative of medicine with another: as chapter 9 and the conclusion discuss, the revolutionary fervor at the end of the 1960s contained many intellectual and cultural crosscurrents and cannot be seen to neatly synthesize the historical forces that shaped it.

Throughout the book, I argue that through these broad social interactions and the spread of therapeutic ideas, revolutions within medicine and psychiatry connected closely to other forces in the cultural sphere. The temptation is to frame postwar culture within a neat metanarrative of Cold War consensus or of countercultural opposition, or to trace the shift from what Rieff calls the "analytic attitude" of Freudian thought to the "commitment therapy" of encounter groups.[40] However, it is better to see cultural production in the twenty-five years following World War II as a varied terrain in which dominant values were sometimes upheld and reinforced, and sometimes questioned and subverted. Rather than echoing the seamless world of classical Hollywood films with tightly codified genres, easily recognizable characters and reassuring endings, postwar culture tended to blur genres, explore alternative identities, and seek pathways rather than resolutions. On this account, we need to replace the image of the passive moviegoer with a view of individuals caught between the comforts of a fixed identity and the sense that selfhood is fluid and unstable—particularly during periods of upheaval and illness.

This theoretical insight helps to root medical experience squarely within postwar culture, rather than in a specialist field of scientific research and clinical practice. Narratives of recovery and healthening were repeatedly challenged by demobilization of the armed forces; concerns over delinquency, dissidence, and psychopathology; and the link between medicine and power. What we find during these twenty-five years is that feelings of entrapment and passivity coexisted with purposeful and active selves, even within narratives of physical illness and psychic fragmentation. Debilitating illness can often reinforce a patient's feelings of helplessness in the face of medical authority, but the illness experience may also help individuals to recognize that social and cultural values are not fixed. As we will see, this conflict is embedded in the tensions between the two postwar therapeutic revolutions, with the inclination to leave decisions to higher authorities contested by individuals and groups who saw themselves as active producers of meaning.

The nine chapters of this book, therefore, adopt a dual perspective, attending both to medical developments and cultural texts that shaped public understanding of health and illness. Repeatedly in these texts, physical and mental illness overlap or mask each other (particularly in the war stories featured in part 1), and the potential for recovery is often problematized by themes of anxiety, paranoia, and subversion. Throughout the chapters, I discuss a number of significant films released between 1945 and 1970, including *The Best Years of Our Lives*, *Pride of the Marines*, *Murder, My Sweet*, *Spellbound*, *Patterns*, *Bigger than Life*, *Tea and Sympathy*, *Shock Corridor*, and *Bob & Carol & Ted & Alice*. I also discuss fictional texts—*Lost Weekend*, *Revolutionary Road*, *From the Dark Tower*, *One Flew over the Cuckoo's Nest*, *Another Country*, and *The Last Gentleman*—and two fictionalized autobiographical accounts, *I Never Promised You a Rose Garden* and *The Bell Jar*, in which illness experiences are framed, explicitly or implicitly, within a medical context. These texts encompass many differences of tone, but as the postwar period progressed, the controlling narrative frame generally became less imposing and explorations of illness grew more searching, thereby enabling writers and filmmakers to challenge the heroic medical model and reveal illness as an irreducible aspect of modern American life.

This twofold focus on medical and cultural developments helps to avoid the pitfall of positioning medical science outside the cultural sphere and also reveals the value of historicizing the tensions between medical knowledge, social practice, and public perception, as illustrated by the anti-stigma debates of the late 1990s discussed in the preface. There is a strong narrative dimension to this book, shifting from clinical control to the possibility (if never the full realization) of personal and social liberation, but it is tempered by an awareness that many problems—both practical and conceptual—that were circulating in the 1940s persisted beyond the 1960s. In this complex terrain, we can position the medical humanities as a version of "cultural science," which draws as much on professional science and medicine as it does on popular representations.[41] This insight is instructive for tracing the conflicting medical currents that flowed through postwar American culture, and that helped to revolutionize both how therapy might be understood and to what ends it might be put.

PART ONE

Fragmentation

1945–1953

1 Going Home

WORLD WAR II AND DEMOBILIZATION

Toward the end of the Warner Brothers film *Pride of the Marines* (1945), blinded war veteran Al Schmid makes his way home to Philadelphia after being badly wounded by a Japanese attack in August 1942 while serving on the frontline, on Guadalcanal in the Solomon Islands. Al is taken to the Red Cross Naval Hospital in San Diego and undergoes surgery for shrapnel injuries and eye damage. During his long journey to rehabilitation, Al struggles with a lack of self-worth, believing that he will be nothing but a burden to his friends; he even asks a Red Cross nurse to write to his fiancée to tell her not to come to the Philadelphia train station, hoping she will forget him. When other wounded soldiers talk of returning to family and friends, he bitterly announces that he will never go back to Philadelphia but instead will live with his brother in Chicago: "I've got no place to go, see." Given that he is totally blind in one eye and has severely limited vision in the other, the irony of the colloquialism "see" is obvious but still startling. Al's war injury makes it impossible for him to see, but it also pushes him into an existential space where it is difficult for him to "be." His comrade Lee Diamond and the Red Cross nurse Virginia Pfeiffer realize that he is mired in his condition and needs to draw on the resolve that a marine would in combat. "Don't stop fighting Al, don't," pleads Virginia as he leaves San Diego on a return train to Philadelphia, where he will collect a Navy Cross for his "extraordinary heroism" as a machine gunner in one of the most significant battles in the Pacific theater of World War II.

Despite the help of his colleagues, volunteers, and professionals—all of whom impress on him the importance of going home—Al can only see pitying hands trying to help. His fiancée, Ruth (whom he first met in a blackout, foreshadowing his blindness), is steadfast despite Al's rejection of her. Just before he boards the train for Philadelphia, the camera cuts to a lonely picture of Ruth praying in church: "He's got to come home where he belongs, he's got to know he's wanted," she soliloquizes, perhaps inspired by the US Army and Navy chaplaincy pamphlet *War-Time Prayers for Those at Home* issued in February 1943. If Al has been unlucky in suffering a permanent injury, then Ruth has also suffered a profound loss. Nonetheless, she selflessly helps him to realize that a sense of home is needed for rehabilitation. This insight is given at twist at the end of the film, when—after the medal ceremony—Al is just able to identify the red hood of a taxi if he strains his eyes. The taxi driver asks "Where to, folks?" When Al simply replies "home," the camera superimposes a shot of the couple over an image of Independence Hall, and we hear the patriotic strains of "America the Beautiful." Al Schmid's homecoming, then, is not merely the tale of a marine's return from injury and despair, but also a therapeutic story about the nation regaining its sense of hope.

This view of the film as a national drama about returning from war is emphasized in the opening voice-over. In it, the working-class Al describes his hometown, Philadelphia, and provides a brief tour of the familiar monuments he took for granted as a child—Independence Hall, the Betsy Ross House, and the Liberty Bell—but by the end of the film these sights have become profoundly symbolic. Al says in the voice-over that the story "could have begun anywhere. It could have begun in your hometown, maybe. And what happened to me might have happened to you." The opening voice-over not only makes the viewer complicit in Al's account, but it also creates a national drama out of a very personal story. In addition, it serves to link the film closely to President Harry Truman's concerns about disability discharges from the armed forces and his stated belief that health is a crucial "part of our national fabric."[1]

The Postwar Medical Scene

In order to explore these intertwining personal and national stories, this chapter examines a number of demobilization narratives that emphasize the close links between physical war injuries and psychological responses to combat. In this way, the themes of fragmentation and therapy in the first part of this book are set against the horizon of war—from the aftershocks of World War II in the first two chapters to the early phase of the Cold War in the third, taking the national story from President Franklin Roosevelt's death in April 1945 through Truman's eight years in the White House to the beginnings of Eisenhower's first term and the end of the Korean War in July 1953.

Demobilization was a taxing process for many disabled veterans, but it was not just disabled soldiers who suffered difficulties. The 1945 mass-market book *Psychology for the Returning Serviceman*, written by army and navy personnel, deals with the mental stress of combat and the return to families, finding a job, and meeting a partner.[2] In a 1946 essay titled "The Homecoming," the sociologist Alfred Schutz observed that many discharged veterans arriving home felt the "magic fruit of strangeness." Schutz noted that 40 percent of the veterans who returned to civilian life through "eastern 'separation centers' did not want their old jobs back and did not want even to return to their old communities," and "on the Pacific coast the percentage was even greater."[3] This estrangement experienced during homecoming is best demonstrated by the three war veterans in William Wyler's popular 1946 film, *The Best Years of Our Lives*. The war affects each of the veterans in the film in different ways, but they each find home life more taxing than the regimented existence they knew in the armed forces.

The year 1946 was very important in the history of medicine. At that time, the Veterans Administration (VA) pushed forward medical research into war neurosis, and a Committee on Veterans' Medical Problems was added to the National Research Council to establish a Medical Follow-Up Agency to investigate veterans' experiences. A series of six public lectures at the New York Academy of Medicine in 1946–1947 on "Medicine in the Postwar World" included three lectures on psychiatry, including one titled "What the Wars' Experiences Have Taught Us in Psychiatry," which aligned personal and social pathology.[4] Perhaps most importantly, in July 1946, nine months after President Truman had outlined his ambitious healthcare plans to Congress, he signed the National Mental Health Act, which focused on funding research, training, and support for states to improve mental health facilities (Alabama, for example, had no preventive mental health program supported by public funds until 1946).[5] In spite of opposition from the American Medical Association, which argued that he was promoting socialized medicine, Truman called for the establishment of a National Institute of Mental Health (which was established in 1949, during Truman's second term), largely in response to reports of dire conditions in state mental institutions.

The twin priorities of the government and medical profession had a potent influence on cultural representations of wounded war veterans. This helps to explain the shift in tone toward the realism of the 1946 films *The Best Years of Our Lives* and *Pride of the Marines* from the sentimentalism of earlier war films such as *Random Harvest* and *Mrs. Miniver*, both released in 1942. *Random Harvest* attempted to address the psychological scars of war, but detailed accounts of rehabilitation were rare in earlier war films, preferring the "For Your Health!" sentiment used as a publicity tagline for David O. Selznick's home-front film *Since You Went Away* (1944). The later films were more closely attuned to the medical complications of war but still retained their patriotism. For example, *Pride of the Marines* ends in 1943 with the war still to be won, and its message is that resolve, the willingness to fight, and guts—the very qualities we see in Ruth's steadfast love for Al Schmid—are needed for the nation to emerge victorious.[6]

There were frequent references to "guts" in combat literature and films, such as when a bilateral amputee veteran in *The Best Years of Our Lives* is applauded for having "a lot of guts." Motivation, courage, and morale were often seen as the key qualities of an effective soldier, but "guts" enabled the soldier to channel anger toward the enemy, epitomized by the phrase "good old American guts" in General George Patton's "blood and guts" speech of June 1944.[7] Although group identity was a theme in World War I, it was emphasized much more in World War II. Therefore, we can approach *Pride of the Marines* not only as a film about the physical injuries of war, but also as one about national homecoming. Returning home from war often marks a moment of narrative and therapeutic closure, but the realities and representations of homecoming in the 1940s were more troubling than that. Many demobilization narratives oscillate between a respect for medical authority and the expectation that soldiers should be self-reliant even after an injury, which complicates the promise of homecoming with the realities of psychological and bodily fragmentation.

Pride of the Marines was one of the first in a group of films that dealt with the demobilization of troops, depicting many soldiers suffering physical disability or war neurosis, or a combination of both. The films were released in the six-year period from 1945 to 1951 and were linked to the work of the VA in addressing social problems of reintegration. This was not just an issue for disabled veterans but for many returning soldiers. For example, the Medical Follow-Up Agency found that 78 percent of canvassed veterans without an obvious disability were having trouble adjusting to work and home life.[8] The VA was eager to increase public knowledge about the obstacles facing veterans mainly because, in the view of the historian David Gerber, national consciousness was "sharply divided": veterans were honored for their bravery in combat but also feared for their "potential to disrupt society."[9] Gerber developed these ideas from *The Veteran Comes Back*, a 1944 study by the sociologist and World War I veteran Willard Waller, in which he argues that the veteran is "dangerous to society not only because he is embittered but because . . . he lacks a stake in the social order."[10]

Waller focused on the "moral irresponsibility" that army life can encourage: the soldier is provided with "food, shelter, clothing, and medical care" and is "emancipated from most, if not all, the controls of civilian life," including family, local community, and the church.[11] The deal, according to Waller, is that if the soldier does his "military duty," then "the army will take care of his needs" and relieve him of civilian obligations. It is not surprising, then, that Joseph in Saul Bellow's first novel, *Dangling Man* (1944), after spending time in a kind of suspended animation, feels a sense of relief when his draft notice finally arrives. But although conscription posed problems for some soldiers, many more experienced difficulties on their release from duty, often feeling cheated that the armed forces had left them unsuited to civilian life: like the "forgotten men" of the previous war, the World War II veteran was often, as Waller describes, "the jobless, womenless, voteless man."[12]

World War II Films and Therapy

One of the central plotlines of *The Best Years of Our Lives* shows Captain Fred Derry returning home to his young wife, only to find that her interest in him ends with his Air Force uniform. Derry can find only demeaning work in his hometown, and he is haunted by bombing raids over Germany. But if he is traumatized (a diagnostic term not explicitly used in psychiatric nomenclature at the time), that fact is discernible only in his depressed countenance and night terrors. The lack of support Derry experienced was typical: although a *Follow-Up Study of War Neuroses* found that 41 percent of veterans were receiving disability compensation for psychiatric disorders arising during the war, only obviously disabled veterans were likely to receive full disability compensation.[13] Those suffering from a combination of organic and psychiatric disorders found postwar life the hardest; as Gerber commented, the "difficulties in adjusting to civilian life" were compounded by the severity of the disability, making regular work and home life taxing for many veterans.[14]

The postwar climate challenged not just wounded veterans returning home, but also the film industry as it grappled with the reintegration of veterans into a changing society. The relationship between the Hollywood demobilization cycle and War Department training films made immediately before and during the war is important for this chapter, helping to identify fault lines in medical and psychiatric developments and in the practical treatment of recruits and veterans. War features that used military consultants or were otherwise linked to the War Department were often not very distinct from training films designed to educate members of the armed forces. There were key differences, though: if soldiers thought that a training film was "too Hollywood," it was unlikely to have the desired educational effect, while "straight" training films lacked a hook to catch a trainee's attention.[15] A number of films produced by the department's Military Training Division succeeded in combining dramatic story lines informed by research in the field of social psychology and effective training methods. For many new recruits, this was part of voluntary education on a level similar to the popular mass-market publication *Psychology for the Fighting Man*, released by the Infantry Division in 1943. Nevertheless, the armed forces' films were carefully constructed to increase morale or—in the case of two training films, *Combat Exhaustion* (1945) and *Let There Be Light* (1946)—to raise awareness about panic attacks and other neuropsychological reactions to combat. *Let There Be Light* (whose working title was "The Returning Psychoneurotics") is particularly interesting, not least because it was directed by John Huston (then a captain in the Army Signal Corps) and because it emphasizes that the psychic damage of combat is as important as its physical toll.

Narrative development was more important for feature films than for short training films, and features were less technical in their medical and military focus, but there was nevertheless a close relationship between the two genres. This is in part because both had a pedagogic mission: training films were designed to instruct recruits, while feature films (at least implicitly) were intended to educate soldiers and the public about the consequences of combat and the support mechanisms that veterans required. In this respect, many postwar features can be seen to have a therapeutic goal: the national mythos of reintegration, in which homecoming and marriage are potent symbols of the "ideology of commitment and community," as Dana Polan terms it.[16] This view is substantiated at the end of *Let There Be Light*, when soldiers at Mason General Hospital on Long Island, having undergone a course of therapy, play baseball to symbolize national reintegration and therapeutic closure. Although Huston was fascinated by Freudian therapy (he made the biopic *Freud* in 1962), I would argue that it is not entirely helpful to read neat resolutions back into films that are otherwise characterized by injury, anxiety, and disorientation.[17] In fact, many of the demobilization films can also be seen to challenge the triumphalism of 1945 in their realistic portrayal of the consequences of combat (it is worth noting that the Department of Defense suppressed *Let There Be Light* for thirty-five years because the film was thought too harrowing for the public).[18]

Distressing graphic images of war were rarely seen in the popular press before 1943, leading the Office of War Information (OWI) to warn other government agencies to release more realistic images of war casualties to prevent public complacency. Even when graphic shots were released, newspapers and magazines such as *Life* remained reluctant to show them.[19] Beginning in 1944, there was a general move in the press and in movies to show more realistic portrayals of casualties—for example, the disturbing images of battle in the Academy Award–winning documentary *With the Marines at Tarawa* (1944)—but censorship was compounded by the insistence in

Hollywood that war films should have happy resolutions. It was not really until the group of demobilization films mentioned above were released that the public were exposed to the medical consequences of combat; even so, tough demobilization films like *Pride of the Marines* (which used technical advisors from the Marine Corps) resorted to home-front sentimentality, thereby suggesting that commitment and love can offset or even overcome profound injury.

On this level, films that end with homecoming and marriage can be seen as a form of therapeutic wish fulfillment, and quite often the soldier who cannot embrace these ideological principles is seen as a maladjusted oddity. Peter Roffman and Jim Purdy adopt this reading in *The Hollywood Social Problem Film*, arguing that:

> The films deemphasize those uncertainties that could potentially question society. Troubling fears of another war or depression, for example, are dealt with briefly and then glossed over or forgotten. The films concentrate instead on more personal and physical traumas . . . [they] begin by showing these difficulties are common to all soldiers, but soon localize them to the neurotic protagonist. While the hero's compatriots quickly reintegrate themselves into the healthy society, he remains defiantly alone in his resentment and insecurity.[20]

The opposition between the "sick individual" and "healthy society" was common in the postwar years, corroborating the belief that homecoming should realign the soldier's values with those of the democratic nation as a marker of health. On this level, demobilization films tend to follow a straightforward therapeutic arc, working through antagonism toward a cathartic resolution. However, this focus on narrative trajectory overlooks unresolved issues that threaten both veterans (disability, instability, and sometimes impotence) and society (intolerance, racism, and violence). The next chapter highlights how such social disruption featured in 1940s film noir, but, as I discuss here, demobilization films of the same period tend to operate dialectically, and thus it is hard to separate disruption and homecoming.

The other key relationship between Hollywood and the military was in terms of directors who were centrally involved in the war effort. Frank Capra, director of the Why We Fight series sponsored by the War Department, was a major in the US Army Signal Corps; the screenwriter for *The Best Years of Our Lives*, Robert Sherwood, was the director of the OWI, while the film's director, William Wyler, was a major in the US Army Air Corps, turning his hand to both war features (*Mrs. Miniver*) and documentaries (*The Memphis Belle*, 1944). Although Hollywood was often accused of distorting or sentimentalizing the war, the films that emerged immediately after its end were marked by harder-edged realism and attention to detail that was similar to British documentary realism. It is difficult to sustain the argument that Hollywood simply became the entertainment arm of the OWI (although certain outlets were closely linked to the agency, such as Walt Disney's wartime propaganda animations), but in more realistic movies produced after 1944, one can see a growing relationship between armed forces training films and war features. It is a mistake to think that the demobilization films focused tightly on war and recovery, because many of them dealt with difficulties faced by returning soldiers and spoke "loudly and bluntly" about social issues, especially bigotry and right-wing intolerance.[21] Gender and race issues also figured prominently in the demobilization films: *Since You Went Away* traces the wartime journey of Ann Hilton (Claudette Colbert) from member of the country club set to industrial welder, while *Home of the Brave* (1949) explores racial tensions and prejudice among US troops. Quite often the films reinforced gender norms and racial prejudices, though—women were depicted as helpers, and black soldiers were rarely trusted to make decisions—whereas the topic of combat exhaustion provided a more nuanced way to explore changing value systems.

Arguably, almost as important as race and gender were the close links that developed in the 1940s between medicine and psychiatry, which meant that demobilization after World War II was treated quite differently from the situation after previous wars. Veterans did not have to be physically wounded for rehabilitation units to realize that they needed help reintegrating into civilian life. Although speedy treatment of neuropsychiatric conditions within the combat zone was the ideal, for most soldiers with combat fatigue, this meant hospitalization or recuperation stateside. Not all soldiers were treated by professionals, and one of the reasons for the War Department's training film *Combat Exhaustion* was the shortage of neuropsychiatrists and the realization that "the burden of recognition and treatment . . . will fall on medical officers without specialized training." Psychiatric treatment often took the form of advice or folk wisdom, frequently pushing the responsibility for rehabilitation onto the veteran himself. For example, in *Till the End of Time* (1946), Gunny Watrous, a rehabilitation officer, says to the young, able-bodied veteran Cliff Harper: "It's kinda tough getting yourself reorganized. . . . But you'll work it out." Such emphasis on self-reliance chimes with the rhetoric of guts and courage, linked here to tough-minded pragmatism. This idea of "reorganization" (the overarching theme of the third section of this book) implies that horizons had to be scaled down for civilian life, relationships relearned, and—for veterans suffering from blindness, deafness, paralysis, or head injuries, as well as those who had undergone amputations—a new set of skills had to be learned. Reorganization also tapped into postwar medical discourse, chiming with the description of combat exhaustion by William Menninger, then president of the American Psychoanalytic Association, as "psychological disorganization" and a profound loss of equilibrium.[22] As this chapter explores, often obvious physical injuries masked neuropsychiatric conditions that were less easy to diagnose or remained latent while the body adapted to injuries.

The equation between "work" and "fight" running through such films as *Till the End of Time*, *Pride of the Marines*, and *The Men* recasts reintegration as a difficult task to which the veteran must apply himself as he would to armed combat. The text shown on the screen at the beginning of *The Men* actually equates battles fought "with club, sword or machine gun" and the greater battle of rehabilitation "fought with abiding faith and raw courage" for those with war injuries. The realism of the demobilization films is also linked to the realistic tenor of postwar politics: the need to be responsible and vigilant were key terms in Cold War philosophy—a fighting faith, as Arthur

Schlesinger Jr. called it—but in the demobilization films, these same masculinized traits implied that veterans must be responsible for avoiding immorality, laziness, and disrespect. However, although a number of demobilization films place this responsibility squarely on the individual, there is also a strong emphasis on collaboration and the need for helpers. Professionals such as doctors, surgeons, and psychiatrists were necessary to treat injuries, but the films often focused on nurses, rehabilitation officers, family members, and friends that help the wounded veteran to deal with his transformed condition. This chapter shows how these tensions play out in the context of World War II, but it also sets up a broader opposition that I trace throughout this book, in which medical authority as a form of therapeutic governance (emphasized in part 2) and the more diffuse therapeutic networks of community (in part 3) mark the cyclical revolutions of the postwar years.

Medicine, Psychiatry, and World War II

One striking characteristic of World War II was the convergence of mainstream medicine and psychiatry. This was not only evident in the US Army Medical Department's expanded use of doctors, surgeons, and psychiatrists, but also in the support mechanisms for wartime families and the representation of the war through cultural and media outlets. In order to contextualize four of the most significant demobilization films released in the mid-1940s that dealt with some of the commonest combat conditions—paralysis, amputation, and blindness (often combined with feelings of exhaustion and loss)—it is important to examine the emerging wartime relationship between medicine and psychiatry.

The psychological and social matrix of 1941–1945 was more complex than that of 1917–1918, even though important lessons had been learned in World War I. For example, the National Committee for Mental Hygiene (established in 1909) had studied soldiers suffering from shell shock; important medical studies of somatic hysteria were released in the 1910s; and, as the historian Nathan Hale Jr. writes, the "human laboratory" of World War I "gave psychiatrists a new sense of mission and an expanded social role."[23] However, although the US Army developed neuropsychiatric support mechanisms for the armed forces during World War I and the interest in psychoanalysis grew significantly between the wars, it was not until World War II that psychiatry and psychoanalysis had a major influence on the therapeutic orientation of medicine, creating what Eva Moskowitz describes as a "psychological front."[24] William Menninger was eager to integrate psychoanalytic and psychiatric institutes, arguing that, despite the "great awakening" of psychiatry during World War I, the emerging field had gone into a lull between the wars and that "misconceptions about mental health and about psychiatric patients were nearly as widespread in 1941 as in 1920."[25] Old techniques had to be relearned; new psychiatric terms such as "operational fatigue" and "combat exhaustion" replaced "shell shock"; and fresh exposure to war brought psychic debilitation much closer to home.

Unlike civilian medicine, military medicine during World War II had as its primary goals preventing disease, preserving manpower, testing recruits' health, and physical rehabilitation. But there was also a vital role for psychiatry, which Colonel Thomas W. Salmon, chief of psychiatry for the Army Overseas, had championed in World War I by emphasizing immediate treatment and expectancy of recovery. It took the prospect of another war, however, to fully develop the infrastructure of military psychiatry. Galvanized by the belief that a second world war was inevitable, a committee on neuropsychiatry was added to the National Research Council in October 1940 to offer advice on national defense, and a psychiatrist was placed alongside medical specialists on each of the 660 regional medical advisory boards. Induction into the armed forces now involved both psychological and physical examinations, and clinical psychologists began working closely with physicians. In January 1941, nearly a year before the attack on Pearl Harbor, psychiatrists started two-day training and orientation seminars for inducting other psychiatrists into medical advisory and army recruitment boards.[26] Tensions persisted between medics and psychiatrists, though; given a choice between an extra surgeon and a psychiatrist, most field hospitals would probably have chosen a surgeon like Chief Surgeon Ulysses D. Johnson, Clark Gable's character in the 1948 MGM film *The Homecoming*, although his values are challenged by the physical damage of war. Part of the problem was that psychiatry in the early 1940s "had no core of tested theory that was accepted by all its practitioners," leading to a wide variety of treatments and therapies.[27] Even so—although the shortage of psychiatrists was of national concern, with only thirty psychiatrists in the US Army as of late 1941 and just three thousand in the United States as a whole—by the end of 1942, integration of the medical and psychiatric professions into military life led to improvements in recovery rates of soldiers. A 1952 report claimed that 98 percent of wounded men recovered during World War II, compared to 90 percent in World War I, with deaths from wounds to the head, chest, and abdomen down by 65 percent.[28]

Important new medical techniques were available, such as antiseptics and oxalic acid to speed up the healing of wounds. In addition, the development of combat gear, such as helmets that were lighter and more resilient, helped reduce the mortality rate. But there were a bewildering array of neuropsychiatric symptoms: many soldiers were removed from the combat zone suffering from anxiety, panic attacks, amnesia, tremors, hysterical paralysis, gastric complaints, or heart conditions.[29] The War Department's film *Combat Exhaustion* offers different statistics, estimating that 20 percent of nonfatal US battle casualties in Italy had developed neurotic conditions and that 40–50 percent of all soldiers in medical care suffered from combat exhaustion.[30] Soldiers forced to retire early from the war were sometimes thought to have a latent weakness that combat had brought to the surface, but by the time of Al Schmid's battle on Guadalcanal in November 1942, an armed forces medical report stated that "the majority of [psychiatric] cases are nothing but a direct result of . . . mental and physical fatigue."[31] As a result, some weary marines were given rearguard duty and others worked in mobile hospitals until they were fit to return to battle. Although leaders realized that prolonged tours of duty would drain soldiers, it was thought that the further a soldier was removed from active service, the greater the chance that he would be unable to return. This led to the implementation of psychiatric aid in overseas hospitals and mental hygiene units in army training camps. However, with only one psychiatrist on Guadalcanal in 1942 (and he acted primarily as a surgeon), it was clear that cases could not be adequately dealt with near the combat zone.[32]

A major event that explored the relationship between psychiatry and war was a conference that was sponsored by the American Psychiatric Association (APA) and held at the University of Michigan in October 1942. One speaker summed up the mood of the conference by claiming that "neuropsychiatric problems arising out of the present war will be the most significant military and economic problems with which the Government will have to deal."[33] Although Presidents Roosevelt and Truman realized that the nation needed to be more responsible for wounded veterans than it had been after World War I, the general feeling was that there were not enough psychiatrists to effectively provide consultation and treatment. Many of the trained psychiatrists were already working with units in the armed forces or in army hospitals, thus leaving few available to help the families of soldiers. The conference called for better psychiatric education, for more clinics and hospitals, and for further research in medical schools and the workplace.

A number of conference papers outlined the available psychiatric training within the armed forces and the role of psychiatrists in selecting "individuals who [were] vocationally fit for service" and for preserving the "mental integrity" of recruits.[34] Speakers noted that some individuals suffering from neurosis or schizophrenia might actually do better in the armed forces than in civilian life, but Colonel William Porter of the US Army stressed the importance of careful selection for therapeutic reasons, identifying a range of "mental deficients" who were unfit for service. He observed that war sometimes ameliorates civilian neurosis but also has a tendency to exaggerate "acute anxiety states" stemming from fatigue, defeat, demoralization, and the inability to channel emotions. Nevertheless, he thought that all these conditions could be successfully treated by sedation, restorative therapy, and hypnosis, as illustrated in the military film *Combat Exhaustion*.[35]

Many of the speakers dealt with the institutional frameworks that aided the selection, training, monitoring, and rehabilitation of soldiers. The discipline of the armed forces and the need for troops to be highly skilled in handling artillery, battleships, and aeronautical equipment meant that the psychiatrist's role was crucial for making decisions about fitness for service. The neuropsychiatric procedure for selecting navy recruits was complex, involving initial surveys, detailed case studies, "indoctrinal lectures by psychiatrists," psychological examinations, and additional tests for marginal cases.[36] But this detailed program masks the reality of many induction experiences: some psychiatrists saw up to two hundred recruits per day and spent only three minutes with each (the APA recommendation was no more than fifty recruits daily and no less than fifteen minutes with each), and many inductees were not properly assessed. The conference offered a more positive picture of neuropsychiatric disorders among the troops than *Combat Exhaustion* but noted that increased anxiety during war ranged from "fear reaction and panic" to "utter demoralization," and from schizophrenia to manic-depressive tendencies, often accompanied by ulcers, gastrointestinal conditions, and enuresis.[37] Common among pilots were nightmares involving crashes, headaches due to oxygen deprivation, volatile blood pressure, loss of appetite or extreme hunger, amnesia, and mild paranoia. It was sometimes possible to diagnose a condition, but at other times there was neither the time nor the methodology required to ascertain whether the root cause was physical or psychological.

The theme of readjustment ran through the APA conference and many speakers agreed that the range of symptoms made it necessary to treat casualties on a case-by-case basis, although it was desirable to standardize procedures for selecting and monitoring troops. However, while doctors were trained to detect tell-tale symptoms such as apathy, drooping shoulders, a pale face, and loss of mobility, they often did not see neurotic soldiers until it was too late. The swift removal of the soldier from active duty was deemed doubly important for safety reasons and because wild or depressed behavior could have an infectious effect on the troops. It was thought beneficial to separate the disruptive soldier from his unit and to ascertain a physical root cause: for example, anoxia (lack of oxygen) often damaged the nerve cells in a pilot's brain, and aeroembolisms caused intracranial pressure and the slowing of motor functions.[38] Although acute forms of loneliness and fear might not have a physical root, a lack of sleep and prolonged exposure to cold were seen as major contributing factors.

The attendees at the APA conference came to two conclusions: there was a more complex relationship between physical and psychological conditions than was often credited, and careful medical screening and treatment of troops were needed in order to facilitate a healthy environment that could aid the war effort. Because substandard psychiatric examinations in 1917–1918 had led to a number of maladjusted recruits and a high demand for hospital beds, by the 1930s proper psychiatric screening was introduced—as endorsed by President Roosevelt in September 1940.[39] At the beginning of the war, confidence was high in the ability of medical screening to ensure that troops were sound in mind and body and to identify inductees who were unfit for service: close to two million men were declared unfit, 12–14 percent of the inductees—which was 11 percent higher than in World War I. Psychological testing was crucial for induction, but the emphasis remained firmly on whether the recruit was physically fit for service. This is neatly illustrated in *Pride of the Marines*, when Al Schmid describes his swift physical induction without any psychological tests. It is also dramatized, more comically, in the Disney cartoon *Donald Gets Drafted* (released in 1942, but set before Pearl Harbor): the air force recruit Donald Duck undergoes an army medical examination, in which the faceless doctors (we see only their hands and voices) dismiss the fact that Donald has nothing between his ears, finds it difficult to read, and is colorblind.

As the two-volume Army Medical Department study *Neuropsychiatry in World War II* (1966) makes clear, it became increasingly apparent that, three years into the war, psychiatric screening was failing "to prevent the appearance of vast numbers of emotional disorders," and psychiatric breakdown could just as well occur in "previously stable personnel as well as those of a weaker predisposition" during combat.[40] The extensive examination recommended by Harry Stack Sullivan, founder of the journal *Psychiatry* in 1937 and president of the William Alanson White Psychiatric Foundation, proved impractical.[41] As the draft accelerated, the nature of the screening changed. After March 1942, it became possible to recruit individuals with neurological disorders for certain forms of duty, particularly men of "marginal intelligence, if compensated for by better than average stability," plus other recruits with "moderate degrees of compulsiveness," speech impediments, and or peripheral damage to the nervous system.[42]

The APA conference emphasized two more key elements. The first was the complex relationship between physical and psychological causes of neurosis, which often included emotional disturbance, hormonal disorders, or irritability of the nervous system. The US surgeon general recommended in 1943 that soldiers whose condition was primarily physical but who also displayed psychoneurotic symptoms should be classified separately from those with combat exhaustion, but in practice it was not always easy to separate physical and psychological conditions.[43] The second element was morale, a theme that echoed the emphasis of Generals Dwight Eisenhower and George Patton during the war; the focus of morale films issued by the War Department; and wartime publicity in the film industry, with its "Our Morale Is Mightier than the Sword" slogan.[44] Morale was generally seen as a crucial ingredient in motivating soldiers and preventing them from experiencing the isolation and fear that can often lead to anxiety and psychosis. Reflecting General George C. Marshall's implementation of a Morale Branch in early 1941 to research soldiers' motivation, Sullivan argued in the concluding presentation in the conference strand on "Psychiatry and the War" that the absence of morale can lead to panic, rage, despair, or apathy, and he stressed the importance of recreation, good food and sleep, comradeship, regular mail deliveries, leave privileges, and welfare for the troops' families. Sullivan avoided abstract terms such as "national morale," but he realized that morale needed improving in the armed forces and on the home front, as well as for veterans—and their families—readjusting to civilian life.[45]

The conference delegates acknowledged the need to improve support mechanisms for soldiers, but they neglected a broader discussion of social workers, pastoral care, and integrated rehabilitation. One reason for this was that the conference occurred fairly early in the US phase of World War II. Nevertheless, the fact that professional groups generally overlooked wider social issues relating to demobilization caused Willard Waller to respond in 1944 with the publication of *The Veteran Comes Back* and Charles Bolté to publish *The New Veteran* in 1945. Both books called for better treatment and support structures than those available in World War I and examined the various levels of social care required to support veterans.[46]

President Roosevelt had unveiled a far-reaching rehabilitation plan to the Senate in October 1942, which would ensure that disabled veterans would "become a national asset"—but for this plan to become a reality, local organizations also needed to make an exerted effort to support disabled veterans.[47] For this reason, toward the end of *The Veteran Comes Back*, Waller outlined five aims of his veterans' program: (1) to restore the veteran to a "competitive position" in society; (2) to reinstate him into the "communicative process" of civilian life; (3) to "help him to overcome any handicaps, physical or mental, which he may have incurred as a result of his service"; (4) to allow him to participate in the "political life of community, state, and nation"; and (5) to encourage him "to overcome attitudes of bitterness and antagonism, and to establish a normal and rewarding relation with family, church, and community."[48] In his far-reaching program, Waller argued that a new "art of rehabilitation" is needed to bridge the spheres of culture, politics, medicine, and industry.[49] It is notable that the demobilization films, which promoted this "art of rehabilitation," focused on the second, third, and fifth of Waller's points, with implications for the fourth point in its intertwining of personal and national stories.

Paralysis, Amputation, and Partial Stories

In September 1946 the American Legion focused its twenty-eighth annual conference on the rehabilitation of wounded veterans, particularly the role that disabled workers could play in business and industry. Featuring the Legion's Rehabilitation Committee, the conference included veterans with severe disabilities, including the bilateral amputee Roger Marriott, a farmer from the San Joaquin Valley. Marriott had begun farming again after his discharge from a hospital in Utah and claimed that his disability was merely an "inconvenience"; he said he could still drive a tractor, do some of the farm work he had done prior to the amputation, and go fishing.[50] Another severely disabled veteran at the conference was First Lieutenant Ralph Anslow, who resembled Al Schmid in losing his sight in one eye and having severe loss of vision in the other. Anslow had also lost both arms below the elbow, but prosthetic devices had been constructed to provide him with a degree of dexterity and autonomy. Partly a showcase for veterans who had come to terms with disability, the conference also addressed welfare issues and the impact of medical advances in surgery and health-care for veterans.

The example of the American Legion conference suggested that many wounded veterans were quickly able to reestablish their lives after the war and that rehabilitation involving surgery, neuropsychiatry, and occupational therapy was broadly successful. Hospitalized veterans (some fitted with prosthetic arms) in the feature film *Since You Went Away* also seem well adjusted, but these examples provide only a partial picture. A *New York Times* report from spring 1946 focused on the material shortages and lack of work opportunities for returning veterans, and a brief image of a young amputee on a train in *Since You Went Away* hints at a psychological disturbance (perhaps dementia praecox or a related psychotic reaction) that is largely masked by the physical loss.[51] Army training films tended to put confidence in a variety of treatments such as narcosis therapy, electroshock and insulin treatment, dietary control, and physical reconditioning. However, if we turn to the group of demobilization films, we see quite a different story: psychiatrists tended to play a subordinate role to physicians, and bodies rather than minds were the most obvious focus.

On the surface, World War II films explored what had been gained by combat rather than what had been lost, particularly as Roosevelt's "Four Freedoms" (the freedoms of speech, to worship, from want, and from fear) had been sanctified by the war. Popular films, such as the government-sponsored *The True Glory* (1945), had a therapeutic goal on a nationalistic level, emphasizing American triumph, focusing on the military leadership of General Eisenhower, and inspiring Mayor Fiorello La Guardia to recommend the free viewings to New York families, claiming that the movie "is not acting—it is the real thing."[52] *The True Glory* is just one example of a resurgence of war films in 1945, but it was the following year—with the release of *Pride of the Marines, Till the End of Time*, and *The Best Years of Our Lives*—that saw a significant shift in cinematic portrayals of the war. These films are notable for their close attention to physical disability and rehabilitation, but they also portray the psychological effects of the war and the variable support networks for veterans.

In the remainder of this chapter, I want to focus on two pairs of demobilization films and view them against the backdrop of President Truman's 1945 proclamation that bolstering the nation's health would be the "most important contribution toward freedom from want in our land."[53] The first pair of films, *The Best Years of Our Lives* and *The Men*, focus on amputation and paralysis; the second pair, *Pride of the Marines* and *Bright Victory*, deal centrally with blindness. Although both amputation and blindness were fairly common among World War II casualties (one British report noted that of 405 men disabled by the war, 200 were amputees, 103 were blind, and 102 had lost vision in one eye), I would argue that these conditions are featured in films because of their figurative qualities in emphasizing the physical and psychological impairment of profoundly injured veterans.[54] In fact, the link between realistic and figurative war wounds was very significant after 1944. The *New York Times* film critic Bosley Crowther claimed in 1945 that fiction films about the war found it difficult to escape the "dramatic extravagance" of Hollywood; his antidote was to follow the British model of "artistic stability and sincerity" or to more factually document the realities of war.[55] Some American directors seemed to heed this recommendation, so much so that the narrative strategies for films dealing with amputation and blindness were as important as the representations of the injuries. I will argue that, although the dramatic spectacle of these films focused primarily on physical injury, psychological maladjustment is central to their narrative trajectory.

David Gerber contends that in medical literature and cultural representations alike, "we find amputees garnering attention vastly out of proportion to their relatively small numbers, and in effect, becoming representative of all disabled veterans."[56] Perhaps one reason why amputees featured strongly in demobilization films is that various medical programs were established in 1944 (at the Columbia University College of Physicians and Surgeons, the New York University College of Medicine, and the Medical College of Virginia) that emphasized the need for fresh techniques to aid physical rehabilitation, including new procedures of amputation. Another reason is that amputation was a visually startling means for exploring the psychological and social consequences of war. Kaja Silverman frames this in terms of loss or lack: "The 'hero' returns from World War II with a physical or psychic wound which marks him as somewhat deficient, and . . . strangely superfluous to the society he ostensibly protected during the war; his functions have been assumed by other men, or—much more disturbingly—by women."[57] From a psychoanalytic perspective, then, the psychological effects of amputation are closely related to the physical loss of a limb or even to castration, threatening the robust structures of masculinity that the armed forces affirmed. To offset the risk of stigmatizing the amputee, demobilization films tended to adopt "a sober, pragmatic point of view" by depicting honest stories rooted in personal accounts of wounded soldiers, but the frequent use of literary source texts was not always that straightforward.[58]

One example of this trend is *The Best Years of Our Lives*, which was adapted from an extended verse narrative, *Glory for Me*, written by MacKinlay Kantor and published in 1945.[59] *Glory for Me* seems an unusual source for a major studio: not only is it written in blank verse, but it follows no particular poetic form that might indicate its genre. The text introduces Captain Fred Derry, the recipient of a Purple Heart for having a piece of copper in his arm from a twenty-two-millimeter shell:

> Strong arm. . . . They sewed it up again.
> He wore a crimson bathrobe only sixteen days,
> For he was young and hard and mean
> And glad to wear the Purple Heart.[60]

Derry is one of three demobilized soldiers in the narrative; he meets the other two, Sergeant Al Stephenson and Seaman Homer Parrish, en route back home to Boone City (an average town) in the Midwest. Although Fred is the first character we meet in the film and his story is given most narrative space, Homer offers the most dramatic statement about the difficulties of reintegrating into civilian life. Both of Homer Parrish's names are significant in this respect, but in Kantor's narrative he is given the surname Wermels and is described quite differently. Wounded by a torpedo, Homer goes into the forces "as a child" but comes out "a monster," with a speech impediment due to a harelip, a high degree of spasticity on his left side, a disoriented brain, and a club foot:

> This was a death—one piece of death,
> Alive on its right side, and dying, jerking on its left.
> It walked with pain and twisted muscles.
> It was so young . . . it had a face without a beard.[61]

This combination of living death and childlike features makes Homer a grotesque character, emphasized by his isolation and his inarticulacy: "He made his sounds alone, and no one listened."[62] Rather than opting for the grotesquerie of *Glory for Me*, the film offers a realistic portrayal of a profound war wound, casting in the role Harold Russell, an actual bilateral hand amputee and not a trained actor. Russell had not been injured in combat but on training duty, and he was fitted with prosthetic hooks that he had become adept at using after a retraining program. We see the hooks only from the wrist down for most of the film, but they are part of two complex metal devices that allow Russell to move, grasp, and push objects (a few years later, new surgical plastics were used to create prostheses). The authenticity of Russell's injury is crucial to the film's aims because, as Gerber argues, he went through experiences of adjustment and social prejudice similar to those that Homer encounters in *The Best Years of Our Lives*.[63] Homer quickly becomes skilled at using his hooks, but it takes him much longer to come to terms with the psychological impact of losing his hands and the stigma of returning home as a war casualty.

One of the reasons for using a range of colloquial epithets to describe war wounds was that psychiatric nomenclature steered away from terms such as psychoneurosis. The phrase "fit for duty" was used as a catch-all phrase to describe physical and psychological readiness, and an army report from September 1944 avoided psychiatric diagnosis entirely, preferring the label "No disease. Temperamentally unqualified for Naval service" in an effort to avoid stigmatizing terms. In the training film *Combat Exhaustion*, a former automobile salesman who has been involved in the North African campaign says "I can't stop from crying like a baby. The blues I guess"; another soldier reports "I feel all in." Terms like "reactive depression" and "operational fatigue" proved useful for characterizing these conditions, but in autumn 1944 the surgeon general called for more education for health professionals, caregivers, and patients, arguing that simply changing the terminology would help neither the advancement of medical knowledge nor the veterans themselves.[64] Whereas Homer in *Glory for Me* seems incapable of understanding his condition (the narrator speaks for him except for a few broken utterances), it is partly the terse vocabulary of the armed forces that prevents Homer in *The Best Years of Our Lives* from expressing his anxiety.

Homer feels comfortable with the hooks only in male company; in contrast, in the domestic sphere and around his fiancée, Wilma (Cathy O'Donnell), he often feels inadequate. He perseveres with the sports he enjoyed before entering the armed forces, but when he sees some neighborhood kids staring at him while he is practicing shooting in the garage, he smashes the window with his hooks, shouting "Look at the freak." The camera emphasizes the condition of dismemberment as it lingers on the broken window that physically separates the hooks from Homer's body. This displaced aggression is taken to another, masochistic level in *Glory for Me*, when Homer's ego disintegration (his brain goes from "man to ape") leads him to attempt suicide. Russell's Homer is not the grotesque character in Kantor's book, but the spectacle of his stumps is "something primal and traumatic," as Silverman argues—not least because the exposure of his amputated arms is delayed until the final part of the film.[65] Only when Wilma threatens to leave him does Homer reveal the mechanism behind the hooks: a gunslinger's brace, without which he is incapable of fastening his pajamas or opening the door. In a tender scene, Homer shows Wilma his stumps and then accepts his passivity as Wilma maternally tucks him into bed.

It is possible to read this scene as a moment of acknowledgment of the symbolic castration of war, or a synecdoche of Homer's story, in which he is cut off (or amputated) from an organic narrative of kinship and marriage. However, it is also a moment when Homer is infantilized: he describes himself as "a baby that doesn't know how to get anything except by crying for it," and he admits all the things he can no longer do.[66] In this narrative of reintegration, then, Homer has to passively give himself up to his caring relatives before he can accept his sense of lack.[67] In this way, *The Best Years of Our Lives* explores—as a study of patients at the Walter Reed Army and US Naval Hospitals that was published eight years later in the *American Journal of Psychiatry* put it—"how the loss of an extremity . . . involves emotional problems beyond the loss itself," often leading to feelings of impotence or uncontrollable aggression.[68]

The ending of the film differs from *Glory for Me* in depicting Homer and Wilma's marriage ceremony, where Homer shows off one of his newly learned skills by using his hooks to place a wedding ring on Wilma's finger. Silverman argues that this moment reinforces Homer's subjugation to the scopic gaze of the wedding guests, but it is better to read this symbolic act as the clearest sign that Homer has come to terms with his amputation, and that he has found the guts to resume a life approaching normality without denying his altered body. However, we need to be careful not to just read this therapeutic ending back into the film, because Homer's aggression and preoccupation with guns lurk in the background. Gerber notes that, in the case of Homer, critics seem reluctant to "perceive a disabled man as an aggressor"; he argues that Homer's rage "is too terrible to contemplate" and too persistent to be entirely overshadowed by the closing wedding scene.[69]

Homer is not the only wounded veteran in the film. Al Stephenson, a family man and banker, finds it difficult to resume relations with his wife and two grown-up children when he returns home. In fact, he barely recognizes his former self, and he resorts to heavy drinking whenever there is a social occasion. The film's focal character, Fred Derry, also suffers from psychic dismemberment, not least because he has no home to return to. Fred is often symbolically positioned between or behind his two war comrades, bridging them in terms of age and degree of maladjustment as he returns to a loveless marriage and a demeaning, low-paying job. He quickly falls in love with Al's daughter, Peggy (Teresa Wright), but the relationship is slow to develop, mainly because Fred had married in haste before being drafted (due to a pregnancy scare in the book). Kantor's narrator describes Fred's physical injury in detail, but his night terrors, depression, and loss of self-esteem reveal a troubled mind and an unwillingness to play along with the fantasy his wife, Marie, has of him being a macho man in uniform. She is not at home when Fred arrives in Boone City, and—after an evening out drinking with Al and Homer—he spends the night at the Stephensons' house. Peggy lets him sleep in her bed (hung with an overtly feminized canopy), but she is awakened when the sleeping Fred relives a bombing raid over Germany. Although Fred is unaware of this moment, Peggy's tenderness as she soothes his brow contrasts starkly with Marie's later reaction to his night terrors: she tells him to snap out of it and to go out more.

The nature of Fred's war experience is not explained until the last phase of the film when, realizing that his marriage has reached a dead end, he leaves town. Awaiting his flight from Boone City, Fred sees a decommissioned fighter plane stripped of engines and propellers; he decides to enter the cockpit, but this only brings back vivid memories of his bombing experience. The scene visually parallels an earlier one in which Al, Homer, and Fred see the panorama of the Midwest landscape on their flight back home, but this time the windscreen is dirty, and the plane seems to be a projection of Fred's abject state of mind. The window prevents us from having a clear view of Fred's face, but it confirms his deep anguish and sense of fragmentation. Silverman reads the moment as one in which Fred's face "seems to have surrendered all consistency, and . . . thus attests to a profound psychic disintegration."[70] She goes on to argue that Fred "never really leaves the scrapyard," but it is significant that a salvage man shakes him from his reverie and, although he is unwilling to listen to Fred's story, he offers Fred a job working with the decommissioned planes. Fred later dismisses the job as one involving "junk," but it gives him the break he needs, and soon afterward Peggy and Fred make a commitment to each other—their embrace closes the film as a therapeutic moment of social reintegration. Although self-reliance is a strong theme in the film, it is through accommodation to others and the willingness to accept female care that Homer and Fred emerge from demobilization and feelings of fragmentation with at least the promise of marital happiness.

The Best Years of Our Lives focuses on the social effects of physical amputation (in Homer) and mental paralysis (in Fred), whereas The Men links these two themes in a more explicitly medical context. Released four years after The Best Years of Our Lives, The Men is an interesting demobilization narrative, not least because it gave the young Marlon Brando the chance to develop his method-acting skills in the demanding role of a paraplegic veteran, with Brando living for a time in a paraplegic unit at a hospital to prepare for the role. Directed by Fred Zinnemann, the film was written by Carl Foreman, who had become a specialist in war injury stories. Foreman was also the author of The Clay Pigeon (1949), the story of a veteran who wakes from a long-term coma to find that he has been charged with informing on his fellow soldiers in a Japanese prison camp; Home of the Brave (1949), based on Arthur Laurents's play dealing with illness and racism in the South Pacific (the film transformed a Jewish soldier into an African American one); and A Hatful of Rain (1957), which looks at the morphine addiction of a Korean War veteran.

Following the opening screen text—which announces that some men have "fought twice," through war and recovery—the camera follows US soldiers moving across a bleak landscape, before it focuses on Lieutenant Kenneth "Bud" Wilcheck (Brando) moments before he is shot from an occupied building. As he falls to the ground, he soliloquizes: "It was a bad shot or else he was impatient. He musta aimed for my head but he got me in the back. . . . I couldn't feel anything from my waist down. I thought I was dying." The film then swiftly cuts from a shot of the prostrate soldier surrounded by flying bullets to the image of an abject and isolated figure lying in bed. The camera moves closer to the bed; the narrator's voice pauses momentarily and then goes on: "I was afraid I was going to die, now I'm afraid I'm going to live. 'Oh, you'll be marching again in a couple of months, Lieutenant Wilcheck.' How many months? How many months? I've lost count. But let's keep it gay. Soldier, repeat after me: 'The war's over now and I'm glad I'm still half alive.'" The voice is initially blank and numb but then becomes more embittered; the camera moves closer, intercutting twisted voices of authority with Wilcheck's bewildered and fragmented thoughts. This opening is almost a direct dramatization of a key line from the 1946 training film *Let There Be Light*, in which the narrator describes anxious and restless soldiers in the hospital wards: "Now in the darkness of the war emerged the shapes born of darkness, the terrible things half-remembered, dreams of battle, the torment of uncertainty, fear, and loneliness."

Wilcheck's prostrate body stirs as an elderly nurse offers him a glass of water and medication. We focus on his face for a third time—the first before he is shot, the second as he struggles on the ground, and the third in profile and half in shadow—as he demands that the light be extinguished. The nurse then leads the viewer from the ward into a seminar on paraplegia, where a specialist named Dr. Brock (Everett Sloane) explains to his audience that any break in the spinal cord caused by a bullet or shrapnel will lead to "immediate and lasting paralysis of motion and feeling in the lower body." The symptoms associated with paraplegia are listed—"pain, muscular spasms, bedsores, paralysis of the bladder and bowels"—but Brock also expresses the belief that they can be controlled with "medical therapy, surgery, proper nutrition, physical rehabilitation, and self-care." His audience is wholly female: there are a couple of nurses, but most of the women are concerned mothers, wives, and friends, including Ellen (Teresa Wright), Wilcheck's former fiancée. When someone asks Brock whether the spine can be regenerated he answers negatively; on the subject of reproduction, he indicates that it depends on the severity of the injury; and on the subject of marital changes, he shows more sympathy, stating: "He isn't different. He's the same man with a spinal cord injury . . . right now he's unhappy, he's depressed, he feels himself totally dependent on others. . . . Is it any wonder he finds it difficult to adjust to the situation?" The fact that we know Wilcheck is experiencing night tremors in the adjacent room gives poignancy to the doctor's response and provides a counterpoint to the stern voices of authority that litter Wilcheck's fevered monologue.

Brock displays a mixture of straight talk and compassion when we see him interacting with other patients, all of whom have spinal injuries. Some of the men have related conditions that have improved with time and care; others with low-level injuries are beginning to use crutches; and still others are close to discharge. The psychological responses are also varied, from passive and meek patients to dissenting voices. One veteran, Norm Butler (Jack Webb), says: "I don't want to be rehabilitated, readjusted, reconditioned, or re- anything. . . . I don't want to take my proper place in society either." Brock jokes with the patients and is almost affectionate at times, but he can also be a stern patriarch, accusing one patient of sabotaging good surgery when he opens healing bedsores by going out against orders, and Brock is intolerant of patients who are unwilling to receive advice and treatment.

The mood changes when Brock leaves the public ward and enters an adjacent area, where Wilcheck lies immobile. The doctor notes that Wilcheck's bedsores and kidneys are improving and that he is nearly ready to leave the bed, after almost a year.

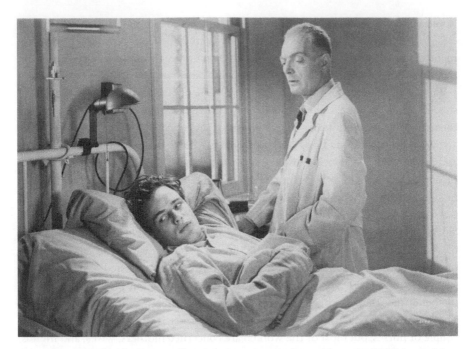

Figure 1.1   Dr. Brock (Everett Sloane) tries to counsel a stubborn Bud Wilcheck (Marlon Brando). *The Men* (Fred Zinnemann, United Artists, 1950).

Wilcheck is sarcastic about using a wheelchair, and he quickly angers when Brock mentions Ellen, Wilcheck's former fiancée. Detecting pathological maladjustment, Brock decides tough measures are necessary, and he stops Wilcheck's medication and has him moved into the communal ward. But Wilcheck not only refuses to join in with other paralyzed vets, he is also aggressive toward Ellen. When she refuses to leave one evening, Wilcheck resorts to revealing his paralyzed legs (not shown on-screen), screaming: "You want to see what it's like. All right, look. I said look at me. Now get a good look, does it make you feel healthy, is that what you want?" The repeated emphasis on looking suggests that the stigma of paralysis most bothers Wilcheck, and his behavior echoes the hidden aggression that often surfaced among veterans.[71] The voices of authority and unease that disturb Wilcheck's sleep early in the film are linked to his aggressive behavior toward Ellen and exacerbate his feelings of inferiority. A honed athlete before his injury, he refuses to spend his new life in a passive state or engaged in low-level activities such as weaving baskets; nevertheless, the scene ends with Wilcheck contemplating a reunion with Ellen, as he mutters in confusion: "I don't know. I don't know."

Wilcheck remains disconsolate for a long time, until Butler provokes him into a more active state. In an extended montage sequence, we then see Wilcheck progress quickly through physical therapy, doing sit-ups, exercising with weights, doing push-ups, and engaging in some occupational therapy. Using a wheelchair is his next step, followed by entering a pool supported by a rubber ring, followed by basketball and working out on the ropes. He is soon adept at using a wheelchair and much more positive about his relationship with Ellen. The quick pace of this montage sequence and acceleration of time offers a direct narrative contrast to the leisurely opening of the film, suggesting Wilcheck's positive reaction to therapy. However, while he seems to adapt well to his paraplegia, he deludes himself into thinking that he can feel his legs again. In the absence of his parents, Brock adopts a paternal role, assuring Wilcheck that "the legs are gone, now the head has to take over. . . . Before you can change the world, you have to accept it how it is without illusions." It is clear that neither Wilcheck nor Ellen is hardheaded enough: he fools himself into believing that he might walk again, and she is naïve about the demands of marriage, dismissing her parents' concerns about her being pushed into the role of a nurse.

In the second of two therapy montage sequences, we see Wilcheck moving to bigger weights, playing basketball in his wheelchair and volleyball in the pool, and walking with the aid of leg braces and parallel bars. He appears to progress without any help, suggesting the return of his self-determination and a willingness to participate in team events. However, when Wilcheck stumbles during his wedding vows, it is clear that he is not ready to accept marriage as a symbol of rehabilitation. Ellen looks shocked, and she panics again that evening when Wilcheck's leg starts shaking uncontrollably as he looks through a photograph album of his prewar sporting triumphs. The pair realize that they have made a big mistake. The scene quickly cuts to Wilcheck wheeling himself back to the ward to rejoin the hospitalized community where, even though the patients are engrossed in watching television, he cannot cope with the fact that they might be looking at him; his pent-up anguish boils over as he violently smashes the ward window with a crutch.

The promise of marital harmony suddenly degenerates into scenes portraying Wilcheck's wild behavior in a barroom brawl and a drunken car crash. Brock realizes that Wilcheck's physical therapy might have been successful, but he remains crippled psychologically. He argues with the hospital administrator that Wilcheck's case should be referred to the recently formed Paralyzed Veterans of America (PVA), a congressionally chartered association founded in 1946 to represent soldiers and service staff with spinal cord injuries. Having accepted the fact that the hospital is his permanent home, Wilcheck is appalled when the PVA decides he should be discharged: "He's well, isn't he? He's married. He's got himself a home. Why isn't he living in it?" When Wilcheck goes to see Brock to protest, he is reminded how hard it is for Ellen to adapt to his paraplegia. Only when Brock admits that his young paraplegic wife had died before they could adjust to their new life does Wilcheck realize how much he has to lose. The doctor does not offer sympathetic counseling. Instead, his final words are: "no-one can do it but you."

The closing scene shows Wilcheck returning to Ellen. Driving with determination, he maneuvers his wheelchair up a cobblestone path to her parents' house, but then he gets stuck when he encounters a set of steps. When Ellen comes out to greet him, they are both uncertain and nervous. Wilcheck points out his resourcefulness in mending a flat tire on his wheelchair and then asks if she wants to go the movies—a literal form of wish fulfillment—before ending with a symbol of homecoming as he accepts Ellen's help in wheeling him into her parents' house. But this apparent resolution—like that of Homer in *The Best Years of Our Lives*—does little to diminish Wilcheck's recent aggression. Both films end by shifting from a fairly realistic portrayal of war injury to a mythic level of therapeutic reintegration. There is much more explicit stress on hospitalization in *The Men* than in *The Best Years of Our Lives*, but the emphasis remains on physical loss and the requirements of reintegrating into civilian life. Too much self-reliance can lead to isolation and pigheadedness; self-reliance needs to be tempered by a willingness to accept the help that, in both films, comes in the form of loving heterosexual relationships.

Blindness and Occluded Stories

"Among the casualties of war," a 1953 VA report claimed, "none deserves more specialized consideration than the blinded veterans."[72] Blindness occasionally figured in cultural responses to World War I, such as Robert Bridges's poem "To the United States of America" (1917), in which the British poet asks Americans to clear "your minds of all estranging blindness," and John Singer Sargent's painting *Gassed* (1919), in which ten blindfolded soldiers trample over dead and dying bodies.[73] However, actual blindness was infrequently discussed in the clinical literature of the 1910s, which tended to focus on shell shock or hysterical responses to combat. For example, Millais Culpin, an expert in psychoneurosis at the London Hospital, argued in 1920 that hysterical blindness arising without organic damage to the eyes is "an excrescence upon an underlying medical condition."[74] Culpin claimed that treatment need not be precise, but the physician should "make the patient believe something effective is being done" by means of "electricity, massage, rest, exercise, [or] drugs."[75] These techniques continued to inform the approach to hysterical blindness, but in World War II this was treated alongside permanent blindness caused by shrapnel and bullets.

By mid-century, the ability to treat blindness was improved by the availability of sulfonamides and penicillin to prevent infections and secondary conditions. However, the stigma surrounding blindness remained high, despite Helen Keller's "Purple Heart tours" of 1944 and 1945—which followed her demystifying autobiography *The Story of My Life* (1903) and the dramatization of her overcoming sensory deprivation (she was blind, mute, and deaf) in the 1919 silent film *Deliverance*. As Frances Koestler argues in her study of blindness, *The Unseen Minority* (1976), although there was a much more "experienced leadership structure in work for the blind" in 1943 than in World War I, a commitment to develop specialist hospitals for those with eye injuries, and the belief that blinded veterans could still be high achievers, the War Department "failed to anticipate how rapidly the number of war-blinded would grow, and how slowly the VA would move to pick up its end of the job."[76] With 230,000 blind Americans even before the war, a 1947 public service pamphlet endorsed by the New York Association for the Blind pointed out that although most people are "by and large . . .

very sympathetic toward" the blind, they "find it hard to believe that a blind person can do anything useful."[77] The pamphlet provided information on a range of optical problems and government aid, applauding naval and army hospitals for "restoring self-confidence in blinded veterans" and treating them as individuals rather than en masse.[78] A 1953 report by the US Bureau of Medicine and Surgery played down blindness, arguing that eye injuries in World War II provided "only a small percentage of the total number of injuries," with only 1,400 US servicemen blinded between Pearl Harbor and the end of the war.[79] According to the report, documented cases included a marine who had been "blinded by a bullet which penetrated his left temple and destroyed both eyes and the bridge of the nose," and courses of "social readjustment training"—including typewriting, Braille, and forms of self-care—started very early. The report noted that a "high degree of individualization" characterized different hospital programs, but it is interesting that the general condition of blindness features prominently in two of the most significant demobilization films to emerge after World War II.[80]

Following up on Dana Polan's argument that blindness is linked to the problematic place of home in the 1940s, we can see that the demobilization films treat blindness both as a metaphor and as an irreversible organic condition.[81] Just as amputation and paralysis are embedded in the narrative structures of *The Best Days of Our Lives* and *The Men*, so visual and social occlusion are pivotal to *Pride of the Marines* and *Bright Victory*. And just as themes of disruption and homecoming intersect in films dealing with paralysis and amputation, so they also emerge in blindness narratives. For example, while the white cane for some blind veterans represented a chance to regain autonomy and independence, for others—like Al Schmid in *Pride of the Marines*—it tapped into their deepest fears and nightmares.

The "Note to the Reader" at the beginning of Roger Butterfield's *Al Schmid, Marine* (1944), the source text for *Pride of the Marines*, highlights the two battles that Al faced: first, the one on Guadalcanal in 1942, where an enemy grenade blew up in his face; and second, the one in which he had to fight his way "back to sanity, health and happiness," foreshadowing the opening screen text of *The Men*, which stressed that many soldiers are twice wounded. Butterfield emphasizes the authenticity of the story, claiming that the book is an oral history that uses Al's "own words, phrases and descriptions." He notes that Al had only 5 percent vision in one eye and a total loss of sight in the other, but he wanted no "special credit" and wished to be seen as "no different from any other young American in uniform."[82] The pride that forms one of the central themes of the film adaptation is evident from the outset of Butterfield's literary account.

Unlike the film version, which shows the young, self-reliant, and fully sighted Al (John Garfield) and his flirtatious relationship with Ruth Hartley (Eleanor Parker), the book begins in the hospital, where we see Al groping for ash trays and learning to light his own cigarettes. Al realizes that he and the other wounded veterans make a "crazy" bunch: one marine struggles to speak with shrapnel in his throat, and another has bullets in his leg and a cast "that smelled worse than anything you ever saw."[83]

Despite their injuries, the comrades have a kind of gallows humor, and the presence of Ruth creates a familial atmosphere in the ward. Unlike the isolated figure in *Pride of the Marines* who is determined to see again, the book tells us very early on that the real Al Schmid has had one of his eyes cut out and shrapnel remains embedded in the other. This framing device has a very different function than the opening of the film (discussed at the beginning of the chapter), emphasizing solidarity and care rather than individualism.

Nevertheless, both stories stress the ordinariness of Al and his active lifestyle. The book also emphasizes his German-Irish family; but in the film, his ethnicity is only implicit until, halfway through, we see him kiss a shamrock on his machine gun which is positioned next to a Star of David that signifies his comrade Lee Diamond's Jewishness. Al is no intellectual, but neither is he a failure. He works hard at the Dodge Steel Company, although he never has much money, and he is very independent until he meets Ruth in the winter of 1940–1941. Initially the radio announcement about the bombing of Pearl Harbor is treated as a joke, but, as soon as he realizes that the United States is at war, Al promptly joins the Marine Corps, with very little evidence of recruitment screening.

After sending Ruth an engagement ring, Al is immediately mobilized, and the film swiftly dissolves from Ruth's voice-over to a battle scene on Guadalcanal. The transition is lengthier in the book, which shows Al becoming friends with Johnny Rivers and Lee Diamond, the soldiers who with him operate a machine gun in a foxhole on Guadalcanal. The middle of the book details events leading up to the nighttime attack by the Japanese and the grenade that hits Al with "a terrific wallop in the face," which is reduced to a dramatic ten-minute sequence in the film.[84] The book conveys Al's sense impressions: the "wet sticky pulp" of his head, the feeling that "somebody had cut off the front of his face with a hatchet," and pains in his arms. But his adrenalin is pumping, and he keeps firing at the Japanese, with Lee (who has been shot in the shoulder) helping him to aim the gun. A note in the book suggests that Al killed over two hundred enemy soldiers that night.

In contrast to the adrenalin-charged marine swallowing his own blood in the bunker, in the next chapter we see Al being carried into a hospital. His face and eyes are "riddled with shrapnel and puffed up with blood and bruises"; a piece of his ear is missing; and he has cuts in his neck, shoulder, and arm as well as a gouge in one knuckle, a gangrenous leg, and concussion.[85] There is little description of the medical team in the hospital, except for an optical specialist, who decides that Al's left eye needs removing due to a severed and infected optic nerve, and Doc Ward, who is presented as both a friend and physician. Al eventually agrees to have the eye removed, and his other wounds clear up fairly quickly, but his emotions fluctuate wildly during his stay in the hospital. He rejects Ruth at one point (after the Red Cross nurse, Virginia Pfeiffer, has written Ruth to tell her about Al's blindness), but he is periodically cheerful when listening to the radio and a visiting comedian, and on receiving Ruth's letters and fan mail about his exploits on Guadalcanal. With his morale and mental health improving, he agrees to use a glass eye and slowly starts to detect color in his one real eye. The story ends conventionally, as Al returns home (he can see the porch steps but cannot count how many there are) to receive his Navy Cross and marry Ruth.

It is noticeable that the role of professionals is kept to a minimum, and the only mention of Al's recruitment test is the line: "The two men in front of him were both turned down—they weren't taking everybody."[86] Apart from the help of the nurse and Doc Ward, Al gets through depression on his own, with only his comrades and Ruth's letters as comfort. Given that the book is an oral history and that Al is absorbed in the physical side of his injuries, the absence of professionals may not be surprising; we are given only passing references to his depression, nightmares, and insomnia during his journey to California and in his erratic behavior toward Ruth. Perhaps if the account had been written in the first person, there would be more attention to fluctuations in mood. Nonetheless, it is striking that the book does not describe any psychiatric consultation during Al's recruitment or rehabilitation.

In contrast to the book's emphasis on Al's unique and heroic story, in his portrayal in *Pride of the Marines*, John Garfield combines Al's unique and typical qualities. The typicality of response reflects the fact that up to 40 percent of casualties evacuated from Guadalcanal suffered from "neuro-mental disease" after prolonged exposure to "exhaustion, fever, malaria, and sudden violent death at the hand of an insidious and ruthless enemy."[87] After Al leaves Guadalcanal, we see the pattern of denial and hostility that characterizes many demobilization narratives: he possesses a sense of humor and a feeling of solidarity with his comrades, but he is prone to dark moods and intolerance, and he is aggressive with the doctors and desperate to preserve his self-reliance, stubbornly refusing to learn Braille. There is more interaction between Al and medical staff in the film than in the book, but his relationship with Virginia is of particular interest because she represents a midpoint between the common sense of the medical profession and the affection of a friend. While it is possible to see Virginia and Ruth as cogs in the micropolitics of the medical establishment, pulling Al back from existential solitude into the family, it is significant that Virginia is a Red Cross nurse.[88] The nonspecialist social worker did not receive much attention at the 1942 APA conference discussed above, where speakers made such dismissive comments as "it is decidedly unwise . . . to expect these heavily burdened workers to carry out a phase in essentially medical treatment."[89] Perhaps the conference delegates were protecting their own profession, but, given the lack of trained psychiatrists, it is surprising that little acknowledgment was given to the contributions of care workers and medical support staff. Demobilization films provide a different view, though. *Pride of the Marines* and *Till the End of Time* both spare narrative attention to figures representing the extended arm of care necessary to rehabilitate wounded soldiers. This is usually a feminized role, blending medical know-how (Virginia reminds Al of his capabilities and limitations) with folk wisdom: "Sometimes when a man has to climb a mountain on his own, he loses his way," Virginia muses.

Virginia and later Ruth are the two people who help Al the most to escape from the isolated world of blindness. Sensory deprivation concerns him less than the fears of stigma and of being a burden to others, dramatized starkly in an expressionistic dream sequence that breaks the film's realistic frame. In fact, the realism is broken twice. The first break is the ten-minute sequence when Al and his two companions are in the foxhole at Guadalcanal; the sounds of Japanese soldiers in the dark and of his wounded companions make Al almost psychopathological, as he fires his machine gun on pure adrenalin. The second break is the extended dream sequence in the hospital, which links back to the Japanese voices surrounding the foxhole. The dream transports Al from Guadalcanal to his arrival at the Philadelphia train station, where Ruth is waiting for him. The couple embrace and then turn to see a blind man slowly walking down the platform with a white cane, dark glasses, and a tin cup. The blind man stops close to Ruth, and we see the couple turn toward him in profile at the right of the frame while he stares straight ahead at the left. Then the figure vanishes, and Ruth turns around in shock—only to stare into the face of Al who is now wearing the dark glasses, which start flashing menacingly like signal lights. Ruth panics and retreats from the platform rapidly in reverse motion. The dream ends when Al awakes, moaning and sweating. He clearly sees the white cane and dark glasses as markers of stigma and a warning of his future life—a haunting image that leads him to ask Virginia to write Ruth to inform her that he will not be returning. Only Virginia's phone call to Ruth provides her with the truth of Al's condition, and it takes a good deal of trickery to get Al back to Philadelphia, where Ruth meets him but does not reveal her identity.

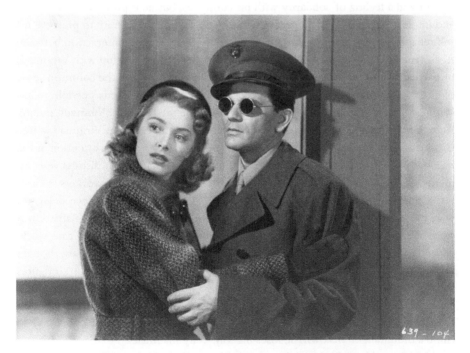

Figure 1.2   Al Schmid (John Garfield) and Ruth Hartley (Eleanor Parker) appear in Al's blindness dream. *Pride of the Marines* (Delmer Daves, Warner Brothers, 1945).

The two women are not the only ones to fulfill a therapeutic function in the film, which reveals the aims of the screenwriter Albert Maltz (who was named as one of the blacklisted Hollywood Ten the following year) of linking Al's story to a broader narrative about national identity.[90] Lee Diamond confronts Al about his self-pity, using his own experience of anti-Semitism to push Al to confront the reality of his injury. Al is slow to heed the advice, though. When Lee contemplates returning to service in the Pacific, Al surprises himself with his violent response: "Get 'em in the eyes, right in the eyes," he growls, before falling silent. He eventually heeds Lee's point that he should not "leave all [his] guts back on the canal, you need them now too," but Al's rehabilitation is incomplete until Ruth has confronted him. He turns aggressive when Ruth finally reveals her identity and rebukes him for not having "enough pride to face the truth" or to "accept being blind like a man." Eventually he comes around, but he worries about no longer being "an ordinary guy," which leads Ruth to appeal to his heroic stand in Guadalcanal: "Don't you realize that every single man that has fought is no longer ordinary . . . it wasn't any ordinary guy who kept the Japs back that night. It's one of the most extraordinary fellas in the world. You. Al Schmid." Not only does she turn Al's condition into something special, but she appeals to all soldiers who have "lost some chips" in winning the war, as Lee describes it earlier. In this way *Pride of the Marines* extends the scope and significance of *Al Schmid, Marine*, transforming a singular war narrative into an exceptional story of national significance.

Baynard Kendrick's novel *Lights Out* (1945) also places a story of blindness within a national framework, providing the basis for one of the last films in the demobilization group. The novel was retitled *Bright Victory* for its Bantam paperback release in 1951, to reflect the title of the Universal film. The story focuses on a veteran's rehabilitation from total blindness after he is hit by a German sniper in North Africa in 1943.[91] It deals much more centrally with rehabilitation than the earlier films, making the wounded veteran the protagonist, rather than one of three in the case of Homer Parrish and Perry Kincheloe in *The Best Years of Our Lives* and *Till the End of Time*, respectively. It also explores the complexities of rehabilitation and reflects Kendrick's interest in the ways in which blindness pushes the body to adapt to partial or total loss of sight—a subject Kendrick had been exploring as a member of the Blinded Veterans Association, which was formed in 1945.

The novel and the film are mostly set at the Valley Forge General Hospital, in Phoenixville, Pennsylvania, which was one of two army hospitals specializing in the rehabilitation of blind veterans. As Koestler notes, the army intended "to keep the soldier in a military hospital until maximum therapeutic benefit has been obtained [leaving] little time for self-pity," including training in deportment and walking, psychological welfare, and relearning motor skills.[92] Valley Forge is portrayed as a safe environment, but it is far from being a place of incarceration: patients move between the wards and grounds at their ease and without posing any threat. In the film, Valley Forge is depicted as being full of well-adjusted veterans, but it is also understaffed, with one physician to attend to 2,000 men.

The initial bewilderment experienced by Sergeant Larry Nevins (played by Arthur Kennedy) when he is wounded is conveyed by Kendrick's subdued description: "Something pinged and hit his forehead with no more shock than a blown pea."[93] Kendrick's hard-boiled tone is not fully adopted in the film, but in both versions Nevins is depicted as a tough guy whose financial security depends on his fiancée, Chris Paterson, and her anticipated inheritance from her businessman father. Nevins's emotions—"Chris was not only pretty; her father owned a barrel factory [in Florida] and lots of good potato land. Might as well have a father-in-law with dough"—are complicated by his wound, leading him into an ambiguous world where his prejudices are severely tested.[94] Once Nevins realizes that he is permanently blind, he enters a self-absorbed state, which is highly dramatized in the film. He initially cannot utter the word "blind" let alone accept his fate, even when a fellow patient advises him to "get a good grip on yourself." This suggests that self-reliance and optimism are essential for dealing with the physical and psychological impact of blindness, as emphasized by a publicity image in which Kennedy, shot in dramatic profile, holds up to his face a walking cane that casts a dark shadow over his eyes. Nevins does not heed this advice, though, and refuses to be optimistic. Half-sedated, he pulls himself out of bed and finds the bathroom, where he futilely scratches and rubs the mirror in an attempt to see himself. Then, in deep despair, he tries to slash his wrist.

Miserable and downhearted, Nevins quickly enters physical rehabilitation. Taught the geography of the hospital by having his hand guided over a scale model,

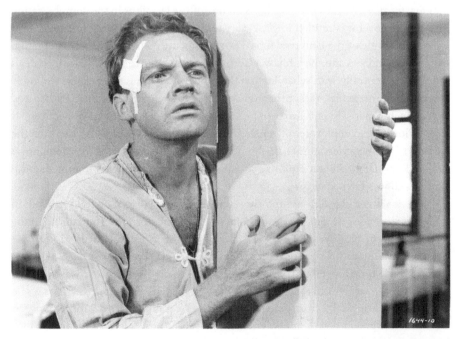

Figure 1.3   A hospitalized Larry Nevins (Arthur Kennedy) struggles to come to terms with his blindness. *Bright Victory* (Mark Robson, Universal, 1951).

he walks with his arm in front of him to anticipate obstacles, and he learns how to feed himself. His rehabilitation is largely physical, but a psychiatrist discusses the psychological dimension of shock with a group of new patients:

> Until these neuroses of panic and despair have been conquered you will not begin the healthy adjustment which will eventually bring you peace with yourselves and with others. . . . So much of your life now depends on you. Yesterday you could see, today you cannot, but tomorrow or some day soon, if you apply yourselves, you'll discover that every part of you was working hard to replace your eyes and you'll be astonished at your success.

The psychiatrist shifts here between physical and psychological registers and is optimistic about the ways in which bodies adapt to sensory loss. But the last line suggests that the focus is primarily on practical adjustments, emphasized by the subsequent discussion of pension allowances for injured veterans.

Nevins finds that he is very adept at obstacle perception and also learns how to get around outside the hospital grounds. But his social life is more of a problem, and he refuses to tell his family about his blindness; only when he realizes that his lieutenant is also blind does he agrees to speak to them. More important, we see Nevins's racist streak early in the film, during his flight home from North Africa with black soldiers. When he makes friends with one African American soldier, Joe Morgan, in Valley Forge, it is only a matter of time before he finds out Joe's race and cuts him dead. This is one of the levels in which blindness operates figuratively. The proximity of black and white soldiers during the war does nothing to erode Larry's perception of the color line, and only when he is truly blind to Joe's racial identity does he treat him as a friend. When he tries to defend his behavior, he is told: "You gonna run into this sort of thing for the rest of your life, Larry. People with no faces, no color. Just voices. Are you gonna ask them what their race and religion is before you decide whether you like them or not?" This quotation provides a clue to the film's underlying message about Nevins's psychological and emotional reeducation, which is treated on a par with his physical rehabilitation.

Nevins is also blind to the feelings of Judy Greene (Peggy Dow), a young woman he meets in a bar who falls for him despite his dismissive behavior. Judy is the sympathetic friend that Nevins needs—at one point he says, "You did it, Judy. You're the doctor that cured me"—but they talk at cross-purposes, and he is incapable of reading her emotions. Nevins assumes that back in Florida financial security awaits him, but after he returns home, he finds that his parents are small-minded, racist, and only able to treat him like a child. They refuse to fully acknowledge their son's blindness, while his future father-in-law wants to sever the ties between Nevins and Chris because Nevins is "no longer an able-bodied man." The couple briefly resume their courtship, but when Nevins stresses the extensive care he needs, Chris decides she is not "strong enough" to cope, and they part.

The film's resolution functions on two levels, linking together twin forms of therapeutic rehabilitation: a job and a caring relationship. Nevins bumps into Judy's brother-in-law at the train station, which leads him to meet a blind lawyer who points out the challenges and rewards of professional life. The lawyer stresses the need for constant toil within a caring environment: he tells Nevins that law school will make any concessions for a student's blindness (very few law books were then available in Braille), but that through blindness he can find inner resolve: "Then one day, like that, you find yourself. It's when you discover that you can concentrate better than the others. That's the one big light in our darkness. That, and someone to love. With those two there's nothing you can't do." Nevins takes away this lesson of resolve and love, guts and care, realizing that the security he has been looking for back in Florida is misplaced. He needs Judy as an emotional anchor, but he also requires security in himself. "I told you I wanted security," he says to Judy. "Well, I was looking for it in all the wrong places. No one can ever give it to you, Judy . . . you got to make it for yourself."

Not only does he promise Judy that he will soon resume his relationship with her, but almost immediately afterward he bumps into his old friend, Joe. Nevins approaches him affectionately; Joe is uncertain at first, but soon they begin to joke as they enter a train carriage together. Holding each other's arms, they sit close to each other, two blind veterans—one black and one white—as the train leaves the station. Not only can reeducation of the senses steer the veteran toward a productive life path, but *Bright Victory* suggests that it can also overcome the blindness to a common humanity that lies beyond skin color. Although other postwar texts—most notably Ralph Ellison's 1951 novel *Invisible Man*—explore racial blindness with greater complexity, *Bright Victory* places strong emphasis on the progressive consequences of cultural reeducation.

The therapy that Nevins receives is partly formal—the physical therapy in Valley Forge and psychiatric advice—but largely informal: a realization that he must be self-reliant and that he has to reeducate his senses to look beyond the myopia of racism and financial security. This part of the story is supported by a later study concerning the psychiatric problems that often accompany the loss of sight and that require "internal reorganization" and a reorientation of the individual's "capacities, his interests, his social position, his body image, [and] his aspirations."[95] *Bright Victory* indicates the need to equip soldiers with the life skills they will need to contend with shifting social, gender, and racial politics, as well as educating all viewers to realize that—in the words of the 1947 public service pamphlet *What Do You Know about Blindness?*—"besides being treated as human beings, blind people want to be treated as individuals."[96] But rather than suggesting that blindness should be treated as a radical difference, the film conveys the message that people who have lost their sight should be nurtured in a supportive environment without undermining their autonomy.

Amputees, paraplegics, and blinded veterans are the most visually dramatic cases in a range of depictions of soldiers who returned from World War II to find themselves misplaced or unable to settle down, such as the exhausted veteran with no home to return to, played by Joseph Cotton in *I'll Be Seeing You* (1944), and the disfigured airman in *The Enchanted Cottage* (1945). Although Judy Greene in *Bright Victory*—like Mary Marshall (Ginger Rogers) in *I'll Be Seeing You* and Laura Pennington (Dorothy McGuire) in *The Enchanted Cottage*—is placed squarely in a facilitating role, the assumption in *Bright Victory* is that Nevins and Judy will "work it out" together. Like Virginia in *Pride of the Marines* and Peggy in *The Best Years of Our Lives*, Judy is obviously helper, lover, and social worker simultaneously, a representative of the people who ensured that therapy was taken out of the hospital wards and into the homes of postwar America.

2 *In the Noir Mirror*

NEUROSIS, AGGRESSION, AND DISGUISE

The demobilization films of the late 1940s and early 1950s constituted an eclectic genre, bringing together elements of combat movie, domestic melodrama, and the social problem film, the last of which emerged in the 1940s before Cold War tensions and the Hollywood blacklist limited the freedom to tackle pressing social issues directly. Although the Office of War Information carefully vetted depictions of soldiers and veterans during the first half of the 1940s, the demobilization films revealed a widespread commitment to depict the realities and consequences of war. But this did not mean that there was a consensus in the mid-1940s about the responsibilities of filmmakers or the film industry. Indeed, in 1945 a public debate on the role of movies revealed deeply divided ideologies. Filmmakers with a social conscience were pitted against the likes of the anticommunist Chairman of the Motion Picture Alliance for the Preservation of American Ideals, James K. McGuinness, who claimed that movies should offer "balm for the spirit."[1] This kind of therapeutic rhetoric provided fuel for Erich Fromm's criticism that Hollywood films were too often like daydreams, "where the real problems of the individual can be forgotten."[2] However, although Fromm shared Theodor Adorno's suspicion of mass culture, they tended to overlook films that dealt seriously with ideas: for example, David O. Selznick's and Orson Welles's interest in psychiatry inflected their cinematic perspectives on World War II.

There is always a danger in choosing a representative cultural form to reflect a national zeitgeist, and the demobilization films are no exception. Many of the films documented the aftermath of war, combining sociological, medical, psychological, and military elements that were sometimes linked to fantasy—such as the dream sequences in *Pride of the Marines* or the healthening narratives of *The Best Years of Our Lives* and *Bright Victory*, discussed in the previous chapter. The demobilization films provide a useful starting point because they engaged directly with postwar medical stories about communal war experiences.[3] But although the films, with their medical subject matter, may seem to reflect the concerns of the immediate postwar years, they represent only a small fraction of the US films produced in the mid- to late 1940s. Only *The Best Years of Our Lives*, which won an Academy Award in 1946, was among the top box-office pictures of the decade, and the musical biopics *The Jolson Story* (about Al Jolson), *Till the Clouds Roll By* (about Jerome Kern) and *Night and Day* (about Cole Porter); the musicals *Road to Utopia* and *The Harvey Girls*; and films set in the 1920s, *Saratoga Trunk* and *Margie*, were among the most watched in cinemas during the 1940s. Therapeutic narratives of the period, then, might more easily be located in these escapist films, in which the troubles of the present are sublimated or disappear. However, this would be to overlook the most distinctive of the 1940s cinematic genres: film noir.

Following from the previous chapter, here I examine the ways in which film noir expanded the range of demobilization stories. Not only do these stories reveal the physical injuries of war to be lingering and diffuse, but they also show that psychological damage arose variously in the form of breakdowns, aggression, and psychopathology. The influence of Freud is at its most explicit in this chapter, with filmmakers appropriating Freudian motifs to explore the neuroses, dreams, and fantasies of characters who are placed under strain by their war experiences. It is clear that World War II was largely detrimental to the mental health of its combatants; less clear is whether the war exacerbated deep-rooted neuroses or whether combat fragmented previously healthy egos. Postwar studies on aggression in the first section of this chapter provide a context for examining representations of psychic fragmentation in film noir. Then I move on to discuss Alfred Hitchcock's film *Spellbound*—arguably the most important treatment of Freudian ideas in 1940s Hollywood—in which war is never far away. The chapter concludes by looking at emerging postwar concerns about psychopathology, which suggests the war unlocked forces that medicine found hard to treat, let alone cure.

Aggression, Exhaustion, and Film Culture

Despite the box-office hits of 1946, cultural historians have frequently returned to film noir as a mirror of a darker national scene in which cynicism and psychopathology reveal a nation struggling with itself. In its name and style, film noir was closely linked to European cinema, but it was propelled in new directions by a number of émigré directors who worked in or on the fringes of Hollywood in the 1940s, including Alfred Hitchcock, Billy Wilder, and Fritz Lang. Critics have noted that wartime blackouts (a *Los Angeles Times* headline on 11 December 1941 read "Los Angeles Blacked Out") were mirrored in the menacing shadows and silhouettes of the noir mise-en-scène, while the retirement in 1945 of Will Hays, author of the Hollywood Production Code, led to a relaxation of screen portrayals of psychological instability, violence, and overtly sexual behavior, coinciding with a lifting on the embargo on graphic images of those wounded in war (illustrated by the Oscar-winning documentary *With the Marines at Tarawa* and the uncensored footage of Nazi concentration camps that the US military supplied to commercial newsreels in 1945).[4] Violence undoubtedly became more common on screen after 1944. What is less certain is whether film noir engaged seriously with public debates about personal conduct and political value, or whether it was too nihilistic a genre to offer more than "sinister mirrors of American angst and moral decay."[5] Nevertheless, in its brooding mise-en-scène, dramatic narratives, and disturbing exploration of violence and psychic fragmentation, film noir amplified postwar concerns and often engaged directly with medicine and psychiatry.[6]

Rather than transporting the viewer into the doctor's office, clinic, or hospital, film noir dealt more directly than the demobilization films did with unstable and potentially dangerous figures at large within society. And while the demobilization films tended to focus on fatigue and film noir emphasized aggression, both genres dealt centrally with marginalized characters who no longer fit in, due to debilitating wounds, alienation, or unemployment. They also responded to broader social pressures as reflected in the 1945 mass-market paperback *Psychology for the Returning Serviceman*, which dedicated a chapter to forms of personal and social conflict. Even though the book underplayed the disruption veterans felt when returning to civilian life, it noted that "when he can't get what he wants [the soldier] wants to fight now. So he finds somebody to fight with, usually some individual or group towards whom he has a long-standing hostility for other reasons. It's the Jews, the reds, the Republicans, the Democrats, the industrialists, the Unions, or the bankers who are to blame."[7]

Psychology for the Returning Serviceman is full of good advice and is sensitive to the issues presented in *The Best Years of Our Lives* (the last chapter of the book is titled "The Years of Your Life"), such as the veteran's return to his family and the problems likely to arise in his relationships. It also touches on social change, class, and race, although there is no mention of gender. But the book does not really grapple with aggressive behavior and suggests that rest and recuperation are all that are needed for a full recovery. This is somewhat surprising, given that studies published earlier in the 1940s had focused on the role of aggression in combat—sometimes released through violence, sometimes turned in on the self, and sometimes provoking hostility toward the returning veteran.[8] Countering the positive message of *Psychology for the Returning Serviceman*, one of the most important books on postwar medicine, William Menninger's *Psychiatry in a Troubled World*, established that individual reactions to war reveal complex patterns—mental, bodily, and psychosomatic—rather than typical or standardized responses. Although specific responses to combat do arise (the violent pounding of the heart, a sinking feeling in the stomach, sickness, and trembling), these were also symptoms displayed by noncombatants, suggesting a continuum rather than a categorical distinction between military and civilian life.

Menninger worried about terms like "effective soldier" because they dealt with function alone rather than with the whole individual, and he was equally concerned about stigmatizing language used to described recruits who displayed "any deviation from maximum effort toward the common objective," including derogatory labels such as "quitter" or "eight ball."[9] Other postwar publications, such as *Men under Stress* (1945), attempted to better examine the particular psychodynamics behind these war experiences, and later books, such as *Breakdown and Recovery* (1959), by the Columbia University professor Eli Ginzberg, dealt directly with both physical and mental problems.[10] Ginzberg's study stemmed from the Conservation of Human Resources Project established by General Dwight Eisenhower in 1950 to "uncover the causes of the major deficiencies in the nation's human resources that World War II revealed."[11] As such, *Breakdown and Recovery* challenged accounts that focused only on psychology by attending to environmental factors that can precipitate an individual's breakdown and recovery.[12] Nonetheless, Ginzberg's seventy-nine case studies lean toward a straightforward moral lesson: "While every man has his weakness he also has strengths. Even if the solider breaks down, a loving family can help him recover, as can a sympathetic government and a growing economy."[13] Whatever therapeutic worth we might attach to this homily, the message clearly glides over a range of related problems.

The narrative pattern in the title of Ginzberg's book stresses the expectancy of recovery, but in the late 1940s Menninger was worrying about the inadequately equipped healthcare system. This was partly because he feared that institutional support was insufficient (the January 1946 issue of *Journal of the American Medical Association* appealed to "physicians interested in neuropsychiatry" to apply for vacancies) and partly because research into neuropsychiatric responses to combat remained in a crude state.[14] The first concern was to address the limited resources available to treat mental illness, as highlighted by Albert Deutsch, by developing mental hygiene institutions in large cities and expanding group-practice training clinics such as the Menninger Clinic in Topeka, Kansas, where the Karl Menninger School of Psychiatry and Mental Health Sciences opened in 1946 to train psychiatrists to treat those wounded in the war.[15] However, combat fatigue came in many forms, and the latency of symptoms meant that in the late 1940s, aggression and trauma were only dimly understood. The Menningers, among others, thought that feelings of aggression did not simply vanish at the end of the war but needed careful management to prevent destructive impulses from taking hold.

Studies of aggression began to appear in the late 1930s, but aggression was linked most closely with the warmongering nations of Germany, Italy, and Japan during the 1940s. For example, the British publication *Aggression and Population* (1946) proposed that aggression is often stimulated by material need or rivalry but is also driven by "the greed and inequalities of a fiercely competitive economic system."[16] That study's central claim is that "our world to-day is advancing at a reckless pace along the path that will lead to the precipice of the unsolved problem of human populations sharing and using the earth's resources."[17] The author, James Dawson, linked aggression to population change, particularly in crowded areas where rival claims over space are most intense—a theme developed by the American-born Alix Strachey, a member of the Bloomsbury group and a Freudian, in *The Unconscious Motives of War*.[18] Dawson saw particular dangers in the population explosion of the baby boom and the growth of African American groups, believing that increased intermarriage in the South was likely to lead to racial conflict. Chapter 7 returns to these issues, but the postwar emphasis on business and scientific technology was more than just a social Darwinist climate in which the fittest would prevail. The general view was that those equipped for yesterday (such as the fighting soldier) were unlikely to keep pace with social change.

This sense of maladaption is illustrated in *The Best Years of Our Lives*. When Fred Derry returns to his old job, he finds that his employer is not impressed with his war record and downgrades him to a marginal status in the workplace. Although Derry's aggression is largely turned inward, we see Homer and Derry ready to pick a fight with a right-wing customer who challenges their patriotic values when he claims that the nation has been fighting the wrong enemy. In this scene the veterans' aggressive impulses are given ideological justification, but in most other ways Homer and Derry are marginal men who are forced to deal with atavistic impulses alone and without medical support—as is demonstrated when Homer smashes the garage window with his hooks, and Derry experiences a traumatic nightmare in Peggy Stephenson's bedroom (see chapter 1 for a discussion of these episodes). The decommissioned fighter jet in which Derry seeks refuge in the junkyard is the underside of the technology boom, but it is also a symbolic reminder that Derry's technical skills as a pilot are redundant in the postwar years.

It is significant that *Aggression and Population* focuses on 1940s military technology—"the aeroplane, the atom and other bombs, the mine and torpedo, quick-firing and ever more powerful artillery, the machine-gun . . . the rocket, even poison gas"—implying that the destructive consequences of aggressive acts were more profound than ever.[19] This chimes with claims that science was threatening to undermine modern democracies, thereby serving as a counterpoint to the triumphant account of postwar science in the major state-sponsored publication, Vannevar Bush's report *Science—The Endless Frontier.*[20] Late in *Aggression and Population*, Dawson turns his attention from national conditions to the individual who finds himself "utterly lost, as only one of so many."[21] Such feelings of anomie led many soldiers and veterans to lash out violently or turn their aggression inward, as fictionalized in the suicide of the young World War II veteran Seymour Glass in J. D. Salinger's 1948 story "A Perfect Day for Bananafish."[22]

An earlier text, *Frustration and Aggression*, published in 1939 under the auspices of the Institute of Human Relations at Yale University, explored the ways in which aggression often stems from frustration. Drawing on Freud's writings on psychic sublimation in *A General Introduction to Psychoanalysis* (1920), the authors of *Frustration and Aggression* nonetheless sidestep Freud when it comes to libidinal drives. This reflects Alfred Adler's split with Freud in 1911, which was mainly because Adler approached aggression in general terms rather than seeing it as rooted in sexual drives (a reservation shared by the Menningers, who were enthusiastic about Freud's metapsychological principles but less persuaded by his theory of infantile sexuality). The authors of *Frustration and Aggression* argue simply that aggressive behavior is normally displayed toward another person or authorities, but fantasies of domination, dreams of revenge, and violent language "undirected toward any object" sometimes substitute for aggression.[23] If frustration is often the root cause, then any situation that prevents closure (or wish fulfillment) puts the aggressive person at risk of exploding outward in sadistic behavior, or turning inward—as illustrated by Salinger's outgoing Seymour Glass, who masks his internal suffering of war trauma until he turns on himself in the final paragraph of "A Perfect Day for Bananafish" and fires "a bullet through his right temple."[24]

Outlets for War Neurosis

Clinicians understood as early as 1942 that combat fatigue and war neurosis were nonspecific terms that hovered around a number of psychiatric conditions. One study of chronic war neuroses by the Menninger psychiatrist Robert P. Knight proposed that, in addition to "a relatively small group of traumatic war neuroses, initiated by specific terrifying experiences," the war made manifest a host of neuroses that, from a Freudian perspective, could be traced back to childhood.[25] But contemporary studies of aggression suggested that wartime experiences might exacerbate or trigger latent neuroses, bringing them to the surface in exaggerated forms and even producing fresh neuroses linked to aggressive impulses that were often encouraged in troops. Within this context, there were many studies of aggression in the late 1940s. In 1949 Anna Freud wrote about aggression in children, and two books by the psychoanalyst Karen Horney (who was born in Germany but based in Brooklyn since the 1930s), *The Neurotic Personality of Our Time* (1937) and *Neurosis and Human Growth* (1950), suggested that aggression was a neurotic mode of moving against others. Horney also chose to avoid the Freudian take on libidinal repression, noting that aggression is sometimes displayed in outwardly provocative behavior but, at other times, manifests itself as self-harm. She detected that the "neurotic personality" reveals itself through aggressive acts ("a propensity to be aggressive, domineering, over-exacting, to boss, cheat or find fault") or submission ("an attitude of easily feeling cheated, dominated, scolded, imposed on or humiliated"), which, by 1950, she had started to link to psychological warfare.[26]

Adler, Horney, and Melanie Klein were among the Freudians who demonstrated an interest in the neurotic roots of aggression. More explicitly, the Viennese scholar Robert Eisler had, in the 1930s and 1940s, studied the relationship between aggression and war, stemming from his time as a combatant in World War I and (as a Jew) his internment in Buchenwald and Dachau during World War II. Eisler linked an anthropological approach to tribal warfare to Jungian ideas of a collective unconscious. Although he titled his 1948 study *Man into Wolf*, Eisler was more optimistic than Freud about ameliorating destructive impulses. Rather than arguing that global warfare was inevitable, Eisler claimed that essentially peaceable human beings become "predatory, murderous and jealous . . . only under extreme environmental pressure" and that corrective social structures can restore the natural order.[27] Despite the social importance of Eisler's message he was not widely read in the United States in the 1940s (he died in 1949 in Oxford, England, before finishing an essay titled "The Sociology of War and Peace"). For this reason, Eisler did not have a direct impact on the mainstream US medical focus on the biological and physiological outlets of aggression, which suggested that anger and fear manifest themselves in almost identical physiological responses, closely linked to anxiety that is triggered by extreme or catastrophic experiences. This is illustrated in the foxhole sequence in *Pride of the Marines*, in which Al Schmid fires repeatedly at the invisible Japanese enemy. Although this appears to be a superhuman act of bravery, Lee Diamond, Al's comrade, suggests later that it might have been psychotic aggression seeking an outlet: either the man turned into wolf, following Eisler's model, or the man reverted to wolflike behavior, as Freud would have argued.

If, as existential thinkers of the 1930s and 1940s proposed, anxiety is part of the condition of being—without root cause or intentionality—then aggression remains metaphysical and nebulous. Yet the links between aggressive behavior and combat experiences suggest that it is physiologically rooted. Behavioral studies on aggression and dominance in animals and testosterone tests at the University of Chicago and the Jackson Laboratory in Bar Harbor, Maine, showed that physiological responses to potentially addictive endorphins were not clearly understood in the years immediately after the war.[28] And although the potential for self-harm was not widely appreciated either, links between pain and physical violence (noted in earlier studies on sadomasochism by Richard von Krafft-Ebing, Havelock Ellis, and Freud) contributed to William Menninger's concern about the lack of integrated support for veterans.

VJ Day and VE Day both promised moments of closure after the bloodletting in the Pacific, Europe, and North Africa, but the fact that many World War II veterans suffered from unresolved anxieties suggested that such therapeutic closure was only partial, or even illusory. Subsequent research into post-traumatic stress, reintegration problems faced by Vietnam veterans in the 1970s, and Gulf War Syndrome in the 1990s have all sharpened clinical and public understanding that the actual and symbolic endpoints of war are very different. Postwar stories, as Karen DeMeester argues, often trace the shift from "violent fragmentation" through ceremonies of "renewal," even though the Hollywood resolutions of the films discussed in chapter 1 rarely tallied with the actual experience of demobilization.[29] It is interesting that "combat fatigue" was widely used to describe the psychic consequences of World War II as opposed to the more dramatic term "shell shock." Medical treatments of the day included the "unique power" of cold to control "pain, shock, exudation, infection, necrosis and the formation and absorption of toxins," and the rhetoric of combat fatigue disguised the real shocks of war.[30] The passivity and expectation of recovery implied by "fatigue" ignore the primitive instincts that combat brings to the surface, which was particularly troubling for veterans suffering from both physical and psychological injuries.

The sense of deflation among some veterans after discharge echoed psychological studies of World War I, perhaps most notably Freud's 1915 essay "Thoughts for the Times on War and Death." Here, Freud proposed that "disillusionment" with the cause of war is often linked to displays of brutality between so-called civilized countries, as well as feelings of betrayal by the state that in times of peace prohibits violent behavior among its citizens: "A belligerent state permits itself every such misdeed, every such act of violence, as would disgrace the individual."[31] Freud's theory was contrary to the model of psychic withdrawal and physical weariness after combat; instead, he detected forms of primal violence legitimized by the state through acts of war. In this way, the state creates a moral maze for soldiers, condoning what would usually be unacceptable behavior, only to leave the solider alone after combat to deal with moral confusion at the point when social values revert back to an antebellum model. On this theme, Jonathan Shay has noted that "character damage"—a combination of mental and physical harm arising through war experiences—often represents "a challenge to the rightness of the social order."[32] Although such "character damage" might offer the individual special insights into the mechanisms of social organization that are usually obscured in times of peace, it is not surprising that aggression is encoded in the aftershocks of war.

Freud's work on war is often linked to what he described in another 1915 essay as "the disturbance that [takes] place in the attitude . . . towards death."[33] In *Beyond the Pleasure Principle* (1920), he framed this disturbance in terms of two basic instincts, most often translated as the "life drive" and "death drive." These instincts are usually held in "precarious equilibrium" but often fall out of balance in times of war, turning into a collective death drive, or what Karl Menninger in *Man against Himself* called "world suicide."[34] These views chimed with a 1947 lecture by Nolan Lewis, the director of the New York Psychiatric Institute, in which he described war as "the explosive expressions of mass emotional illnesses."[35] Although Lewis looked to peace for an answer (perhaps influenced by his role as psychiatric consultant at the Nuremberg War Crime Trials the previous year), Freud believed that for civilized societies to function, they must bury or tame these instincts, even going so far as to deny or repress death.[36]

The psychiatrist Gregory Zilboorg usefully summarized the Freudian position in 1943, stating that when the death instinct is "projected outward it appears as aggression."[37] But just as love can be twisted into forms of narcissism or the disintegration of the ego, so aggression, when it "turns away from reality and hurls all its force onto our own selves," can lead to melancholia, alcoholism, and suicide.[38] The Freudian model does not clearly show how self-harm could be linked directly to war neurosis, but studies in the late 1930s and 1940s connected self-blame directly to Freud's 1917 essay "Mourning and Melancholia," concluding that "self-castigation may be a displaced form of inhibited direct aggression."[39] We will see in the reading of Alfred Hitchcock's *Spellbound* later in this chapter how the amnesiac protagonist turns frustration—and possibly murderous impulses—into self-harm, or what might be described as a version of the death drive. It is also interesting that during and immediately after World War II there were a number of depictions of self-harm as forms of rerouted aggression. The most notable of these representations is the alcoholic and self-destructive protagonist of Charles Jackson's 1944 novel *The Lost Weekend*, which Philip Wylie described as a triumph of transmuting "medical case history into art."[40]

It is useful to briefly examine *The Lost Weekend* because it encodes a number of related themes that are central to this chapter. Jackson's novel was published in the year that Congress considered reinstating prohibition, the year that alcoholism was dubbed one of the nation's major public health problems as reports spread of drunkenness among officers and soldiers stationed in the Pacific.[41] In his account of alcoholism spiraling out of control, Jackson drew on his own experiences but also on clinical literature, such as Karl Menninger's accounts of self-destructive behavior in *Man against Himself.*[42] The context of its writing is important for an understanding of *The Lost Weekend*, and it is worth noting that the release of the film adaptation in 1945 coincided with the waning of the Hollywood Production Code, which since 1934 had prohibited "the use of liquor in American life, when not required by the plot or for proper characterization."[43] The psychological triggers of alcoholism were still dimly understood, although Alcoholics Anonymous (ten years old in 1945) was treating 15,000 members, the recently formed National Committee for Alcohol Hygiene in Baltimore was campaigning for increased public awareness of alcohol dependency, and medical research on cirrhosis of the liver was advancing at a good pace.[44] Whereas the veterans in *The Best Years of Our Lives* drown their postwar blues in alcohol, Don Birnam's drink problem in *The Lost Weekend* is fueled by a lack of any defined social role and feelings of self-pity. "I've never done anything," he exclaims. Wylie described Birnam's condition as "adult infantilism," predicting that the novel would become a textbook case for Alcoholics Anonymous (in fact, Billy Wilder consulted that group's literature when making his film version), but it is Birnam's feeling of redundancy that offers an oblique commentary on the marginality that many soldiers felt.[45] Jacqueline Foertsch has argued that Birnam is "psychologically deranged by alcohol instead of traumatised by social factors, such as the war," and Erin Redfern focuses on the libidinal implications of the "knotted logic" that leads Birnam to equate homosexuality with pathology.[46] Nevertheless, increased alcohol consumption among veterans lingers in the background of the novel and film.

Studies of alcoholism and addiction from the late 1930s revealed a social dimension to untamed instincts. One study from 1937, based on thirty cases of adult male alcoholism treated at the Menninger Clinic, claimed that "alcohol addiction is a symptom" of an underlying personality disorder "rather than a disease" in itself.[47] It is not clear whether Birnam suffers from clinical maladjustment or infantilism, but his feelings of marginality fuel his addiction, driving him to robbery to sustain his habit and leading to what a contemporary clinical study described as "alcoholic insanity."[48] Tom Dardis and John Crowley have pointed out that although many writers in the 1920s—including F. Scott Fitzgerald, William Faulkner, Ernest Hemingway, and Eugene O'Neill—drank heavily,[49] two signs of the increasing social recognition of alcohol were the first Broadway production in October 1946 of O'Neill's play *The Iceman Cometh,* in which the characters drink in order to cling to their dreams and a 1945 article on the "Psychiatric Orientation of the Alcoholic Criminal," which claimed that "criminality is closely associated in the personality field with alcoholism."[50] The authors of this article—a Johns Hopkins University psychiatrist, Robert Seliger, and a Maryland psychotherapist, Victoria Cranford—link the rise of alcoholism in the 1940s to broader social patterns: "We understand the effects of our national expansion, restlessness, heterogeneity, industrialism and economic growth on the incidence of alcoholism to be enormous, owing to mass and individual insecurity and change in nearly all spheres of life."[51] Seliger and Cranford do not mention the war explicitly (nor do they directly equate alcoholism and aggression), but it is very clear that they see a link between alcohol dependency, social insecurity, and criminal behavior. The authors suggest that individuals must be more responsible and "not expect the community or the state to administer to all their wants and desires," but those in positions of power also needed to change: "Society must assume its responsibilities on a realistic basis to help provide environments that do not tend to produce retarded or warped personalities."[52]

More broadly, contemporary studies of alcoholism and self-harm linked internally directed aggression to psychopathology, as reflected in the Freudian theory of the death drive and Jean-Paul Sartre's argument in *Being and Nothingness* (1943) that the self often attempts to reduce itself to nothing through masochistic practices.[53] This exploration of aggression and postwar identity played out in a range of cultural representations in the late 1940s, especially prominently in the dramatic and spatially complex mise-en-scène of film noir—in which the isolated individual is placed under various strains. But the interest also linked to a longer history of pathological case studies, the most prominent being Edward Kempf's major clinical study *Psychopathology* (1920), which examined a broad range of psychotic behavior displayed by patients being treated at St. Elizabeth's Hospital in Washington, D.C., during the 1910s, including a number of wartime cases.[54] The energies of World War II are sometimes explicitly evoked in 1940s films relating to combat fatigue, psychopathology, or criminal behavior stimulated by the conditions of war, and sometimes they operate on a more subtle level. Within this context, this chapter focuses on the complex nature of anxiety—linked to aggression and self-harm, and often symbolized in film noir through the image of the mirror.

The Returning Soldier and Film Noir

There has been much debate about the exact relationship between the emergence of film noir and World War II. In *Wartime*, for example, Paul Fussell argues that, unlike the heroism of World War I, the 1939–1945 war gave rise to "a whole new literature of fear."[55] In the drive to encourage fearlessness among recruits, a soldier's "failure to control" visible symptoms of anxiety was frowned on by military leaders, but these uncontrollable fears nonetheless filtered through late 1940s culture.[56] The discussion here focuses on film noir as a crucible for exploring medical concerns in the wake of World War II, when anxiety and neurosis were perhaps more widespread than ever before, before moving on in the next chapter to examine the dangers to ego identity precipitated by the early Cold War.

Film noir directors were fascinated with the darker recesses of the human mind and were inspired by the hard-boiled detective fiction written in the 1930s, notably stories by Raymond Chandler and Dashiell Hammett, which were licensed for film adaptations during the war. Film noir grew from a handful of movies in the first half of the 1940s to over twenty-four a year between 1946 and 1951. Its themes and plots usually revolve around mistaken identity, crimes of passion, jealousy, irrational violence, and criminal behavior.[57] War victims sometimes appeared explicitly, as in the bleak postwar film noir *The Blue Dahlia* (1946), written by Raymond Chandler, in which Lieutenant Commander Johnny Morrison (Alan Ladd), having returned from the Pacific, becomes the prime suspect in the murder of his adulterous wife. Interestingly, in the first draft of the film, Morrison's friend Buzz Wanchek (William Bendix), who has a metal plate in his head because of a war wound and experiences blackouts and anxiety attacks, was scripted as the murderer, but the War Department forced Chandler to revise the plot to avoid depicting an injured war veteran as a psychopath. In the released version, the veteran becomes the victim of another's crime, whereas in the RKO film *Crossfire* (1947), a member of a group of demobilized soldiers commits a murder in a story of racial intolerance and anti-Semitic aggression. Described as part of a wave of "cynical tough guy films," *The Blue Dahlia* and *Crossfire* both portray innocent veterans as murder suspects.[58] But *Crossfire* goes far beyond the loss of innocence; it depicts the hate killing of a Jewish man who—unbeknown to Montgomery (Robert Ryan), the murderer—had fought on the same side as him during the war.

Just as Norman Mailer's war novel *The Naked and the Dead* (1948) was to present racism and anti-Semitism as rife among American soldiers in the Pacific, so the roots of hatred in *Crossfire* are much deeper than combat reflexes. Nevertheless, it is the violence of war that creates the moral and psychological turbulence that leads to social crossfire. Montgomery is shown to suffer from personality disorder, which the film is careful to associate with a deeply rooted anti-Semitism rather than explicitly with war anxiety. As David Spiegel has argued, "the linking of personality disorders to posttraumatic symptomatology did not constitute a challenge to the importance of early life developmental difficulty and dynamic conflict in the etiology of neuroses. However, it had the disadvantage of scapegoating emotional casualties of combat, in essence blaming the victims rather than the combat trauma for the disorder."[59] Partly due to the Defense Department's control over cinematic representations of war, but also to protect injured veterans who might be otherwise be stigmatized as psychopaths, *The Blue Dahlia* and *Crossfire* touched on raw nerves without fully laying bare the complex etiology of murderous personalities.

One of the most distinctive wartime films to shed light on the noir treatment of physicians and psychologists is *Murder, My Sweet*, called *Farewell, My Lovely* (the title of Chandler's 1940 novel, from which it was adapted) when it was first released, in 1944. Three of the film's key personnel—the director Edward Dmytryk, screenwriter John Paxton, and producer Adrian Scott—were to suffer at the hands of the Hollywood blacklist, but there is nothing explicitly ideological about this story featuring Philip Marlowe. It involves a wild goose chase in search of a lost jade necklace, harbored by its predatory owner, the femme fatale Helen Grayle (Claire Trevor). The narrative takes place in the darkened spaces of Los Angeles, but, given the film's release in 1944, the war is the implicit backdrop for a convoluted story of doublecrossing, violence, and corruption. Marlowe (played by Dick Powell) is both of this world and set apart from it, aligned with the only honest character, Ann Grayle (Anne Shirley), about whom Marlowe is nevertheless suspicious.

Three elements of *Murder, My Sweet* are directly related to medical issues. The first emerges in the opening scene, which begins with a blindingly bright light but then shows Marlowe in a shadowy and smoky room, being interrogated about a murder committed using his gun. Marlowe is blindfolded, but we do not know why until the end of the scene, when we see that his eyes have been scorched by a fired bullet. Blindness does not feature here as explicitly as it does in demobilization narratives, but a darkening lens provides a visual metaphor for a story centered on ignorance of other people's motivations.[60] On three occasions Marlowe loses consciousness, and the description of one occasion—"a black pool opened up at my feet. I dived in. It had no bottom. I felt pretty good—like an amputated leg"—suggests that tropes of blindness and amputation threaten Marlowe's hard-boiled façade.

The second medical element is dramatized through the film's antagonist. The sophisticated Jules Amthor (Otto Kruger) introduces himself as a "quack" psychologist. When Marlowe responds with bewilderment, Amthor continues: "You mean there are some things you don't understand. I've often credited the private detective with a high degree of omniscience." The patriarchal Amthor accuses Marlowe of displaying "abrupt transitions . . . characteristic of your generation," before bragging that he is ahead of his time "in the field of psychic treatment." The film juxtaposes Amthor's sophistic psychology with the terse pragmatism of Marlowe, whose actions are comparable to those of a combat veteran who gets his hands dirty without clearly seeing his surrounding situation. As we might expect, throughout the film's narrative, sympathy lies with Marlowe, mainly for his earthiness and refusal to overintellectualize.

The film's third and most explicit engagement with medicine is a famous setpiece montage. The encounter with Amthor ends with Marlowe's capture. Almost strangled by the massive hit man Moose Malloy (Mike Mazurki), Marlowe is drugged by a physician, who continues to haunt Marlowe in a "coked up" dream sequence that features superimpositions, swirling shapes, and disorienting camera movements. Within this montage, Marlowe stares at the outsize faces of Amthor and Molloy

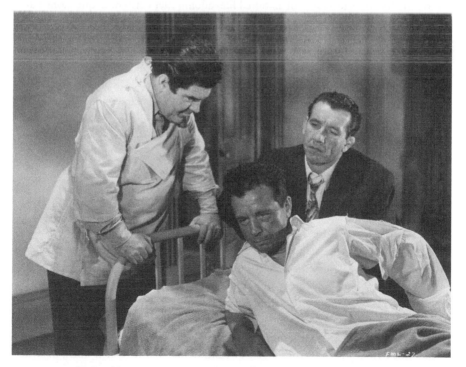

FIGURE 2.1   Philip Marlowe (Dick Powell) struggles to regain consciousness after being drugged. *Murder, My Sweet* (Edward Dmytryk, RKO, 1944).

before trying to open a long line of receding doors, pursued by the physician with a huge hypodermic needle. When the needle reaches him, Marlowe again descends into blackness. He awakens to another blinding light, but it does not bring lucidity as he cannot rid himself of the cobwebs that fog his mind and literally cover the screen.

Not only are two seemingly respectable characters—Amthor and the doctor—portrayed as untrustworthy crooks, but they characterize a world in which no one can be trusted. On escaping from captivity, Marlowe again encounters Ann Grayle, who suggests that he has "no clear idea" of what he is doing. "I don't think you even know which side you're on," she proclaims, to which Marlowe replies: "I don't know which side anybody's on. I don't even know who's playing today." If the war is not explicitly evoked in the film (partly because this dialogue is lifted from Chandler's story), it offers critiques of "taking sides" in wartime and of medical competency—from the quack psychology of Amthor to the "narcotic poisoning" administered by the physician which transports Marlowe into a world of "crazy things."

This reading of *Murder, My Sweet* is a good example of the broad interest in medicine and psychiatry among postwar film directors and scriptwriters, but there were also palpable tensions at the time, as medical professionals and social theorists worried that films were oversimplifying or distorting neuroses. From his Los Angeles vantage point in 1951, Theodor Adorno was concerned that "depth-psychology, with the help of films, soap opera" and a standardized "culture industry," was starting to invade the "deepest recesses" of national life, adding that existential questions ("terror before the abyss of the self") were being subsumed by a fad for psychological types.[61] The clinical psychologist Vincent Daly was also concerned that popular culture was distorting complex psychological patterns:

> Unfortunately, many novelists, movie producers and pseudo-scientific magazine writers have pictured mental therapy in a glamorous, and sometimes horrible, manner. Before you read any further, it would be very advisable to cast any conclusions which you have formed from reading popular magazines, newspapers, and popular movies, from your mind. Psycho-therapy can be discussed intelligently only by trained workers and while many of the popular writers may be sincere, they are all forced to give a distorted picture, because the true medical facts cannot be discussed anywhere save in a medical journal.[62]

Daly's short 1950 work, *Understanding Mental Illness*, addresses the reader in straightforward language, suggesting that the nerves can "rebel" after a sustained period of extreme emotions. His intention was to educate his readers, advising them not to feel estranged if they find themselves admitted to a hospital and to be wary of simplistic representations of illness—advice that was particularly relevant to veterans suffering from combat fatigue.

Before returning to the themes of aggression and psychopathology, it is useful to examine two key scenes from a pair of sentimental World War II films, in which noir elements jar with melodrama. The sentimentality of many home-front movies contrasts with the hard-boiled cynicism of film noir, but there are significant overlaps:

melodrama remains omnipresent in the tough-guy film *Crossfire*, for example, and noir elements creep into some of the most sentimental of war films. The two scenes analyzed here reflect contemporary medical concerns and illustrate the ways in which masochism (in the first example) and aggression (in the second) are played out on the screen. Both cases reveal connections between film representations and medical ideas, but they also highlight the limitations of cinema when it comes to war trauma, with the films resorting to platitudes about good advice and self-improvement.

The first scene derives from Selznick's sentimental war production *Since You Went Away*, directed by John Cromwell in 1944. The film, based on the popular 1943 novel by Margaret Buell Wilder, traces the lives of a New England family on the home front while the father is at war. All the female family members help with the war effort, including Jane Hilton (Jennifer Jones), the eldest daughter, who volunteers for the WAVES to help wounded and immobilized soldiers recover (Jones herself was a volunteer nurse during the war). Up to the point where Jane hears that her fiancé, Bill Smollett (Robert Walker), has been killed in action she attends to the physical needs of injured soldiers. However, after she hears the news about Bill, the film shifts its emphasis from bodies to minds, with Jane's personal loss reflected in the story of a convalescing marine. We initially see Jane wheeling the bandaged marine, Danny Williams, around the hospital grounds. But Williams is not a passive victim of combat, and his disgust with war contrasts with Jane's ideals about the honor of serving. When she asks, "Would it help you to talk about it?" (referring to his war experiences), he replies flatly: "I hate the ocean." We assume that Williams's hands have been wounded either in combat or training, but given his delicate state of mind, the burns might easily have been due to self-harm.

When we see next see Williams, he is being treated on the analyst's couch by Dr. Sigmund Golden, an army psychiatrist whose professional credentials are displayed next to a paperweight bearing a quotation from Carl Sandburg: "America, thy seeds of fate have borne a fruit of many breeds." The consultation room offers a direct contrast in tone and lighting to the pastoral hospital grounds: within the darkened space, a light shines on the patient's agitated face as Golden peers over at him and speaks in a thick Central European accent. The doctor and patient are first seen through an interior window, a partition that visually separates Williams's head and arms from his prostrate body. He says despairingly: "Me in the merchant marines? That was a joke in the first place. I've always hated the water, ever since I was a kid." Then he recounts two incidents: the first when his brother pushed him off a pier as a child, and the second when he was rebuked for being "yellow" (or cowardly) in battle just before his brother was killed. The inference is that the patient's acute fear of the water is closely linked to his brother's death. Golden tries to convince Williams that he is not a coward; that his service was noble; that understanding this will help him overcome his fear of water; and, echoing Roosevelt's first presidential address of 1933, that successful therapy will mean he "won't even be afraid of being afraid."

Midway through the therapy session, we see Jane approaching the room. Cautiously, she places her head between two sliding glass doors just as Williams says about his brother "that was the last time I ever saw him." The parallel to Jane's loss of her fiancé is obvious, but the shot of her head between the two glass doors also echoes the separation of the patient's head and body minutes earlier. As Golden leaves the room, Jane looks toward Williams as he stares blankly into space, with the tacit assumption that rest and recuperation are all he needs. When Jane asks about the patient's well-being, Golden replies: "In time. In time. He is a fine young man. He must have another chance at life. We must work to give it to him." When Jane comments that the patient's burns have nearly healed, the psychiatrist adds, "Yes, his burns, but his most serious injury—that, I am afraid, will take more time." "The injury to his mind?" Jane asks, naïvely. "No, not to his mind—to his confidence in himself and others," Golden replies, and he recommends that the patient rebuild his life "all the way back and all the way forward." This is neither a Freudian thinking back to the site of childhood trauma nor an existential re-imagining of the patient's life world, but an attempt to reestablish the psychic cohesion of a beleaguered soldier. The scene sets up the expectation that it will explore the recesses of the neurotic veteran's mind, but it fizzles out into good advice and morale boosting.

The second scene is from another sentimental Selznick production, *I'll Be Seeing You* (1944), which deals centrally with the psychological wounds that Zach Morgan (Joseph Cotton) has suffered in combat. The film draws parallels between Zach and Mary Marshall (Ginger Rogers) who, unbeknown to him, is on a week's Christmas leave from prison. Zach's condition is a textbook case of nervous exhaustion, as described the following year in the mass-market *Psychology for the Returning Serviceman*: a hypersensitivity to noises, worry about relationships, an inability to fight back, and conflicting emotional states that are "extremely hard to control or remove."[63] Nervous, quiet, and uncertain, Zach is not being treated by a military or civilian psychiatrist, but we see his condition improve as his relationship with Mary develops, culminating in a joyful New Year's dance. But the elation is only short-lived. Only seconds after the couple kiss on the way back from the dance, an aggressive neighborhood dog leaps toward Zach. He freezes, with his arm hiding his face, but he is forced to fight the dog. Man and beast roll in the street, the one almost indistinguishable from the other, before the owner arrives to pull the dog away. Given that we see no direct scenes of war combat in the film, this violent street fight comes closest to identifying an external enemy. Otherwise, Zach's fight is wholly internal.

In the following scene, Zach returns to his lodgings in good spirits, sure of his love for Mary, and ignorant of her approaching return to prison. He wishes himself and a portrait of Lincoln a happy new year and then waltzes joyfully with an overcoat as his imaginary partner. He soon becomes dizzy and collapses exhausted against a dresser. The mood suddenly changes, as he rubs his face and tries to focus on the mirror. Initially his face is blurred (implying a weakened ego); then it is distorted, when he drags his fingers down it. As he sinks into a semi-fugue state, we hear him speaking softly and reassuringly in an interior monologue:

Hold on, Zach. Hold on. Hold on, Zach. Hold on. You're just a little tired, that's all. You just got through a lot of excitement. That fight with the dog took a lot out of you. That's why you're sweating. It doesn't mean anything. Sit down, Zach. Sit down. Sit down, Zach. Sit down. That's it, sit down. Take it easy. Don't get scared, Zach. Don't get scared. Maybe it is one of those things. They told you it might happen.

The repetitious internal voice is his way of reestablishing psychic cohesion. As the music becomes more dramatic and the shadows more threatening, Zach sinks into a chair and tries to loosen his tie and jacket. His heart races, and he begins to have trouble breathing as he staggers toward the bed. And then the voice returns:

Hang on, Zach. Hang on. You know what you're going to have to go through. It's sure banging away. It doesn't sound that loud. You're just thinking it does, that's all. The doc told you there's nothing wrong with your heart. Beating fast like that doesn't mean anything. This is it. You thought for a minute that it wasn't, but it is. You're in for it now. . . . You know what's coming now. It's tough to get hold of yourself, Zach. Better call for a doctor to get the hypo reading, or maybe a tub.

A series of intense close ups on Zach's eyes, sweating forehand, and agitated hands clutching his shirt is accompanied by the sound of a dog barking, before that noise fuses with the sounds of military planes and gunfire. The light in the room intensifies and then becomes blinding as the sound of gunfire suddenly becomes louder. A voice returns. It's not Zach's, but Mary's voice: "Zach. Zach. Zach. Zach, you've got eight days to believe. Eight days. You must believe. Must believe. Must believe. Must believe." The words help Zach. He stops sweating and rises from the bed. The light in the room becomes steadier, the music triumphant, and he stands up, pronouncing: "I made it."

There are a number of important factors here. First, the use of noir devices (lengthened shadows, dramatic lighting and music) to amplify Zach's anxiety do not easily fit into the film's sentimental frame and its vague allusion to his medical condition. Second, the fact that Zach tries to be his own therapist is reminiscent of the voices we hear in Bud Wilcheck's head at the beginning of *The Men* (see chapter 1). In the absence of a therapist or doctor, Zach reassures himself through repetition, using simple and direct language and internalizing the advice given to him by military doctors. Third, it is evident that Zach cannot cure himself; the fight with the dog reawakens the trauma of warfare (or perhaps even deeper impulses from childhood) and precipitates his relapse. It is only when the calm and encouraging voice of Mary blends with his own repetitions that he manages to come out of the panic attack. The endpoint of the scene takes the form of a religious conversion, as Zach looks into the light in a rapturous way. The power of love, then, has the capacity to overcome his trauma.

In the very next scene, we see Mary's cousin, Miriam (Shirley Temple), inadvertently telling Zach about Mary's prison sentence (the result of accidental manslaughter when her lecherous boss tried to assault her), which threatens the purity of the couple's mutual feelings. The film appears to be heading toward a tragic conclusion, as Zach departs by train and Mary returns to the grim women's state prison. But at the end, we see Zach silently emerge from the shadows. He and Mary embrace and express their love for each other, before the film ends with the choral strains of Jerome Kern's romantic ballad "I'll Be Seeing You."

These two scenes, from *Since You Went Away* and *I'll Be Seeing You*, offer different therapeutic trajectories: the first involves a psychiatrist and suggests that conflict resolution is a long way off, as the patient's masochistic impulses cast a shadow over doctor's recommendations; and the second is a form of self-therapy guided by the light of love. Nevertheless, both scenes emphasize the importance of physical environment. The contrast between the relative freedom of the hospital garden and the threatening shadows of the psychiatrist's room in *Since You Went Away* is stark, but spatially the patient's confinement is total. The shots in which both Williams's and Jane's heads are separated from their bodies suggest that war violently fractures spaces, making bodily and psychic cohesion impossible. The apartment scene in *I'll Be Seeing You*, when a joyful re-creation of the New Year's dance breaks down into bodily sweats parallels an earlier street scene in which romance gives way to the aggressive attack by a vicious dog. Zach's room paradoxically becomes both smaller, as the walls seem to press in on him, and larger, as he struggles to muster the courage to move to the bed. In the two films, rooms restage the events that led to combat exhaustion: for Williams, the experience of seeing his brother die triggers his own childhood fears; and for Zach, the secondary trauma of the dog's attack blurs with the primary trauma of war. Williams's neurosis appears to be harder to cure, given that it is rooted in primal fears—unless, that is, Zach is masking his real anxiety with an undisclosed war incident.

These scenes suggest that the mise-en-scène of film noir helps to play out temporal stories on a spatial plane. This, as Edward Dimendberg argues in *Film Noir and the Spaces of Modernity* (2004), is a crucial element of the noir aesthetic that presents a world of "harassed working-class protagonists, petty criminals, seedy gambling joints, [and] ramshackle urban neighborhoods" that are "akin to a modern version of purgatory."[64] The threatening environment is even more acute for neurotic and psychotic protagonists; it is often impossible to ascertain whether the environment is a projection of psychological damage or whether bewildering spaces undermine the character's cohesion. This is a central aspect of Dimendberg's argument: "centripetal and centrifugal space, tendencies toward concentration and dispersal, recur and often overlap through film noir."[65] Dimendberg relates this spatial rhythm to urban development during and after the war, but it generates another level of meaning that grapples with the mixed messages that many returning World War II veterans faced as both war hero and combat victim. This symbiotic relationship between spaces and identities is more acute in the representation of war casualties. Maladjustment is not just about victimhood: aggression, violence, and psychopathology are also frequent responses to film noir topographies, in which protagonists are hemmed in or unable to act. In other words, noir spaces are both geographical and existential zones in which self-knowledge and ontology are thrown into question. If the noir mise-en-scène is an anti-therapeutic environment in which no one can be trusted, it also suggests that space itself is important for understanding the therapeutic trajectory of postwar culture.

Space, Psychopathology, and Film Noir

Just as the demobilization films focus on the relationship between psychic episodes (primary trauma, combat damage, and postwar neurosis) and the spatial dynamics of illness and recovery, so film noir makes explicit the links between space and psychology. The topographies of film noir are both real—threatening alleys, darkened rooms, seedy bars, empty warehouses, deserted riversides—and figurative, dramatizing the kinds of psychic and social conflicts we have seen in *Since You've Been Gone* and *I'll Be Seeing You*. This creative use of space is part of the fabric of film noir, but it is also directly linked to its cinematography: night shots, high-contrast lighting, intense shadows, occluded vision, and disguise all intensify the twilight world of noir. It is significant that many noncinematic discourses of the 1940s engage with theories of space and spatiality—a parallel I will deploy in order to analyze film noir as a cultural space in which medical and psychiatric questions were explored.

One such discourse is the development of European phenomenology. The facts that film noir had some of its roots in France and that European existential thought was in vogue in the 1940s strengthen these connections. The French philosopher Maurice Merleau-Ponty, for example, focused on the concepts of the body as object and subject in his 1945 study *The Phenomenology of Perception*.[66] Rather than separating body and mind from each other in the Cartesian tradition, Merleau-Ponty proposed that consciousness arises from embodied subjectivity. Perception of an object or another subject cannot be clearly separated from the environment, leading Merleau-Ponty to assert that any act of perception contains within it traces of the subject's body in the world. Thus, we cannot divide the perceptions of the mind from bodily perceptions; sense and thought become mutually informing. The phenomenological world for Merleau-Ponty lacks the clarity of rationalist thought, but it is also an open world in which significance can be forged through direct experience.

For some this might prove to be a world of freedom, but, as Erich Fromm discussed in his influential work *Escape from Freedom* (1941), modern individuals are devious in finding ways of relinquishing liberty, often born out of the insecurity of isolation. Sometimes this escape is characterized by blind trust in authority (Fromm argued that authoritarianism is sadomasochistic), but at other times, it is expressed through destructive impulses that become "a passion within a person" and "always succeed in finding an object."[67] Although Fromm (like Adler and Horney) played down Freud's emphasis on libido, he sensed that the fear of freedom links an internal death drive to external surroundings. According to this view, when the "growth and expression of man's sensuous, emotional, and intellectual capacities" is blocked, then individuals often turn "towards destruction" and nurture "hostile tendencies" that are directed "either against others or against oneself."[68] Fromm continued to develop this line of thought into the 1970s, but his emphasis on isolation and the thwarting of creative energies struck a chord with cultural explorations of aggression and self-harm in the 1940s. And although Fromm did not address contemporary combat directly, the experience of war (particularly in Central Europe) closely informs his study.[69]

More explicitly, the solitude of noir protagonists stems directly from the experiences of war casualties. A 1945 report, "Psychiatric Casualties among Officers and Men from Normandy," claimed that "men are more deeply influenced by solitude and the pull of group ties, and whereas [a private] will break down after the loss of a comrade the officer tends to break down because of the feeling of loss of power to exhibit his responsibility."[70] The causes of breakdown relate not merely to combat fatigue, but also to a loss of status within a group. The report also notes that cases of amnesia were less profound in World War II than in World War I, and hysteria was less frequent due to "the elimination of dullards from front-line service."[71] Other reports in the *Bulletin of War Medicine* are less sanguine about war casualties: one noted that anxiety was often compounded by worries over "future employment, postwar security and fear of further injuries," and another described traumatic psychoneurosis caused by a frightening experience, often manifesting itself in a "recurrent dream which recapitulates the traumatic event."[72]

A range of 1940s films explored wartime amnesia, most notably the RKO film *Dangerous Moonlight* (1941), the adaptation of James Hilton's novel *Random Harvest* (1941) in which the war casualty Charles Rainier (Ronald Colman) suffers from such profound combat fatigue that he cannot remember anything about his identity or his life, and Alfred Hitchcock's *Spellbound* (1945), a loose adaptation of Francis Beeding's gothic novel *The House of Dr. Edwardes* (1927), which moves beyond the war into the realms of psychoanalysis and criminality. Jonathan Freedman has noted the close link between the investigative mode of film noir and psychoanalysis, arguing that "the psychoanalyst is narratively merged with the detective in discovering a single repressed trauma whose unveiling—usually accomplished through the successful decoding of a dream—simultaneously frees the patient of neurotic symptoms and brings a crime to an end."[73] The example of Marlowe in *Murder, My Sweet* shows the detective working alone to piece together fragments; his allies are only temporary and usually motivated by self-interest. The arch-rationalist Amthor is shown to be corrupt, and Marlowe must use a mixture of intuition, behaviorism, and reason to solve the case—just as a psychoanalyst might in tracing the cause of a neurosis.

There is more, though. In *Murder, My Sweet*, Marlowe literally turns from detective or analyst into a patient, when he is drugged by Amthor. Film noir sleuths are by necessity hard-boiled and pragmatic, but Marlowe's vulnerability reinforces Ray Pratt's reading that noir protagonists are often forced "to recognize repressed and hidden aspects of their own pasts," implying that epistemological and ontological questions are inseparable: in other words, the crime that needs solving blurs with the identity that needs interrogating. Pratt argues that "at a deeper level the protagonists themselves are represented as first having to trace out, discover, and experience for themselves the nature of the largely unknown or inadequately understood systemic forces that either wish to contain or . . . eliminate them."[74] There is nothing specific in Marlowe's dream that helps him to solve the mystery, but the dream reinforces the view that those in authority—empowered by reason, medicine, or violence—are not to be trusted. Self-reliance is the order of the day.

Film directors made noir stories "more terrifying and exciting for the audience" by plundering clinical case studies to create worlds in which characters are neurotic and boundaries dissolve between normality and pathology.[75] In 1944 the director Joseph Mankiewicz wrote to Karl Menninger, stating that "I am convinced that the next period of years will bring psychiatry in general, and psychoanalysis in particular, into great prominence as a most important source of literary, dramatic and motion picture material."[76] These links between psychiatry and culture were already in place by 1944, bridging the investigative modes of psychoanalysis and noir epistemology as the analyst-detective risks himself in the pursuit of dangerous knowledge. Some critics, such as Robert Warshaw, were skeptical about whether films such as *The Best Years of Our Lives* could offer a "true presentation of reality," but film noir took viewers in the opposite direction, toward disturbing psychic landscapes and dangerous topographies.[77]

Film noir tended to privilege a male worldview, often distorted and paranoid—particularly in films made after 1947, when Cold War fears of hidden enemies overshadowed the hard-boiled stories of Chandler and Hammett. It is easy to interpret femmes fatales, such as Cora Smith (Lana Turner) in *The Postman Always Rings Twice* (1946), as a projection of male anxieties about impotence or unrequited desire. Even in such films as *Leave Her to Heaven* (1945), *The Locket* (1946), and *The Dark Mirror* (1946), where strong female characters—the femme fatale Ellen Berent (Gene Tierney), an alluring kleptomaniac (Laraine Day), and the mysterious twins Terry and Ruth Collins (both played by Olivia de Havilland)—reveal criminal streaks and deeper psychic complexity than their male counterparts, underlying anxieties nevertheless revolve around masculinity.[78] These anxieties recur through 1940s culture, as they do in Salinger's story "A Perfect Day for Bananafish," in which Seymour Glass calls his wife "Miss Spiritual Tramp of 1948," and in Philip Wylie's best-selling *Generation of Vipers* (1942), which rails against a culture of "momism" and echoes contemporary theories that alcoholism in men can often be traced to an "over-indulgent, over-protective" mother and a "cold and unaffectionate father."[79] At a time when Alfred Kinsey was carrying out primary research for the 1948 *Sexual Behavior in the Human Male* (see chapter 6), this widespread worry about masculinity encouraged screenwriters and filmmakers to develop Freudian readings of frustrated (or perverted) sexuality. Nevertheless, the medical and psychiatric patterns of many noir films (for example, incest in *Leave Her to Heaven* and the doppelgänger complex in *The Dark Mirror*) suggest a broader engagement with medical conditions, only some of which had psychosexual etiologies. Although war is not always an explicit backdrop to the noir films of the 1940s, many of their male protagonists seem to be caught in a death drive resulting from the destabilization of the social or sexual order.

In some cases, the links between film noir and psychoanalysis are explicit—and there is no clearer case of this than *Spellbound*. Rather than dealing with the quackery of psychics, as do *Nightmare Alley* (1947) and *The Amazing Mr. X* (1948), *Spellbound* reflects the fascination of Selznick, its producer, with psychoanalysis—which, as a cultural mode, fluctuated between the twilight worlds of film noir and the optimistic promise of healing. Selznick employed his Californian analyst May Romm (an expert on fetishism and exhibitionism) as an advisor on *Spellbound* to lend the movie authenticity. Romm had been recommended to Selznick by Karl Menninger while he acted as a consultant at the Los Angeles Psychoanalytic Association, but—after Joseph Mankiewicz warned him about the new project ("the psychoanalysts at the sanitarium are almost without exception maladjusted men"), Menninger wrote to Selznick to express his unhappiness about the film's distorted depiction of analysis.[80]

As one of the key therapeutic postwar institutions, the Menninger Clinic formed the basis not only of the group practice in *Spellbound* but also of Vincente Minnelli's 1955 film *The Cobweb*, adapted from the 1954 book by William Gibson. Although he was a long-time contributor of a health column in the *Ladies' Home Journal* and understood the need to allay "exaggerated and often superstitious fears" of mental illness, Karl Menninger was eager to ensure that therapeutic techniques were not distorted through popular culture.[81] Selznick had consulted Menninger on the depiction of combat fatigue in *Since You Went Away*, but the Kansan analyst was unimpressed by the depiction of dysfunctional analysts and insanity in *Spellbound*.[82] Mankiewicz was so concerned about *Spellbound* that he pressed Menninger to use his influence within the American Psychiatric Association and the American Psychoanalytic Association to "consider *now* what can be done, in some way, to control—or at least temper—the presentation of their respective sciences . . . and to prevent, if possible, the resultant disrespect and distrust that may be generated in the minds of millions of people."[83] The exchanges between Mankiewicz, Menninger, Selznick, and Romm have led some critics to argue that *Spellbound* is a pointed critique of therapeutic culture. For example, Freedman argues that Hitchcock used the film to undercut Selznick's love affair with psychoanalysis by reviving "the determinedly despairing Freud . . . for whom the vicissitudes of the psyche and hence of culture itself are governed by the indominability of the death-drive, the inevitability of repetition-compulsion, the interminability of analysis, and the impossibility of cure."[84] Such Freudian elements were dispersed widely through late 1940s culture. The baroque dream sequences in the 1944 film adaptation of the musical *Lady in the Dark*, for example, suggest that Freudian culture had moved far from its clinical roots. In *Spellbound*, however, Hitchcock manages to sustain a fairly robust psychiatric framework, so much so that it is difficult to agree with Freedman's view that the film critiques or satirizes therapy.[85] The film clearly has satirical elements, but its genesis, script, and themes do not deliver a single message. More persuasively, *Spellbound* explores the phenomenology of psychoanalysis, addressing the cluster of issues—aggression, psychopathology, crime, isolation, disguise, and space—discussed in this chapter.

Set in Green Manors Clinic, in Vermont, the film begins with dramatic orchestral music and a wind-swept, wooded landscape. Then it cuts to the doors of the clinic, while a long text (one of Selznick's signature techniques) scrolls down the screen, equating psychiatry with "modern science" in its desire to "open the locked doors" of the mind and expressing the confidence that "once the complexes that have been disturbing the patient are uncovered and interpreted, the illness and confusion disappear . . . and the devils of unreason are driven from the human soul."[86] This not only places therapeutic hope in the psychiatric cure, but it also characterizes therapy as a rational instrument with the capacity to dispel "illness," "confusion," and "unreason." This rationalist rhetoric might lead us to think that the narrative will offer solutions in the name of "modern science," but instead it links a plot concerning the murder of the psychiatrist Anthony Edwardes (due to succeed the current proprietor, Dr. Murchison, as the head doctor of Green Manors) with a case of a paranoid amnesiac, John Ballantine (Gregory Peck)—who, for reasons as yet unknown to him, has taken the place of Edwardes and swiftly becomes the murder suspect. The story is complex because it blurs an unfolding romance between Ballantine and Constance Petersen (Ingrid Bergman), with Dr. Petersen playing the roles of detective and psychiatrist as she tracks down the true murderer and protects Ballantine from the law.

Petersen is characterized as a workaholic and somewhat repressed psychiatrist until she meets Ballantine masquerading as Edwardes, the author of *The Labyrinth of the Guilt*

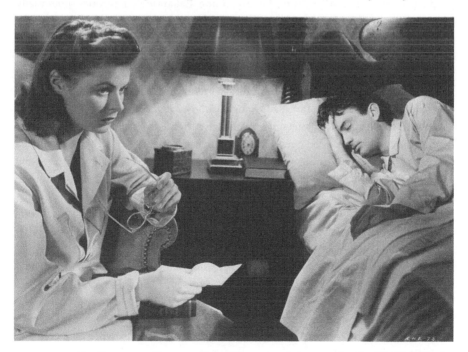

FIGURE 2.2   Dr. Constance Petersen (Ingrid Bergman) tries to unravel a psychiatric case as John Ballantine (Gregory Peck) sleeps in *Spellbound* (Alfred Hitchcock, United Artists, 1945).

Complex—a book that, as Selznick noted in his September 1944 letter to Menninger, gives a direct clue to Ballantine's condition. After a nighttime confrontation, the couple enter a new psychic labyrinth in which Petersen's professional distance is compromised by her attraction to Edwardes—symbolized by a exuberant image of a series of opening doors when they first kiss.[87] When Edwardes/Ballantine collapses while operating on a patient (who has assaulted another patient and attempted to kill himself, suffering from delusions of patricide), Petersen realizes that the man she is falling in love with is not Edwardes. Trusting in his core of goodness, however, she follows Ballantine to New York as he flees from the clinic when he realizes his false identity.

One of the film's key conflicts is between Ballantine's manifest and latent personalities. Normally a gentle and unassuming character, in the presence of Petersen his gentleness is almost infantilized, but we later find out that his nervous exhaustion derives from being shot down while serving on the Italian front during his time in the Army Medical Corps. The sound of gunfire accompanies Ballantine's reflection on his wartime experience in Rome, as he recalls being hit by a fighter jet and having to bail out of his own plane. He cannot remember clearly whether he deserted the army, but his hatred of killing does not tally with his occasional violent outbursts against Petersen when she suggests that "your guilt fantasies were probably inflamed by your duties as a soldier." The film makes no other references to the war, but it is an important context (especially as the film was released the same year as the Selznick production *Since You Went Away*) for explaining Ballantine's neurotic—potentially psychotic—condition.

At the beginning of the film, we see two patients: Norma, a young and glamorous woman, and Harry, the patient who tries to kill himself—an act that precipitates Ballantine's first breakdown. The two patients imply that seemingly normal behavior masks a series of destructive impulses: Norma's nymphomania and Harry's delusions of patricide. These patients foreshadow increasingly dangerous phases in Ballantine's paranoid behavior, which Petersen's psychiatrist friend and mentor, Dr. Alexander Brulov, refers to as "a loaded gun." This is most clearly manifested in a noir sequence in which Ballantine sleepwalks during a stay at Brulov's house in Rochester, New York. Peering at himself blankly in a bathroom mirror while shaving (we do not see the reflection of his face, just a shadow), the somnambulistic Ballantine becomes anxious when his eyes light on the white porcelain sink, which reminds him of the scene of Edwardes's death. Seeking an escape into darkness, he wanders through the dimly lit house holding the razor, with the potential of harming himself and the sleeping Petersen, whom he hovers over with the blade before descending the stairs to meet Brulov, who is working late. Unbeknown to Petersen, Brulov has already detected Ballantine's neurosis. Brulov keeps the patient talking while he secretly prepares bromide in a glass of milk that sends Ballantine into a deep sleep. One distorted camera view, close up to the bottom of the glass, reveals the drug's swift work as well as Ballantine's psychic distortions.

A professional disagreement about Ballantine's condition takes place the following morning between Brulov and Petersen, who is surprised at her former teacher's detection. The psychiatrist is dismissive of the charade: "The moment I see you with a husband whose pupils are enlarged, who has a tremor of the left hand, who is on a honeymoon with no baggage, and whose name is John Brown, I know practically what is going on." Petersen, by this time deeply in love with Ballantine, claims that Brulov's diagnosis of schizophrenia is based on a preconceived understanding of the mind rather than the individual patient. Brulov is again dismissive, stating that she is a "schoolgirl in love" who is functioning on "the lowest level of the intellect" and allowing her emotions to cloud rational diagnosis. Petersen requests more time to conduct an analysis of Ballantine, but Brulov warns her how dangerous Ballantine's amnesia might be: "Should [we] sit and hide for half a year waiting to find out if he will cut your throat, my throat, and set fire to the house?" The disagreement revolves around two opposing views: the first is based on rational "modern science" and sees the potential harm of a patient that Brulov is sure is a killer; the second is emotionally sensitive to the patient's condition, but also potentially naïve in Petersen's desire to exonerate Ballantine. However, her care can alternatively be interpreted as embodying what Karl Menninger called the transformative power of therapy, which serves to reorganize destructive energy into "constructive channels."[88]

We might be tempted to read the film as a playing out of the two-cultures debate: the argument that cold science can deal only with fixed medical categories, while emotional entanglement can never lead to a therapeutic solution. Jonathan Freedman's reading of *Spellbound* rests on the film's negative examples of psychiatrists, as well as Brulov's almost comic dismissal of that "Freud stuff as a lot of hooey." However, although we might wish to place Brulov in this negative camp for his rebuke of Petersen, the two therapists are productive counterparts, particularly when it comes to analyzing the film's most famous sequence: Ballantine's dream.

We have already seen numerous examples of Ballantine's fear of white shapes. When free association fails to work in therapy, Brulov and Petersen coax the patient into sharing his dream, which is rendered both visually (courtesy of Salvador Dalí's surrealist artwork) and in words by the patient, with commentary from the two analysts. It is a more complex sequence—both visually and analytically—than anything that appears in many noir films, involving numerous symbols, images of violence, and a fantastic mise-en-scène, some of which was cut from Dalí's original commission. The inclusion of a snow sequence and a masked murderer in the dream lead Petersen to realize (with Brulov's help) that Ballantine's anxiety is provoked by sled tracks in the snow outside. The primary trauma does not prove to be his war experience, but rather a childhood tragedy when his brother is killed accidentally, caused by the young John sliding down a banister and accidently impaling his brother on a sharp railing. This childhood trauma had been transferred onto the recent murder of Dr. Edwardes at a ski resort; it transpires (although it is not revealed at this point in the film) that Dr. Murchison has killed the real Edwardes so he can retain his place as proprietor of Green Manors. The film leads us to believe that this masquerade stems from Ballantine's witnessing the murder and then unconsciously adopting the persona of Edwardes to mask his transferred guilt.

As soon as Ballantine recalls his childhood memory, his biographical details return to him—including his real name and why he went to the ski resort, due to "nerve shock" on returning from war. Neither the therapeutic sequence nor the reenactment on the ski slope is analytically convincing, but they provide compelling examples of personal identity being shaped by environment: the double trauma of childhood and adult murders, as well as the experience of war. This is not the end of the film, though. Although Petersen thinks the analysis is "all cleared up," she has ignored certain aspects of the dream. Neither she nor Ballantine knows the identity of the masked murderer, but it is noticeable that Ballantine's incipient aggression and tendency to sleepwalk clear up after the initial analysis of the dream. This does not prevent Ballantine from being arrested as the most likely suspect in the murder case. Brulov again dismisses Petersen when she expresses her determination to fight on, and she relies on intuition to identify the masked man as Murchison. On returning to Green Manors, the proprietor actually helps Petersen to interpret the remaining details of Ballantine's dream, before turning a gun on himself rather than accept defeat or capture (he turns the gun toward the camera and shoots himself in an uncanny mirror image).

Ballantine is largely absent from the closing sequence of the film, but the unmasking of his identity is as much an unraveling of an institutionalized mystery as it is of the patient's active remembering. The spatial continuum of the film—linking Green Manors to Brulov's house, Ballantine's dream sequence, and the ski resort—suggests that illness cannot be compartmentalized or fully treated on the analyst's couch. Psychopathology does not lie with Ballantine (he is proved innocent of two murders), but with the corrupt proprietor of Green Manors. This suggests that illness is an institutional and communal problem, deeply bound up with social behavior rather than locked within the recesses of the self.

From Neurotic to Psychopath

Film noir often plundered clinical case histories for sensational plotlines, but this chapter has shown numerous crossovers between postwar medical discourses and cinematic representations, with primary or secondary causes often related to combat experiences. *Spellbound*, in particular, brought to public attention the psychoanalytic interest in the irrational mind, but it also tapped into the widespread postwar interest in criminality and psychopathology. This linked back to Edward Kempf's 1920 clinical study *Psychopathology* but more directly reflected the increasing number of psychopathic patients admitted to state mental hospitals in the mid- to late 1940s. Of the patients admitted to those hospitals in 1952, 1,717 (around 17 percent) were diagnosed as having psychopathic personalities (1,460 were men); by 1958 the number had increased to nearly 18,000.[89] The statistics from wartime records suggest that of the 10 percent rejected from the armed forces, 29 percent were deemed to have psychopathic personalities (which works out to 3 percent of the total rejections), while of the 450,000 "neuropsychiatric separations from the army," 30 percent were in the category of "nonmedical discharge," which included the diagnosis of "psychopathic personality."[90] It was widely recommended that all psychopaths should be hospitalized to protect other people, they should be supervised by a psychiatric specialist, and they should be housed within an institution "with a minimum of firm authority and regulation" but protected "to a maximum extent, from difficulties arising out of poor judgment and moral indiscretions."[91]

This perceived affinity between psychiatric disturbances and crime grew in the 1940s. One cinematic example is Montgomery, Robert Ryan's character in the RKO film *Crossfire*. A contemporary reviewer described Montgomery as "the bigot, the fanatic—loud-mouthed, self-assertive, narrow, cruel. Here is the Klansman, the bandit, the lynch mobster—the American fascist in the flesh."[92] It is easy to stereotype such an anti-Semitic character as a member of the "lunatic fringe" (as the film's producer, Adrian Scott, called him), particularly as the medical roots of Montgomery's deeply ingrained prejudices are not explored.[93] Postwar films often quite crudely portrayed rampant racism and sadistic intent—for example, the vicious racism directed against an African American soldier in the 1949 film adaptation of Arthur Laurents's play about anti-Semitism, *Home of the Brave*, or the psychopathic killer in another medical noir film, *The Spiral Staircase* (1945), who targets women with disabilities— but many text-based contemporary studies took a more nuanced view of crime.

The "psychiatric-psychologic" volume *Crime and the Human Mind* (1944) begins with the words: "Crime is a many headed monster. Its tentacles reach far and embrace all walks of human life."[94] Written by the Columbia University psychiatrist David Abrahamsen, the book was just one example of the growing interest in psychopathology and criminality. That interest was confirmed by the publication of the Howard University psychiatrist Benjamin Karpman's four-volume *Case Studies in the Psychopathology of Crime* (1933–48), documenting research at St. Elizabeth's Hospital. Based on a series of case studies of the "criminally insane," the multivolume work places great hope on the use of psychoanalysis to "cure" what Karpman describes as "emotionally sick people."[95] Rather than basing a diagnosis on the circumstances of the crime (or identifying a single root cause), Karpman uses personal materials such as letters and dream accounts to identify patterns that might account for psychopathological behavior.

Not all accounts were as positive as those in *Case Studies in the Psychopathology of Crime*, and definitions of the psychopath varied widely. Psychopaths were often placed within the "lunatic fringe" or portrayed as masters of disguise, fueled by FBI Director J. Edgar Hoover's widely reported "war on the sex criminal" in the late 1930s.[96] The southern psychiatrist Hervey Cleckley wrote an influential book called *The Mask of Sanity* (1941) that was based on observations of hospitalized male patients and that classified the psychopath as the opposite of the nervous type, characterized by emotional callousness and a disregard for the moral consequences of crime. From the outside, the psychopath may seem normal, but Cleckley argued that he or she hides destructive urges behind the kind of appealing façade often explored in noir narratives. Rather than positioning the psychopath among the dispossessed or socially marginal, Cleckley detected a "fragmented personality" lurking behind the mask of normality—the psychopath as businessman, scientist, or psychoanalyst—putting the individual "at the mercy of phantasies indistinguishable from what is real."[97] Not only was *The Mask of Sanity* influential within psychiatric and criminological circles (several subsequent editions of the work were published), but it gave rise to increased interest in personality disorder, culminating in *The Three Faces of Eve*, the 1957 film adaptation of Cleckley's study.[98] It also suggested, as Zilboorg argued in 1951, that criminality was now almost always seen in psychoanalytic terms.[99]

In 1954 Walter Bromberg wrote about "the sardonic, snarling mask of the psychopath, behind which lies the frightened, lonesome face of a neurotic character," perhaps referring to the 1953 case of the rejected scientist Bayard Peakes, who aimed to "kill some physicists" at Columbia University but ended up murdering a secretary working at the American Physical Society.[100] In 1963, three years after the release of Hitchcock's signature film, *Psycho*, *The Encyclopedia of Mental Health* called "psychopath" a "label so variously defined and so loosely envisaged" that it is often referred to as a "wastebasket diagnosis," good only for "personality disturbances that do not neatly fit into other categories."[101] If it had been written in the 1950s, the *Encyclopedia* would probably have used "psychopath" as a normative term, diagnosing psychopathic individuals as deviants and categorically different from others, but in the early 1960s it asserted that psychopathology was a matter of degree rather than of kind. The *Encyclopedia* did not recommend discarding the term, but it noted that "many psychiatrists have found it a condition easier to recognize than to describe." Echoing *The Mask of Sanity*, the Encyclopedia claimed that the condition was often associated with the confidence man or fraud, leading to duplicitous and conniving behavior: "a supreme egotist—parasitic, sadistic, heartless, craven, and eely, with infinite capacity for victimizing others, and with seeming indifference to the pain and loss he habitually inflicts, except for the cruel satisfaction he sometimes derives from his malignant ill-doing."[102] Rather than someone who lives close to a family or neighborhood, the psychopath is a "wanderer seeking new and unexplored territory," often criminal in behavior but sometimes childlike and immature. This recalls the links made in the 1910s between criminality and dementia praecox, but it also reflects the currency of the term "homosexual panic," which was introduced as a diagnostic category by Kempf in *Psychopathology* and was included as supplementary term in the first edition of the *Diagnostic and Statistical Manual of Mental Disorders* in 1952.[103]

These elements are evident in the portrayal of two psychopathic characters played by the depressive and alcoholic actor Robert Walker in early 1950s films, both of which borrow heavily from film noir. In 1949 Walker returned to Los Angeles after having undergone a six-month course of treatment at the Menninger Clinic for prepsychotic depression and following bouts of heavy drinking.[104] After making his name in Hollywood for playing gentle and comic characters, Walker was cast against type in Hitchcock's *Strangers on a Train* (1951) as the enigmatic but sadistic killer, Bruno Anthony, whose elaborate plotting casts a dark shadow over his victims. The second of Walker's characters, in *My Son John* (1952), is the intellectual John Jefferson, who returns from Washington, D.C., to his small childhood hometown harboring un-American ideas. The two narratives contribute to the postwar trend of linking sexual dissidence to criminality, relating to contemporary medical studies associating alcoholism with homosexuality—a trend that quickly became a stereotype, as noted by the New York sociologist Edward Sagarin (under the pseudonym Donald Webster Cory) in *The Homosexual in America* (1951), and as depicted in *The Lost Weekend*.[105] What makes the characters in *Strangers on a Train* and *My Son John* disturbing is that their sexual orientation and the psychological triggers that shape their actions are left indistinct. In *Strangers on a Train* (the film was adapted from a Patricia Highsmith novel, and Raymond Chandler worked on an early draft of the script), Bruno Anthony is a remorseless psychopath, an endlessly manipulative figure that Fromm later termed the "exploitative-sadistic" type in *An Anatomy of Human Destructiveness* (1973). In contrast, John Jefferson in *My Son John* is disconcerting because he cannot be labeled as a clinical type or simply dismissed as a psychopath or criminal (Walker died before the film was completed, from an injection of the sedative sodium amytal administered by his psychiatrist).

Chapter 6 will return to a discussion of the links made in the 1950s between psychopathology, sexual dissidence, and criminality. For now, it is important to note that it is the ways in which anxiety and aggression seep into everyday life that marks their progression beyond noir themes and characters into postwar culture as a whole. From representations of adolescence in *The Catcher in the Rye* (1951) and *Rebel without a Cause* (1955) to the development of a postwar theater of neurosis (as explored in the 1955 study *Freud on Broadway*), and from two increasingly neurotic detectives played by James Stewart in Hitchcock's *Rear Window* (1954) and *Vertigo* (1958) to the World War II veterans who experience pressure in the workplace in two 1955 novels adapted for cinema, *The Man in the Gray Flannel Suit* and *The Blackboard Jungle*.[106] In these examples, everyday environments are deeply anti-therapeutic, facilitating anxiety crises triggered by weakened egos or the absence of family or social support.

The French analyst Jacques Lacan's theory of "the mirror stage" (first presented at the International Psychoanalytic Conference in Zürich in 1949 and published in the *Revue française de psychoanalyse* that same year) did not prove influential in the United States until after Lacan's work was translated into English in the mid-1960s. However, the many instances of mirrors being deployed in cinematic representations to highlight psychic fragmentation, to unmask a character in disguise, or to dramatize violence are important aspects of postwar culture. War was not always the context for explaining "personality disorganization," as a 1958 study called it, or the ways in which everyday life triggered neuroses or violent behavior.[107] Nevertheless, the anxieties and aggression stemming from World War II overlapped with Cold War fears and the experience of the Korean War for a new wave of soldiers, which suggests that war defined the horizon of American illness well into the 1950s.

3   *Ground Zero*

SCIENCE, MEDICINE,
AND THE COLD WAR

Writing fifty years after the end of World War II, Tom Engelhardt warns us against simply seeing 1945 as a triumphant year, claiming that "the end of victory culture" did not begin with the Vietnam War but soon after 1945, when "the pleasures of victory culture" and "the horrors of nuclear culture" became close companions.[1] The privileged players of the Cold War were government agents, scientists, and policymakers, but nuclear and communist fears percolated throughout American culture, from civil-defense activities to science-fiction stories of mutation and alien attack aimed at children and teenagers.[2] In the government-sponsored film *Duck and Cover* (1951), for example, Bert the Turtle demonstrates nuclear safety procedures for schoolchildren. But in November 1952 the recently formed Committee for the Study of War Tensions in Children argued that Bert was actually provoking anxiety among some children, rather than simply teaching them a precautionary drill.[3] The adult world of responsibility was, according to Engelhardt, linked closely to primitive fears and childhood fantasies. Although the primary role of medicine at mid-century was to keep disease and minor family illnesses at bay—a cure for one strain of the common cold was announced in 1957—medicine and psychiatry wore a frightening mask during the Cold War, linked closely to secrecy and science.

One reason for this view was that everyday life had become more medicalized than before the war. Although President Harry Truman's 1947 plan to socialize medicine failed, largely because of opposition from the American Medical Association and its members' suspicions of the British National Health Service (established in 1948), Truman's administration invested heavily in medical education and health services across a spectrum of activities. The politicization of medicine was satirized in a series of Herblock cartoons in the late 1940s and early 1950s, but nothing slowed the growing trend to redefine "forms of behaviour once understood in a moral or religious context, such as alcoholism, juvenile delinquency, and homosexuality . . . as medical issues to be treated by drug regimens and psychotherapy."[4] Such modes of medicalization were a mixed blessing, leading to the recognition of hitherto neglected psychiatric complaints—codified in 1952 in the first edition of the *Diagnostic and Statistical Manual of Mental Disorders*—but also to tighter social and medical controls over behavior, particularly at times when the Cold War heated up.

The Cold War might seem like a very different time, ideologically and culturally, than the aftermath of World War II. But it is important not to forget that Americans' fears of attack had begun with the bombing of Pearl Harbor and had been given a nuclear twist when Truman gave orders to drop atomic bombs on Hiroshima and Nagasaki in August 1945. The theme of fragmentation explored in the previous two chapters is also germane to the early Cold War years, when rumors of espionage, invasion, and contamination heightened anxieties and, in some cases, psychological traumas. Science, technology, and medicine were all highly regarded at mid-century, but they were arguably more likely to exacerbate Cold War fears than to end war or cure disease. This chapter discusses these fears within the context of the early Cold War, the Korean War (1950–1953), and studies on psychological warfare of the time. It also discusses the postwar intellectuals Norman Mailer and Lewis Mumford, who, by the late 1950s, had started to criticize the centralization of power and covert mechanisms of social control in everyday life.[5]

Such concerns have been foregrounded by recent readings of the Cold War, such as Ron Howard's film *A Beautiful Mind* (2001), in which the mathematician John Nash's schizophrenia is directly linked to the paranoia stimulated by the fears of hidden enemies. Nash was one of the more heroic scientific figures to emerge during the Cold War years—thanks to his work on game theory—but he could also be seen as one of the era's victims. The facts that Nash's paranoid schizophrenia first manifested itself in 1958 and that he was admitted to McLean Hospital in spring 1959, while working at MIT but liaising regularly with the RAND Corporation and the Department of Defense, implies that his illness was directly exacerbated by Cold War logic. *A Beautiful Mind* exaggerates the parallels between social and clinical paranoia, but it supports the belief that the military-industrial complex (as President Dwight Eisenhower called it in his farewell address of 1961) had started to impinge—sometimes overtly, in federal warnings, and sometimes imperceptibly—on all citizens, whether they knew it or not. Ellen Leopold has argued that Eisenhower's "Atoms for Peace" speech to the United Nations in December 1953 garnered international support for a peace initiative, but it also benefited US manufacturers and justified nuclear development. From one perspective, "Atoms for Peace" was the president's attempt to allay international fears and to "solve the fearful atomic dilemma" by pledging that "the miraculous inventiveness of man shall not be dedicated to his death, but consecrated to his life."[6] However, as Leopold argues, it also underpinned a new phase of Cold War secrecy in terms of nuclear development— secrecy that, as this chapter shows, was deeply damaging to public health during the late 1940s and early 1950s.[7]

Medicine, Ethics, and the Cold War

If demobilization films and film noir explored the psychic and bodily fragmentation of conventional warfare, as discussed in the previous two chapters, then we have to shift perspective slightly to understand the phenomenology of the Cold War. The support networks enshrined in Truman's September 1945 healthcare message to Congress and the Veterans Administration's commitment to support soldiers and their families are harder to locate in the early Cold War years, when a Republican-controlled House and Senate between 1946 and 1948 limited Truman's health reforms, and when anticommunism and containment had started to dominate foreign and domestic agendas. It is easy to overplay paranoia about communism and what has been called the "mass psycho-political hysteria" during the McCarthyite phase of the Cold War, but there is enough evidence from the late 1940s and early 1950s to suggest that public mistrust of institutions began early in the Cold War years.[8] Indeed, in 1947 some Republicans were suspicious that Truman's plans to socialize health insurance (which he revived for his 1948 election campaign) meant that communists were working inside the health sector "in furtherance of the Moscow party line."[9] Although Truman defended national health insurance in October 1948 by asking "Is it un-American to visit the sick, aid the afflicted, or comfort the dying?," Cold War anxieties fed off the fear of invisible threats—what J. Edgar Hoover called "an indoctrinal spray seeking to control every part of the member's heart, mind, and soul."[10] And whereas combat fatigue could often be allayed by rest, Cold War fears were more insidious because they made invisible the sense of external threat recently experienced in the combat zones of Europe, North Africa, and the Pacific. At least there were practical steps that could be taken against a known and visible enemy, but an invisible enemy was more dangerous—and not just to the nation's armed forces.

The precise relationship between national and individual psychology is tricky to establish, even within a historical context. For example, in *Psychopathology and Politics* (1930), the political scientist Harold Lasswell tried to map national character onto an individual's "personality system." In this respect, Lasswell shared with the British psychoanalyst Edward Glover an interest in the psychology of national governance, evident in Glover's *War, Sadism, and Pacifism*—which first appeared in 1933 and was republished after the war to trace the broader contours of national psychopathology.[11] Despite the ongoing interest in this field—including titles such as *World Tension: The Psychopathology of Foreign Policy* (1951) and *The Russian Mind* (1953)—it is reductive to suggest that an individual's mind is determined by national and international policy, even though, in the case of *A Beautiful Mind*, John Nash's schizophrenia appears to be the direct result of a schizoid Cold War policy. The temptation is to blur the registers between the individual and the political, national, or regional. Taking up this theme in 1951, Gregory Zilboorg argued that "we are apt to fall into a little confusion whenever we wish to draw a close parallel between imperialistic statesmanship and psychotic self-centeredness."[12] The prevalence of this trend does not make its conclusions necessarily true—including the vogue for exploring the psychopathology of Hitler or Stalin—but it reveals a cultural nexus into which Cold War psychiatric and medical practices need to be placed.

Another example of this trend can be found in a 1966 report by the Group for the Advancement of Psychiatry, which noted that during the Cold War, actual "warfare becomes a less and less satisfying outlet for the release of aggressive impulses or combat heroism"; instead, war becomes "impersonal and mechanized," as "the best soldier" is transformed from the "hero" to the "automaton."[13] In this environment the professions of psychology and psychiatry—and medicine, more generally—took on a different hue, becoming potential resources for strengthening Cold War resolve. Good therapists should ensure that their patients' feelings of dehumanization are checked or overcome, but "the new features of time, space, magnitude, speed, distance, irreversibility, and automation" described in the group's report were not so easily avoided.[14] What would normally be conceived of as maladaptive responses—an "increased emotional distance," a "diminished sense of personal responsibility," the "increasing involvement with procedural problems to the detriments of human needs," or the "inability to oppose dominant group attitudes and pressures"—might actually be upheld as strategically useful patterns during times of ideological war.[15] Members of the Group for the Advancement of Psychiatry did not think that their profession had been perverted by encouraging such maladaptive responses, but they did believe that Cold War pressures had contributed to a climate in which the social, ethical, and therapeutic orientations of psychiatry were thrown into conflict.

This range of unseen threats had three distinct impacts on American life: first, anxiety about the risks and effects of invisible nuclear radiation; second, the fear of communist spies in the government, entertainment industry, and even, some argued, in the health sector; and, third, the suspicion that professionals whose job it was to help people were actually working to promote unquestioning conformity. Medicine and psychiatry were widely seen as social goods, but some commentators had an uneasy feeling that the health profession was working against individuals, turning more of them into patients and creating a culture of dependency that compromised personal freedom. In this respect, at the beginning of the 1940s Erich Fromm had argued in *Escape from Freedom* that the individual's reliance on authority often means that freedom is abandoned as anxiety producing or even as a false goal.[16] Rather than replacing authority with positive concepts of freedom as Fromm recommended, adapting a childlike dependency on medical authority can offer comfort in unsettled times. But when an authority shows that it cannot be trusted, this bond is jeopardized.

This mounting crisis of authority could also be seen in the medical arena. Responsibility was one of the key factors in President Truman's attempt to reform the healthcare system in 1947–1948, alarmed as he was by the armed forces' high rejection rate of drafted Americans. However, when Truman's plans were scuppered by the American Medical Association, many people felt that the goal of healthcare had been lost in a struggle for political high ground.[17] It is clear that Truman's health reform plans suffered at the hands of organized medicine—although, as the next chapter discusses, Truman was following the same broad principle of organization that President Eisenhower upheld during his two terms in office. In many respects, Eisenhower extended Truman's containment policy into the domestic sphere, but if Eisenhower promoted organization as an antidote to communism, then it gave rise to the suspicion that individuals were alone and potentially defenseless in the face of institutions that had their own secretive strategies and vested interests.

The emphasis on science and medicine during the Cold War is central to understanding the direction of state-sponsored research, university funding, and laboratory projects. This was stressed in a 1959 conference at West Point, in which five hundred army scientists discussed the importance of science in military affairs, but detailed evidence of the co-opting of medicine for ideological ends was not readily available until the mid-1990s, when President Bill Clinton established an Advisory Committee on Human Radiation Experiments to investigate the claims and rumors of testing on humans in the 1950s. Back in 1948, the health crusader Albert Deutsch was celebrating the fact that conscientious objectors had "submitted themselves as voluntary guinea pigs for wartime medical experiments that sped up important life-saving and disease-fighting discoveries."[18] However, documents declassified in the 1990s tell a different story. Eileen Welsome published a Pulitzer Prize–winning report about plutonium injections administered to twelve "nuclear guinea pigs," while other research has revealed that thousands of experiments to investigate the effects of radiation burns were conducted on American citizens with federal backing between 1944 and 1974.[19] Questions of bioethics are closely linked to the covert nature of these experiments. In the case of the flash burn experiments in Richmond, Virginia, the initial motivation of the surgical consultant Everett Evans was to enable medics to treat burns in case the Soviets dropped a nuclear bomb on American soil. Burn therapy had been treated seriously since 1941, with emphasis placed on preventing infection and ensuring that the patient received the correct vitamins rather than simply treating the surface wound.[20] The problem with Evans's experiments was that, although most of the subjects were volunteers and received financial rewards for participating, there were profound ethical considerations at stake in testing flash burns on the arms of poor black college students, hospitalized patients, and prisoners in the state penitentiary. Even though the press put a positive spin on medical research using prisoners, the practice was particularly troubling as it contravened the 1947 Nuremberg Code, a code of ethics established to prevent a repeat of the atrocities practiced by the Nazis—such as blast tests on prisoners of war in Buchenwald—and to ensure that research subjects gave voluntary consent and were made aware of the hazards of any experiments.[21] By the mid-1950s the American Medical Association and the National Institutes of Health were emphasizing these hazards as a "primary concern" when it came to approving new medical projects. Nevertheless, the medical historian Susan Lederer argues that experiments such as Everett Evans's burn research might have been fired by "cold war zeal" rather than "scientific arrogance," although Evans had not fully considered the human cost or ethical implications.[22] The fact that no US court cited the Nuremberg Code until 1973 was, George Annas contends, based on the fact that no medical experiments resulted in lawsuits prior to the early 1970s and that "the Nazi experiments were considered so extreme as to be irrelevant to the United States."[23]

The close relation between medicine, the social sciences, and the military after World War II gives weight to the notion that psychiatry and medicine were increasingly locked into the military-industrial complex, rather than representing a set of ideas and practices designed to help individuals regain or sustain their autonomy. The loss of autonomy concerned the likes of Erich Fromm, David Riesman, and Norman Mailer. For example, the category of the "other-directed individual" that Riesman outlined in his influential *The Lonely Crowd* (1950) was thought to be susceptible to external influences to a degree rarely experienced before World War II (as discussed in chapter 4). Despite these critical voices, in the late 1940s many people thought that military investment brought prestige to psychology: a 1952 study, *Psychology in the World Emergency*, for example, described the potential gains in the field of social psychology for "the selecting and training of leaders, the organizing and managing of teams, the predicting and influencing of attitudes."[24] Evidence of the political and military stake in medicine and social-scientific research can be glimpsed in a memorandum signed by Secretary of Defense Charles Wilson in February 1953 to establish a protocol for the use of human subjects in scientific experiments, and in the establishment of a committee on medical sciences to ensure distance between "Pentagon policy" and "physician-investigators" contracted by the Department of Defense and thus foster a culture of independent research.[25]

Nevertheless, psychologists involved in screening recruits and medical researchers extending their atomic experimentation beyond the realm of animals (most often mice, pigs, and dogs) were still just bit players in the Cold War power game. *Psychology in the World Emergency* describes the situation well: "Not only are the military services taking the lead on problems of personnel selection and classification but they are also sponsoring the major studies in the fields of learning, training devices, proficiency measurement, attitudes, leadership, management problems, operating procedures, systems analysis, and job design."[26] Predating Eisenhower's "Atoms for Peace" speech by a year, this volume suggests that state-sponsored psychological and medical research was necessary to safeguard national security. The problem, for critics on both the left and the right, was that once ideological issues began to encroach on independent research, scientific findings were liable to be appropriated or distorted for political ends.

The symbol of US military strength during the postwar years, the Pentagon (completed in 1943) was also a symbol of the alliance between the military and government that matched the might of the Kremlin. Although the design of the Pentagon was based on a rational system of geometry, one *New York Times* writer in 1943 pictured the military headquarters in distinctly organic terms, calling it a "mammoth cave" and "the gigantic brain cell of the Army."[27] In the middle of the Pentagon's giant labyrinth of numbered corridors is an open space, which colloquially became known as "ground zero" during the Cold War. The Soviets reputedly had missiles trained on the Pentagon's ground zero, which contained a café that workers visited every day for breaks and lunch. Whether or not this rumor was true, it suggests that even during their leisure time, workers were subject to the logic, surveillance, and jeopardy of the Cold War.

Military strategy was based on the attempt to contain communism in Southeast Asia and behind the iron curtain that divided East and West Europe, together with the development of nuclear weapons that would be deployed only after provocation. The philosophy of containment was not dreamed up by the Pentagon, but by the statesman George F. Kennan in his famous "Long Telegram" of 1946 (published a year later as "The Sources of Soviet Conflict"), while he was working for the Department of State. Some detractors, such as Walter Lippmann, thought that containment policy might turn out to be a wild goose chase across the globe, trying to stem communism wherever it arose, but the Cold War philosophy of being wary and vigilant at all times followed from Kennan's work with the government up to 1950.[28] It is important to differentiate between the official policy of containment and the anticommunist fervor that threatened political equilibrium in the late 1940s and early 1950s: the first was a systematic policy, and the second was a shame and blame culture fueled by Joseph McCarthy's accusations of communism, often with scant (or even no) evidence or based on past (and sometimes fleeting) affiliations with the Communist Party. Thus, the vigilance urged by Kennan was often clouded by supposition and rumor, while the line between what was considered necessary propaganda, which raised awareness of nuclear dangers and promoted American values in Europe, and so-called deceitful propaganda, based on accusations and fears of hidden enemies, became blurred.

During the early Cold War there was little hard evidence to suggest that the Pentagon was involved in a campaign to cover up scientific and medical testing conducted in the name of national security. But there is enough evidence in terms of operational research and weapon systems, as Lori Bogle argues, to indicate that the military was entrusted with building "a resolute national will" by using "new psyops"—or psychological operations—both at home and abroad in the struggle against communism.[29] While Radio Free Europe and the Voice of America helped to spread democratic propaganda abroad, "psyops" were linked to covert operations and occluded methods of agitation, often veering into the realm of public diplomacy.[30] Critics have tended to treat the word "warfare" with some skepticism when it is used "in the absence of overt hostilities."[31] However, Christopher Simpson cites the US Army's Joint Strategic Plans Committee's 1948 definition of "psychological warfare" (information that was officially classified until the late 1980s) as a technique that employs all

> moral and physical means [as a] weapon to influence the mind of the enemy. . . . In this light, overt (white), covert (black), and gray propaganda; subversion; sabotage; special operations; guerrilla warfare; espionage; political, cultural, economic, and racial pressures are all effective weapons. They are effective because they produce dissension, distrust, fear and hopelessness in the minds of the enemy.[32]

After consulting other previously classified National Security Council documents Simpson adds that "plausible deniability" was upheld "to permit the government to deny responsibility for 'black' operations," implying that the Cold War really did lead to a culture of secrecy.[33] We will see later in this chapter how closely psyops were linked to both sides in the Korean War, but it was not only psychology that became part of the covert milieu of the Cold War.

If one scans mainstream newspapers from the mid-1940s and 1950s, one finds little evidence to specifically link scientific and medical experiments to the dealings of the Department of Defense. However, information declassified later in the century suggests that up to half a million Americans were subject to medical testing in the twenty-five years after 1940. Not only did evidence arise about the burn and plutonium tests discussed above, but there were also reports of other experiments: boys at the Fernald School, in Massachusetts, had been fed radioactive cereal; cognitively disabled children had been infected with a hepatitis strain at Willowbrook State School (Robert Kennedy described the institution as a snake pit in 1965); children at the Children's Hospital in Washington, D.C., were given experimental diet pills and drugs for skin diseases; it was rumored that the Army Chemical Corps had released mosquitoes carrying yellow fever near black communities in Georgia and Florida; and a radiologist at the University of Cincinnati experimented with total body radiation on cancer patients in a study funded by the Department of Defense.[34] Some of these reports are in dispute, but previously classified information suggests that children, the poor, the disabled, and African Americans were the most vulnerable to covert experiments.[35] What is clear is that the Department of Defense Reorganization Act of 1950 and the Pentagon's desire to distance itself from the Nuremberg Code and the 1948 Declaration of Geneva—established to reaffirm the Hippocratic Oath and to prevent a repeat of the human experiments carried out by the Nazis—brought medical, psychological, and scientific experiments under the umbrella of national defense.[36]

On this reading, if the Pentagon was the Cold War symbol of the United States as a strong fortress, then it was also a "megamachine," as Lewis Mumford described it in *The Pentagon of Power* (1970), in which the "new controllers of human destiny" are "untouchable: unchallengeable: inviolable" in their "underground control centers."[37] Mumford was particularly worried about new forms of irrationality that advanced technology might precipitate, sending the populace back into a "primitive state" severed from narratives that connect past and future.[38] This questioning of centralized power and reliance on advanced technology grew slowly at first and then more rapidly in the 1960s, by which time Norman Mailer was identifying the Pentagon as the supreme symbol of authority in *Armies of the Night* (1968), its "geometrical aura" reflecting the nation's "schizophrenia." Mailer thought that the Pentagon might appear to be a geometrical rational construct on the outside, but that it hid powerful and potentially "insane" forces within.[39]

Nuclear Fallout

Following the discussion of the promises and dangers of Cold War medicine in the previous section, this section examines the ways in which medicine and psychiatry in the late 1940s and early 1950s inflected nuclear fears, before I move on to discuss the strategic deployment of psychological operations (or "psyops") during the Korean War. The texts discussed here are drawn from journalism, film, fiction, a television interview, psychiatric studies, scientific reports, and public lectures, and their variety indicates how serious and widespread questions of prevention and treatment became during the early Cold War years.

As discussed in chapter 1, "Medicine in the Postwar World" was the theme of a high-profile lecture series presented at the New York Academy of Medicine in 1946–1947, which emphasized "the application of atomic research to medicine" and the use of antibiotics to control infectious diseases as the two major postwar medical achievements.[40] In one of the lectures, Arthur Solomon of the Harvard Medical School outlined the use of radiation therapy for leukemia, thyroid cancer, and polycythemia vera ("an overactivity of red blood corpuscle formation"), noting that "red and white blood cells are particularly sensitive to radiation, for many of the citizens of Hiroshima have died from aplastic anemia."[41] Without hesitating to contemplate the nuclear blasts at Hiroshima and Nagasaki, Solomon suggested that a combination of chemotherapy, radiotherapy, and research into the "basic reactions that take place inside the human body" presents an "enchanting vista of the atom in medicine," which, "like the microscope itself, will enable us to penetrate to regions hitherto beyond human sight."[42]

Solomon's lecture is a classic example of the "grand march of medicine" model, but he seemed impervious to wider social forces and ignorant of arguably the most important cultural text in the mid-1940s to express nuclear fears: John Hersey's *Hiroshima*, first published in the *New Yorker* on 31 August 1946 as a feature entitled "A Reporter at Large, Hiroshima." The editors noted that the entire issue was devoted to "an article on the almost complete obliteration of a city by one atomic bomb, and what happened to the people of the city," fueled by the realizations "that few of us have yet comprehended the all but incredible destructive power of this weapon, and that everyone might well take time to consider the terrible implications of its use."[43] Hersey's piece was interrupted only by the *New Yorker's* regular cultural listings, including a diverse mixture of films: the triumphalist war film *Henry V*, with Laurence Olivier; a film about the Italian underground, *Open City*; the postwar spy film *Notorious*; and three film noirs, *The Big Sleep*, *The Postman Always Rings Twice*, and *The Strange Love of Martha Ivers*. Against this eclectic mixture of triumph and despair, the issue juxtaposes a cover portraying a harmonious mixed-race community with a feature on the most devastating explosion of the twentieth century.

The original intention was to run the 30,000-word piece over four issues of the *New Yorker*, but Hersey persuaded the editors to change their minds, and there was a great deal of secrecy leading up to the piece's publication. The response was phenomenal: all copies were bought almost instantly; the Book-of-the-Month Club was eager to send a free copy to its members; and an ABC radio serialization was broadcast in September. This unprecedented public response was partly because hardly anyone in the United States had previously read stories of the Hiroshima survivors, and partly because Hersey had come to public attention as a World War II war correspondent (including on Guadalcanal, which formed the backdrop of his 1943 *Into the Valley*). *Time* and the *New Yorker* had sent Hersey to Japan with great expectations, but what they received was a dispassionate account focusing on six Hiroshima residents: a personnel clerk, a physician, a widow with three children, a German missionary, a surgeon, and a Methodist pastor—subjects whom Hersey chose because they had interesting stories rather than because they represented the city. Nevertheless, the choice of two physicians and two religious men lends gravitas to the stories, indicating that the bomb cut across the city, affecting professionals and ordinary citizens alike. Dr. Masakazu Fujii, for example, the prosperous proprietor of a "private, single-doctor hospital" containing a great deal of modern medical equipment, sees his hospital toppling into the river while he "like a morsel suspended between two huge chopsticks" is thrown into the river surrounded by "the remains of the hospital" and "materials for the relief of pain."[44] Hersey's flat tone reveals ironies—a doctor swimming in a river of anesthetics—but his point here is to bluntly emphasize how a doctor could suddenly lose his hospital and potentially his life.

In contrast to the responses of the artists Jackson Pollock, Mark Rothko, and Barnett Newman to the dropping of the bomb—Pollock proclaimed that "it seems to me that the modern painter cannot express this age, the airplane, the atom bomb, the radio, in the old forms of the Renaissance or any past culture"—Hersey offered a more domesticated journalistic account.[45] The aftermath of the blast is brought home through factual statements and realistic storytelling, and Hersey's decision to use a "flat style," as he later told the historian Paul Boyer, was an attempt to offset the drama of the bomb.[46] *Hiroshima* did more than offer a sustained eyewitness account; it resurrected the individual's story from the historical immensity of the blast. Perhaps more clearly than Engelhardt's thesis (outlined at the beginning of this chapter) that triumph and despair became inseparable, Hersey suggests that obliteration and survival are keynotes of the atomic age.

These twin themes of obliteration and survival are embedded in the most important wartime scientific experiments. The secrecy surrounding the Manhattan Project and the experiments at Los Alamos have become part of the folklore of the 1940s, especially given that two of the chief scientists, Niels Bohr and Leo Szilard, were calling for international cooperation to control the discovery and to demonstrate "the bomb's explosive power before all nations," while J. Robert Oppenheimer was arguing for international arms control in his role as chair of the Atomic Energy Commission (AEC) in 1946.[47] These three scientists realized that uncomfortable moral questions went beyond the boundaries of pure science, reaching some of the primitive impulses that the bomb was to symbolize for abstract expressionist painters. Even before the bomb was dropped, Rothko and Adolph Gottlieb were claiming that "all primitive expression reveals the constant awareness of powerful forces, the immediate presence of terror and fear, a recognition and acceptance of the brutality of the natural world as well as the eternal insecurity of life."[48] Nuclear technology might have the beneficial capacity to create an alternative energy source (as Eisenhower suggested in his 1953 "Atoms for Peace" speech), but the bombing of Hiroshima revealed the kind of brutality and insecurity that Rothko and Gottlieb spoke about three years before Hersey's publication. As *Hiroshima* makes clear, terror and fear had shifted from the combat zone into everyday life. Although President Truman announced in August 1946 that the bomb had been used "to shorten the agony of war, in order to save the lives of thousands and thousands of young Americans," nuclear fears brought life and death into close proximity long into the 1950s, as reflected by a myriad of cultural forms.

Boyer points to a 30 June 1946 episode of the Mutual radio show *Exploring the Unknown* (1945–1948) that focused on the potential for a full-scale atomic war—to which we can add the 20 December 1947 episode, "The Dark Curtain," featuring Veronica Lake, which dealt with mental disorder, psychotherapy, electroshock therapy, and lobotomy—as examples of the "frightening fare" of postwar popular culture. Boyer argues that the "surge of fear" was at first "a spontaneous and authentic response to the horror of Hiroshima and Nagasaki," but that this soon gave way to a culture of manipulation: "In their efforts to use grass-roots pressure to shape public policy, atomic scientists, world-government advocates, and international-control advocates played upon profound national unease. The politicization of terror was a decisive factor in shaping the post-Hiroshima cultural climate."[49] But this tone was very different from the widespread support in the American press for the dropping of the bomb as the symbolic end to war. Diana Preston estimates fewer than 2 percent of six hundred editorials opposed using the bomb, and where concerns were expressed, they tended to be less about fallout or radiation and more about the bomb's "future use elsewhere and specifically against ourselves and our children," as an editorial in the *New Republic* described it.[50] However, the fact that the blast affected people in very physical ways—causing burns, mutilation, sickness, and mass obliteration in Hiroshima and Nagasaki—meant that the bomb blighted the lives of ordinary citizens more than the Truman administration or the press acknowledged. A US Army documentary, *Atomic Medical Cases* (1949), shot in the weeks following the bomb blasts, provides a clinical but informative look at the casualties of the bomb (including a number of medical subjects), but few people outside the military would have seen this film. This underlines the importance of Hersey's account in turning the public's attention toward ordinary people, not by resorting to sentimentalism but by focusing on everyday details. Boyer describes Hersey's style as "so uninflected it struck some readers as heartless," but that enabled Hersey to give "the same weight to horror, heroism, and mundane banality."[51]

However, the ramifications of the atom bomb for comprehending sickness and health were more diffuse then anyone—scientists, government, and members of the public alike—acknowledged at the time. The War Department was interested in health studies such as its medical branch's October 1945 report, *The Effect of Bombing on Health and Medical Care in Germany*—on the Allied bombing of thirteen German cities during 1943–1944—which documented loss of life and the more "subtle, long range effects" of communicable diseases, hospitalization, sanitation, and nutrition.[52] And, following initial research in the autumn and winter of 1945, during the American occupation of Japan, an Atomic Bomb Casualty Commission was set up in 1946 as a joint initiative (endorsed by Truman) between the US National Academy of Sciences and the Japanese Health Institute. Between 1946 and 1974, the commission investigated the genetic impact of ionizing radiation in Hiroshima and Nagasaki, and this work continued until 1990 under the aegis of the Radiation Effects Research Foundation, partly funded by the AEC that Oppenheimer had chaired in its early days. Initial problems of flooding in Hiroshima and an overly bureaucratic Japanese government were compounded by the problems inherent to genetic research. A 1991 report called *The Children of Atomic Bomb Survivors* makes clear that the research was necessarily long-term because genetic abnormalities are often recessive, and symptoms would not necessarily arise in the first generation after the bomb blast.

Some investigators were deeply concerned that health workers would become secondary victims, contaminated by the primary victims of the blast. Nevertheless, scientists were very interested in recording information on pregnancies (over 75,000 in Hiroshima and Nagasaki between 1948 and 1954) and infant mortality from neonatal complications (even though only half of the infants were autopsied). Although everything within two kilometers of the blast was destroyed, data was collected about the frequency of leukemia and the prevalence of radiation-induced cataracts which were experienced by 2.5 percent of survivors within a thousand meters of the hypocenter, but sometimes with a latency period of up to two years.[53] However, the primary focus of the research was on visible congenital abnormalities in children, with one 1947 report noting that "there is no general agreement as to what proportion of cases of abnormal fetal development is genetically determined, and what proportion is due to nongenetic factors."[54] Although the harmful effects of radiation were obvious, it was tricky to assess to what extent ionizing radiation contributed to birth defects and miscarriages.

It was also almost impossible to gauge the quantity of radiation that a particular parent had been exposed to, or even how many bomb victims died from radiation alone, as oppose to a sublethal dose linked to other physical injuries. Additional factors had also to be considered: the facts that Hiroshima had been hit by a uranium bomb and Nagasaki by a plutonium bomb, and that Japan introduced more liberal abortion laws in the early 1950s that led to a decline in the birthrate, to name but two. The long-term research of the Radiation Effects Research Foundation benefited from technological developments and advances in recording genetic information, but the results were inconclusive. An article published in the *American Journal of Human Genetics* in 1990 reported: "Humans are less sensitive to the genetic effects of radiation than has been assumed on the basis of past extrapolations from experiments with mice."[55]

This account of US and Japanese scientists working together on the project hides more antagonistic views. The first studies of the Atomic Bomb Casualty Commission focused on genetic defects in children of the blast's survivors and had to contend with "grossly exaggerated predictions concerning the fate of their children."[56] Despite the emphasis on the democratic potential of science during the US occupation of Japan, scientific and government agendas were often at odds: it was important to begin research as soon as possible after the bomb blast, but excessive bureaucracy led to an eighteen-month gap before pregnancies were first registered, in December 1947.[57] Although the authors of *The Children of Atomic Bomb Survivors* report claimed that "we were never, in Washington . . . or in Japan, aware of any political pressure meant to influence the organization of the study or the way the data were analyzed," medical findings on the genetic collateral of the bomb could easily be used for nonscientific purposes. Within this context, from 1949 onward, classified research sponsored by the Department of Defense and the AEC (including the 1949 US Armed Services report titled *Medical Aspects of Nuclear Energy*) examined the biomedical effects of radiation sickness based on n the assumption that a Cold War enemy might use atomic weapons against the United States.[58]

In addition, tensions between Japanese and American scientists were inevitable, particularly as the occupying forces placed controls on Japanese scientific investigations (Japan did not regain investigative freedom until after the signing of the San Francisco Peace Treaty, in September 1951).[59] A report released by the Japanese Committee for the Compilation of Materials on Damage Caused by the Atomic Bombs in Hiroshima and Nagasaki in 1979 pointed out that an assessment of physical damage, such as blast injuries, thermal burns, keloid scars, cataracts, gingivitis, depigmentation, hemorrhaging, leukemia, and longer-terms effects of radiation in prenatal illness and genetic mutation overlooked profound psychological issues that could not easily be quantified: "The shock intensified their suffering. . . . Psychologically, the victims were burdened with almost inconsolable hopelessness and anguish—which have been termed 'keloid of the heart' and 'leukaemia of the spirit.'"[60] The initial impact of the bomb was physical obliteration, but it also destroyed the soul of the cities.

The American psychiatrist Robert Jay Lifton also shifted the focus from bodies to minds. Lifton—like Jackson Pollock and other artists and thinkers—saw the aftershocks of the atom bomb as devastating to all humanity, rather than something that concerned only the Japanese. Writing in 1963, Lifton claimed that "since these consequences now inhabit our world, more effective approaches to the problem of human survival may well depend on our ability to grasp the nature of fundamentally new relationships to existence which we all share."[61] Existential themes and fears impinged on the depiction of veterans and criminals in film noir (as discussed in chapter 2), but the violence, horror, and absurdity of Hiroshima had an even greater existential charge.

Lifton lived in Japan and conducted research on the psychological consequences of Hirsohima in the 1950s, but his extended treatment was not published until 1967 as *Death in Life: Survivors of Hiroshima*. Lifton's approach derived from psychoanalysis, but his rhetoric was shot through with existential ideas. For example, he wrote that after the atomic bomb blast in Hiroshima, "there was a widespread sense that life and death were out of phase with one another, no longer properly distinguishable—which lent an aura of weirdness and unreality to the whole city," a statement that resonated with Barnett Newman's claim that the atom bomb brought with it a new sensibility that threatened, or even eradicated, conventional morality.[62] Lifton was careful not to impose his own psychological prejudices on Japan, but he sensed that the bomb had created an "unnatural order" and had changed the "rules" separating life from death, leading to the obliteration of those living close to the epicenter, as well as a psychic "closing-off" among survivors as they contended with inexpressible feelings of emptiness, guilt, and self-hatred.

Nuclear Fears

In New Orleans in October 1949, President Truman's Assistant Secretary of State, William Walton Butterworth, launched the Thirteenth Annual Congress of the International Society of Surgery by reminding his medical audience that "sickness, drudgery and want are no longer the inevitable lot of humanity."[63] Butterworth's emphasis was not on the power of the atom bomb, but the hopes that medicine offered to the postwar world, such as advances in the use of penicillin. In order to foster a close relationship between the government and medical science, Butterworth told his international audience that the State Department had established an advisory group to do just that. Butterworth's celebratory tone reflected other publications in the late 1940s, including the two-volume *Advances in Military Medicine* that praised "the increase in number and quality of preventive and therapeutic resources" that "will redound to the future health of all nations."[64] The creation of the World Health Organization in 1948, Truman's desire to develop an equitable healthcare system, a new emphasis on nutrition and vitamins, and advanced care for disabled veterans were all aspects of this more enlightened medical attitude.

The immediate effects of radiation sickness from the dropping of the atom bomb had diminished by the time Butterworth made his speech. However, the long-term effects of radiation in Japan were only just starting to be understood. It took twelve years for the Medical Treatment Law for Atomic Bomb Survivors of 1957 to be implemented in Japan, a system that would give atomic survivors two free health examinations each year (80 percent of the survivors participated). There was no need to introduce such measures in the United States because there had been no atomic attacks in that country—indeed no border attacks of any kind since 1941. Even though Truman was considering using the bomb on North Korea "in a situation of necessity" (as he admitted when questioned by the press on 30 November 1950), Butterworth's argument that atomic power was a "feeble agent" in the face of surgical advances, nutritional education, and the widespread use of antibiotics ran through medical publicity of the 1950s.[65] Nevertheless, it was hard for many Americans to remain unaffected by the threat of nuclear war.

Delivering his Nobel Prize speech only ten days after Truman's press conference, the novelist William Faulkner spoke about a new mentality that had been awakened by the atom bomb and a new attitude toward life and death. Perhaps Faulkner was exaggerating when he said that young American novelists had forgotten how to write with the "heart" because they were preoccupied with the pressing question of "when will I be blown up?"[66] But he refused to accept the fact that the atomic threat would usher in the "end of man," stressing his belief that "the poet's voice" was a social pillar that helps humanity "to endure and prevail." Or perhaps this new attitude affected only the survivors of the atom bomb attacks and their descendants? Lifton did not believe that to be the case, arguing that the atom blasts had created a new "A-bomb man" in Japan, changing "the survivor's status as a human being" and turning the survivors into social outcasts, often with physical stigmata.[67] However, on the whole, the resentment and anger felt by Japanese survivors did not have much effect on American national sentiment. Truman was still defending the use of the atomic bomb in 1958; and even Eleanor Roosevelt, visiting Hiroshima in June 1953, was cagey about whether the bomb should ever be used again as a weapon.[68] Lifton noted that many Japanese survivors saw themselves as guinea pigs in, and even the racial victims of, a US experiment, but the fact that Japanese writers could find words to respond to the bomb's impact suggests a degree of resilience that challenges Lifton's belief that the Japanese cities were lost in existential darkness.[69] Accounts such as Michihiko Hachiya's *Hiroshima Diary: The Journal of a Japanese Physician* (1945) and Yoko Ota's *City of Corpses* (1950) suggest that meaningful words were possible in response to the bomb.[70]

There were no direct equivalents in the United States, however, with heroic war stories, domestic dramas, and consumerist narratives offering more obvious directions for young writers and filmmakers. Although articles such as "What the Bomb Really Did" in *Collier's* (March 1946) dealt with the physical effects of the bomb, its destructive potential arguably did not fully register until the film *On the Beach was* released in 1959, two years after Nevil Shute's novel of the same name was published. As the essay "Mental Health and Atomic Energy," published in *Science* in 1958, made clear, even though nuclear power might be "uncontrollable" because radiation is "invisible, unheard, [and] unfelt," many writers and filmmakers were slow to represent nuclear fears.[71]

Many of the earlier films dealing with nuclear issues were sponsored by the government or the military, including *Duck and Cover* and an instructive twenty-minute color film made by the Armed Forces Special Weapons Project, called *The Medical Aspects of Nuclear Radiation* (1950). This film attempted to explain radiation and to dispel some of the "falsehoods" in the media, stressing the safety of nuclear science, the wisdom of medical authorities, and the expectation that "radiation patients" can be effectively treated through blood transfusions and penicillin. The film suggests that media distortions about hair loss, impotence, and genetic mutations are understandable as symptoms of "man's fear of dangers that he cannot sense, a fear fanned into widespread misunderstanding by sensational speculation about what radiation can do." The narrator counters these fears by shifting the viewer's attention from a gentleman's wristwatch with a radium dial to footage of a giant atomic burst to ensure that nuclear concerns are kept in proportion. He claims that most deaths and injuries in Hiroshima resulted from the impact and heat of the blast rather than radiation sickness. In fact, the narrator estimates that such sickness represented only 15 percent of the danger of an atomic bomb blast but caused 85 percent of nuclear fears. The film calls for realism, caution, and preparedness (healthy eating, cleanliness, and vigilance), arguing that "sound medical practice demands not only a knowledge of the way harmful agents operate, but an accurate estimate of those agents."

With the intensification of the Cold War after 1948 and growing fears that the Soviet Union possessed the hydrogen bomb, which could do ten times more damage than its atomic cousin, fears increased. We should not look to official texts to gauge these fears, though, but to cartoons and comic strips (which the psychiatrist Fredric Wertham was claiming were harmful to children, as discussed in chapter 6), as well as to popular films. The same year that Japan introduced free medical tests for survivors the science-fiction film *The Incredible Shrinking Man* was released, which neatly illustrates the diffusion of atomic fears through popular culture. Adapted by Richard Matheson from his book *The Shrinking Man* (1956), this low-budget film examines the effects of radiation on Scott Carey (Grant Williams), a white-collar worker, after he experiences a strange cloud while sailing, presumably in the Pacific. The delayed response to a nuclear storm (or pesticide, as is assumed later) causes Carey to shrink, slowly at first—his white-collar shirts, symbolizing his middle-class status, become too big for him—and then seemingly without end. Carey's doctor initially dismisses his concerns, but as the shrinking continues, he is referred to specialists who eventually make the connection between the exposure and his medical condition. However, they are powerless to arrest or reverse the process. The reliance on, but also the impotency of, medicine is illustrated in one of the film's publicity shots, in which Carey sits atop a medicine bottle, with other bottles of potions, pills, and a glass with a medicinal spoon dwarfing his diminished body.

The result is that Carey's marriage becomes meaningless, and he takes up residence in a doll's house, where his anxiety is proved well-founded in an attack from the family cat. The story revolves around fears of domestic containment and the struggle for marital power (symbolized by the doll's house) as much as nuclear contamination. Pushed into a cellar and out of earshot of his wife, Carey drops into an almost alien landscape, where previously familiar domestic objects become strange and where an encounter with a spider (perhaps a nightmarish version of his wife) leads to a fight to the death. Although Carey survives (in the novel he narrates the story in flashback), we leave him at the end of the film as a mere speck in the darkness. Rather than existential despair, Carey comes to realize that although his comfortable suburban trappings are no more (his wife has left; his house and job are useless to him) he has become one with the universe. We might read this ending as Carey's being forced to confront ground zero but, as the film historian Mark Jancovich notes, he is also compelled to entirely reorient his values. Carey had previously assumed that "zero

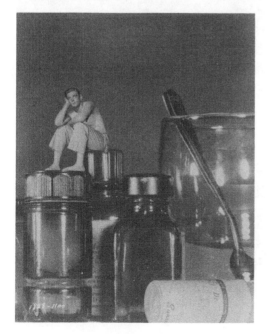

FIGURE 3.1 Grant Williams as Scott Carey contemplates his diminished size, surrounded by ineffectual medical cures. Publicity still for *The Incredible Shrinking Man* (Jack Arnold, Universal, 1957).

inches means nothing," but he realizes that at a microscopic level, the world has a new and often overlooked fascination.[72] The opening titles of *The Incredible Shrinking Man* accompany an abstract image of a mushroom cloud, but the film ends with a version of eco-mysticism in a world that is almost post-holocaustic.

Popular culture dealt with the atom bomb with a mixture of levity—the phrase "sex bomb" and songs with such titles as "Atomic Cocktail" (1946), "Atomic Baby" (1950), and "Atom Bomb Baby" (1957)—and concern: the Bermudan band the Talbot Brothers sang the calypso "Atomic Nightmare" (1957), in which the listener is warned to try to outrun the atomic fallout. Fears of nuclear destruction very quickly became stock in trade for science-fiction films, from *The Day the Earth Stood Still* (1951), in which a humanoid alien, Klaatu, reminds the earth of the might of nuclear power; to genetic mutation films such as *The Thing from Another World* (1951) and *Invasion of the Body Snatchers* (1956), in which a small-town doctor, Miles Bennell, becomes a fugitive in a Californian city where humans have been replaced by unfeeling clones born from alien pods. In this uncannily familiar world, body and mind come under attack from irresistible biological forces (what Bennell calls "a malignant disease spreading through the whole country"), making it hard for the fugitive doctor to hold on to his sanity. While the Army film The *Medical Aspects of Nuclear Radiation* ends with the claim that mutations can sometimes be advantageous, there were hundreds of B movies in the 1950s that connected fears of invasion to mutations or clones.

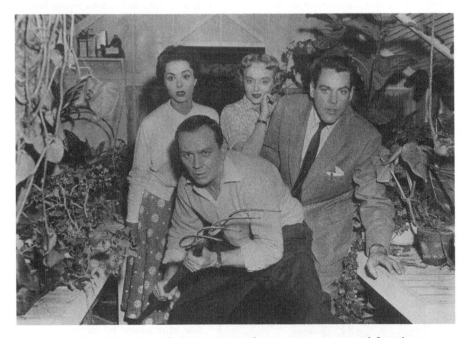

FIGURE 3.2   Dr. Miles Bennell (Kevin McCarthy), wearing a tie, and friends contemplate a biological invasion early in *Invasion of the Body Snatchers* (Don Siegel, Allied Artists, 1956).

The Day the Earth Stood Still stands out from many of the Cold War films in dealing seriously with the social factors that inflamed nuclear fears, even though its director, Robert Wise, claimed that the film was made only for entertainment. It opens with a spaceship landing at the center of a baseball diamond in Washington, D.C., and then shows how media stories can run like wildfire, mutating as they spread. The military quickly surround the spaceship, but there appears to be no leader who can respond when one soldier shoots Klaatu as he offers the humans a strange object that turns out to be a symbol of peace. The federal government also lacks a commander: Klaatu is visited in a hospital by a government agent who tells him flatly that it would be impossible to bring together an international delegation to listen to his message that the world is in danger unless it mends its ways. The fact that a political figure—a bureaucrat, at that— arrives at the hospital suggests that medicine is in the service of government rather providing places of refuge built on sound medical practice. Klaatu escapes from the hospital and, as a humanoid, moves anonymously among Washingtonians. Realizing that his chances of convincing the world's political leaders to organize a summit meeting are nonexistent, he tracks down the respected physicist Dr. Barnhardt (who bears a passing resemblance to Albert Einstein) to help him convey his message.[73] The power of Klaatu and his gigantic robot accomplice Gort to make the world stand still for a minute reveals the pettiness of human affairs, but Klaatu is turned over to the military through a mixture of naïveté on behalf of a young boy, Bobby, and the scheming of his mother's boyfriend. The film demonstrates the possibilities of nuclear power as a source of fuel for Klaatu's spaceship, but it ends with the warning that unless all nations and their political, military, and medical institutions mend their ways, a higher authority, represented by the robot Gort, will enslave the world. This message about the importance of international collaboration and the fostering of a culture of openness was very apposite for 1951, but it was a message interlacing peace with threats.

What was not widely known at the time, largely because of the secrecy of the Los Alamos experiments, was that above-ground nuclear testing had been occurring on a regular basis in the Southwest. The first nuclear explosion in Alamogordo, New Mexico, in July 1945 was treated with almost religious reverence; Oppenheimer drew his responses from John Donne's sonnets and the Hindu Bhagavad-Gita, reputedly claiming that the bomb, Trinity, gave off "the radiance of a thousand suns." Between that moment and 1963, when President Kennedy announced the end of above-ground and underwater explosions in the Limited Nuclear Test Ban Treaty, the United States produced 216 nuclear explosions, most of them in the Southwest or the Pacific. The fact that almost as many explosions were carried out by the Soviet Union—an estimated 214 between 1949 and 1961—indicated the necessity for an international accord, as the two giants of the Cold War tried to outpace each other with scientific research. Talks actually began in 1955, but it took seven years of negotiation before the treaty was concluded in 1963, with Kennedy announcing that "America's weapons are non-provocative, carefully controlled, designed to deter, and capable of selective use."[74]

Public concern about nuclear fallout was also growing in the mid- and late 1950s, some of it fanned by science-fiction films with their images of mutations and

distortions in size, from the shrinking man of Jack Arnold's 1957 film to the emascu-
lating threat of *Attack of the 50 Foot Woman* (1958) and the radioactive spill that gave
rise to the leviathan in *Behemoth the Sea Monster* (1959). Some of the above-ground
tests created fallout from small particles and gases that spread far from the Nevada
test site, such as the April 1953 controlled explosion, Simon, which produced fallout
that drifted as far as New York State, or the massive blast of Bravo in Bikini Atoll
in the Pacific Ocean (March 1954), which covered two neighboring atolls and their
inhabitants with fallout. Bravo became an international incident, and it led to urgent
discussions. These talks later gave rise to the Limited Nuclear Test Ban Treaty, which
permitted only underground testing—and only if the resulting debris would not
extend past the boundaries of the state in which the explosion occurred.

The scale of actual destruction in the United States was not really gauged by
reports on Hirsohima, nor could the actual threat of nuclear attack be assessed
through its sublimations in science fiction. More recent studies of fallout and reports
by "atomic veterans" working on nuclear test sites—often called ground zero—
provide a very different picture than that offered by the historical record. In *Voices
from Ground Zero* (1996), F. Lincoln Grahlfs estimates that a quarter of a million military personnel were involved in the nuclear testing in Nevada and the Pacific Ocean
or were exposed to residual radiation by working in Hiroshima and Nagasaki in the
months after the bomb was dropped. In the 1970s more than six thousand claims
were filed with the Veterans Administration for medical complications resulting from
veterans' nuclear work, and fewer than fifty of the claims were rejected because they
provided no evidence "linking radiation exposure to health damage."[75]

Accounts questioning the received wisdom about atomic testing were published in the mid-1980s as part of a critical vanguard that intensified its questioning
during President Ronald Reagan's first term in the White House. This was largely
a response to new information that came to public attention in the 1970s, such as
reports on increases in the incidence of leukemia and cancer in Utah, one of the
states downwind from the Nevada test sites. The reports actually started to appear
in the 1960s but, in the case of a 1965 report prepared for the AEC on cancer in Utah,
the file was opened only in 1979, following a government investigation.[76] Howard
Ball documents in *Justice Downwind* (1986) that the radioactive effects were widely
experienced in the bodies of miners and farmers (many of them Mormons), as well
as blighting livestock and crops. Although the effects of the nuclear tests were not
officially revealed for some years, even in the early 1950s experts knew that above-
ground tests were unsafe and that prevailing winds were carrying radioactive particles some distance, as happened with the May 1953 test bomb Harry (sometimes
called "Dirty Harry"), the effects of which were downplayed by the AEC. The only
warning in a series of press releases was to inform motorists to close their car windows and vents; they were reassured that fallout would be at "non-hazardous levels," even though radiation readings were off the scale in the downwind town of St.
George, Nevada.[77] Part of the reason for such misinformation was arguably a lack
of concern about the mountain populations of the Southwest: the photojournalist

Carole Gallagher emphasized that people living downwind from the tests were described secretly by the AEC as a "low-use segment of the population."[78] A number of books in the 1980s and 1990s focused on the drift of nuclear fallout and the legal actions that citizens and pressure groups started to take in the 1970s, but Gallagher's study, *American Ground Zero* (1993), offers a series of oral histories of workers and victims of the blasts, with unforgiving photographs of those suffering from cancerous tumors, leukemia, and long-term intestinal problems.

Perhaps because few people were interested in discovering the truth in the early Cold War years, the CBS journalist Edward R. Murrow—forever trying to shake the public out of its complacency—interviewed Oppenheimer in January 1955. The interview took place six months after lengthy hearings in which Oppenheimer had been branded a security risk by J. Edgar Hoover, and the AEC decided that he had "fundamental defects of character," prompted by his outspoken concerns about the development of the hydrogen bomb.[79] After some initial pleasantries, Murrow asked Oppenheimer about the possibility of total nuclear destruction, and he replied at length:

> You can certainly destroy enough of humanity so that only the greatest act of faith can persuade you that what's left will be human. This is a matter on which much, much, much more should be known. It is important to say what we know and to say what we don't know. The genetic problems, the problems that might happen in the future to the human species as a result of having radioactivity in the body or having radiation outside, the geneticists don't know enough to be sure enough of that. We do know what happens if you are near a bomb explosion, we know that from experience and common sense. The things we know ought to be in the public domain . . . the things that aren't known should be talked about because one of the ways to get things found out is to have it clear that we don't know the answers and, also, one of the ways to give people the kind of responsibility and humanity which we would like to think we have is to recognize when they don't know something.[80]

In this interview Oppenheimer, one of the key figures in the Manhattan Project, expressed his deep concern for the future of humanity. This might have seemed melodramatic at the time, but he displayed a profound sense of humility about what is not known. When asked how the "poor civilian" can keep up with science, Oppenheimer claimed that everyone is ignorant, saying that scientists know only a few "patches" and "spots" in "a sketchy way," and he spoke of having affection and respect for other human beings. Instead of searching for absolute knowledge—a quest that pragmatists like John Dewey had been warning against for years—Oppenheimer recommended that we look for "virtual connections, these casual and occasional connections which make the only kind of coherence we have." Oppenheimer had grown suspicious of populist politics, but in this case he believed that intellectuals should be actively engaged in the world instead of working in a hermetic environment.[81] Rather than the profundity that accompanied his description of the Trinity bomb, nearly a decade later Oppenheimer talked about connectivity and a "lacework of coherence," which suggests that meaning is open and provisional rather than closed and complete.

The key for Oppenheimer was not the purity of science or the sophistication of medicine, but ensuring that knowledge is not sealed off from a public that might otherwise be swayed by the audacious claims of someone like Senator Joseph McCarthy. Little information was available in 1953 about the damaging effects on health of the nuclear tests in Nevada, and the New York State Health Department and the AEC both thought the level of radioactivity would be "negligible."[82] When Murrow asked him about nuclear testing two years afterward, Oppenheimer's response was cagey, using a double negative: "I'm not unworried about it." A great deal of data could not be published for security reasons, but Oppenheimer and fellow Los Alamos scientists were concerned that political secrecy was hindering research: "The trouble with secrecy is not that it inhibits science . . . the trouble with secrecy is that it denies to the government itself the wisdom and resources of the whole community." Oppenheimer remained worried that public information had degenerated into propaganda, and as an antidote he called for "a free and uncorrupted communication" as "the heart of living in a complex and technological world."[83] He did not undermine the importance of science and medicine, but he wanted to ensure that technology is the servant of humans rather than their master. He shared with a number of Cold War critics (including Lewis Mumford, Reinhold Niebuhr, and Erich Fromm) the belief that the emphasis on scientism or "technics" was backward-looking and likely to create a new tyranny. Technics does not offer a direct cure for the sick body, nor can it by itself ameliorate the disturbed mind. In fact these thinkers believed that it has the potential to place the individual at the mercy of an impersonal system that denies freedom and autonomy.

Oppenheimer's humanism is clearly evident in his interview with Murrow, and it can be aligned to the realistic stance adopted by many intellectuals in the late 1940s and early 1950s. But he did not come down on the side of either the arts or the sciences, as other figures in the two-cultures debate (discussed in the introduction to this book) tended to do. Although the former Librarian of Congress Archibald MacLeish tried to rescue poetry in an age of science, writing in 1960 that "to learn to live in the new universe the scientific outlook has discovered for us is at least as difficult as to learn not to die in it," Oppenheimer implied in his 1955 interview that there are no easy therapeutic answers.[84] Instead, he pointed to a fundamental connection between the arts and sciences: "Poets and scientists understand each other as creators, though scientists may not like the poetry and poets in general will regard the scientist as dull and trivial."[85] Bridging the two cultures may, once again, prove to be the answer.

The Korean War and Mind Control

The atom bomb blast provided a dramatic end to World War II in the Pacific theater, but the conflict that the United States faced only five years later returned the nation's focus to Southeast Asia. The Korean War tends to be overlooked because it lacks the strong narrative of World War II and the breadth of media representations of the Vietnam War. Nonetheless, it was a vital hot point in the Cold War that led to significant developments in technology, healthcare, and therapy. These developments illustrate both the benefits and dangers of postwar medicine, and—as the final section of this chapter makes clear—the Korean War was successful in terms of medical treatment on one level, but deeply damaging to soldiers and prisoners on another.

In terms of military healthcare, techniques learned in the previous war for treating the soldier as close as possible to the combat zone were refined during the Korean War, based on expectations of recovery: clearing stations four miles from battlefields were used for minor surgery; mobile army surgical hospitals (MASH units) positioned ten miles from the front specialized in neurosurgery, spinal cord surgery, and repairing damaged blood vessels; and hospital ships were based around Japan. Colonel Albert J. Glass of the US Army Medical Corps had championed the notion of the expectancy of treatment during World War II, and he played a significant role in the Korean conflict, ensuring that soldiers could regain active roles in the war. Glass was a key figure in linking medical and psychiatric discourses; he detected a much lower rate of psychological breakdowns in Korea than in World War II, partly because screening processes had become more rigorous, but also because a "brief respite from battle" to relieve fatigue was deemed to be more important than searching for "magical routines, drugs, or psychological explanations of the past and present."[86] For Glass, the physician's capacity to reassure his patient and to maintain focus on the present were more important strategies in military medicine and psychiatry than delving into the "remote past [to] explain the present breakdown."[87]

Many hospitals in Korea suffered from poor conditions and overcrowded wards, which compounded an epidemic outbreak of hemorrhagic fever in June 1951, and the Korean healthcare system was decimated after the war, leaving a country full of illness.[88] However, from a US perspective, the Korean War was in many ways a success on the medical front, particularly for those soldiers suffering physical wounds. Of those treated for injuries, only twenty-three soldiers out of every thousand died, a fact that was particularly remarkable as there were fewer medical personnel for every hundred soldiers in the Korean War than in World War II. The development of better protective clothing and body armor, studies of wounds and frostbite, and the equality of pay and conditions for women and men in the Army Nurse Corps were all major achievements made during the Korean War. The physician Howard Rusk, writing in 1953, thought that these medical achievements were remarkable given the difficult environment, poor sanitation, extremes of temperature, and "hordes of refugees who jammed the roads and formed a mobile source of infection" in Korea.[89] General George Armstrong, the surgeon general of the army, cited six reasons for medical success in the war: (1) the availability of penicillin and antibiotics; (2) the availability of blood supplies; (3) the mobility of the sixty-bed MASH units; (4) specialist army training programs that began in 1946; (5) rapid evacuation of the wounded via helicopters that had been adapted to serve the needs of the patients and medical teams; and (6) well-equipped hospitals based in Japan, to which patients could quickly be taken.

The fact that the US Army worked alongside other allied forces and support units underlines its success, as does the statistic that army helicopters successfully evacuated over 20,000 casualties and helped to reduce the mortality rate to the lowest level ever for a significant war.[90] But these success stories do not erase the realities of the war, which was largely a series of skirmishes around the thirty-eighth parallel as the troops of Communist North Korea, with their Chinese allies, were kept from moving south by the South Koreans and their Western allies. The wrangles between General Douglas MacArthur and President Truman over military strategy suggested that no one quite knew who was running the campaign, apart from ensuring that it was a limited war that would prevent communism from spreading throughout Southeast Asia. The facts that Korea was an alien environment for nearly all the Allied soldiers, that very few of them knew the local language, and that they had inadequate training and clothing for the winter conditions they faced meant that the war was a lot tougher than the medical success story attests. George Barrett, a *New York Times* reporter stationed in Korea, noted that many of the US soldiers acted mechanically, with "an almost robot-like disinterest . . . that is in disturbing contrast to the assertive individualism of the World War II soldier."[91] This mood of bewilderment, indifference, and disjointedness detected by Barrett, particularly among the youngest soldiers (the average age of the troops was in the early twenties), tallies with the poet William Childress's depiction of Korean soldiers in his retrospective poem "The Long March" (1972), which describes troops who "dumbly follow / leaders whose careers / hung on victory."[92] Although soldiers could be treated and healed in this war, they had only a temporary respite before they resumed their duties; and those who were too severely injured to return to combat often had their disability claims disallowed. Thus, the Korean War can be considered as a conflict in which medicine was subordinated to the higher authority of political and military leaders, making decisions that were often at odds with each other, particularly as the army and White House disagreed over war strategy.

Korea was never an atomic war, but there were reports that Truman was developing biological weaponry (there is little evidence that such weapons were used in combat, even though some Koreans suffered from respiratory anthrax). In their book *The United States and Biological Warfare* (1998), Stephen Endicott and Edward Hagerman detail declassified documents and supporting photographs that reveal that biological weaponry was being explored by the Truman administration before the Korean War. Information about biological weapons was bought from the Japanese after World War II in exchange for immunity from prosecution for war crimes, offering the United States a deadly arsenal that it could use if war broke out with the Soviet Union. On this view, not only was secret experimentation ongoing prior to the outbreak of the Korean War, but the military were preparing to use biological weapons in December 1951—although the experiments ceased in 1953 when it became clear the weapons could not be delivered effectively.[93]

There were many charges made against the US government, not only by the North Koreans and Chinese. One impassioned charge was made in a public letter by Istavan Rusznyak, president of the Hungarian Academy of Sciences, that was published in *Science* in spring 1952—when warfare in Korea was at its most intense. Writing from Communist Hungary, Rusznyak stated that all Hungarian scientists were "profoundly shocked to learn of the horrible fact contrary to all human feelings that the United States forces fighting in Korea have used bacteriological weapons to exterminate the peaceful Korean and Chinese peoples," and he urged Americans "in the name of the lofty ideals of science and of the moral principles of mankind to raise your voices in protest against this ghastly deed."[94] Unsurprisingly, the president of the US National Academy of Sciences, Detlev Bronk, refuted Rusznyak's claims and stressed that the independent International Committee of the Red Cross (ICRC) was investigating such charges made against both sides in the war, but he noted that "the Communists so far have rejected the proposal of the ICRC" for further investigation. Overall, Bronk saw such accusations as part of a campaign to "incite passions and hatred" rather than promoting scientific truth.[95]

The charges did not end there, though. Following the initial exchange between the two men, *Science* published a second letter that Rusznyak sent Bronk. In this, Rusznyak claimed that the facts of "bacteriological warfare . . . are known to all who live in countries with an unfettered press" based on photographs, a report from the International Federation of Democratic Lawyers, declarations from foreign correspondents, and a document from the World Peace Council. The letter cast doubt on the independence of the ICRC and charged that the National Academy of Sciences had either been "grossly misled or stand[s] too much in awe of one or other of the thought-control agencies that limit the freedom of thought in your country today."[96] An editorial note followed this second letter but offered no direct response, simply stating that the National Academy of Sciences was committed to pursuing the accusations further by establishing a "commission of impartial persons expert in bacteriology, entomology, and epidemiology."[97]

This exchange is evidence that any claim to have the facts of the matter during the Korean War was met with charges and countercharges of propaganda, and scientific facts were subordinated to political ideology. Endicott and Hagerman not only reveal experimentation with biological weaponry but also claim that the Truman administration "lied to both Congress and the American public when it said that the American biological warfare program was purely defensive and for retaliation only."[98] They relied on Chinese reports and declassified British and Canadian documents, which made connections between "the presidential office, the Department of Defense . . . the military services and the medical, scientific, academic, and corporate communities."[99] According to this information, the Chemical Corps of the US Army led the tests with chemical weapons, including poisonous gases and napalm, but there were also experiments with biological weapons such as bacteria, toxins, fungi, viruses, and parasites (some causing anthrax, smallpox, undulant fever, and bubonic plague), and their delivery in the form of cluster bombs, leaflet bombs, aerosol sprays, and guided missiles. One general in the Chemical Corps went so far as to claim that this was "public health and preventive medicine in reverse," leading to death rather than life, but in the name of a greater good.[100]

Whatever the reality of the biological experimentation, it has been proved that the Office of Strategic Services (incorporated into the Central Intelligence Agency in the mid-1940s) was experimenting with mind control during World War II, testing the use of marijuana, mescalin, and LSD as truth drugs, as well as the debilitating effects of electroshock treatment. Other allied and axis countries were conducting similar experiments. In response to the atrocities of the Nazi concentration camps, the Nuremberg Code was adopted in the late 1940s to ensure that participation in any such tests was voluntary. The ten-point code of ethics did not directly inform Pentagon policy until 1953, however, and with perceived threats from communist countries mounting the Central Intelligence Agency began to conduct more widespread experiments in 1949, not always using volunteers.[101] In light of these trends, if the Korean War seemed at first like a conventional conflict of bodies, the fact that both the Americans and Chinese were conducting their own forms of psychological warfare places it clearly within the Cold War context. The University of Pennsylvania, University of Washington, Tulane University, and McGill University (whose Allan Memorial Institute for Psychiatry made the *Feelings of Depression* film that is discussed in chapter 4) all took part in experiments (linked to the CIA in the case of McGill) with drugs, sensory isolation, shock treatments, "psychic driving," hypnosis, narcotherapy, and, in some instances, "brainwashing," as the journalist Edward Hunter named it in 1951.[102] Primarily linked with Chinese and Soviet practices, brainwashing quickly became part of Cold War rhetoric.

Articles started to appear not long after the end of the Korean War which suggested that, under the leadership of the US Army's Psychological Warfare Division, psychiatry was being used "perversely to produce drastic changes in men's fundamental attitudes and beliefs," as Major Henry Segal, chief of the neuropsychiatric evaluation team in the Army Medical Corps in the Korean Communication Zone put it: "Psychiatric principles and techniques were being utilized . . . destructively in a deliberate, coldly calculated, highly systematized attempt to produce a state of mental aberration detrimental to the individual concerned and of value only to the Communists."[103] The US investment in psychological warfare was based on evidence that brainwashing techniques had been carried out on American prisoners of war, following reports from some of the 1,400 prisoners which suggested that emotional isolation, political indoctrination, and social-psychological manipulation had often gone hand in hand.[104]

To gauge the truth of such claims, Segal surveyed reports of sixty-eight repatriated US prisoners who had been taken to the Evacuation Hospital in Seoul. The reports noted that among the former prisoners of war "talk was shallow, often vague, and with definite lack of content"; they had "large memory gaps"; they appeared "suspended in time"; they were "incapable of forming decisions"; they displayed "little if any spontaneous talk of home, family, or future"; and the "entire group demonstrated an incredible degree of cooperation with the medical authorities."[105] Despite these symptoms, Segal concluded that any attempts to indoctrinate allied soldiers had been "quite ineffective" because few prisoners ever "converted to Communism"—but perhaps that had not been their captors' intention, given the former prisoners' "confusion, unceasing anxiety, fear, needless death, defection, disloyalty, changed attitudes and beliefs, poor discipline, poor morale, poor *esprit*."[106] One columnist, reporting on Segal's findings, noted that the prisoners of war claimed that US troops had used germ warfare against the North Koreans and Chinese, but many of them felt "it was all right for us to do that in a war," especially given the suspicion that the Chinese were chemically inducing mental disorders in their prisoners.[107] This cauldron of military, political, and psychiatric ideas gave rise to the myth of the "Manchurian Candidate," a term made famous by Richard Condon's 1959 book (adapted for screen two years later), in which a brainwashed American soldier returns to the United States as a communist agent.

Prior to his psychiatric studies in Hiroshima, Lifton had gone to Korea and Hong Kong to examine reports of brainwashing among repatriated soldiers. His first article on the subject, "Home by Ship," was published in April 1954, six months before Segal's survey.[108] Lifton was convinced that mind-control experiments had been conducted on American prisoners of war, noting that press coverage of brainwashing was often unhelpful, "sensationalist in tone, distorted because of inadequate knowledge, or obscured by the strong emotions which the concept of brainwashing seems to arouse in everyone."[109] The problem with mind control is that its history is difficult to disentangle from its mythology, and, as Lifton wrote, "its aura of fear and mystery has become more conducive to polemic than understanding."[110] In Southeast Asia Lifton found a complex web of ideas and ideology involving prisoners of war as well as those attending colleges that taught communist and revolutionary ideas.

Lifton interviewed American, European, and Chinese subjects and realized that generalizations across the three groups were very hard to make. What he found in his Western subjects after they returned home was a sense of disconnection and unrest and a form of repetition compulsion—symptoms evident in Rod Serling's television drama *The Rack* (1955), which portrays a US Army captain, Edward Hall, who had been tortured and brainwashed by North Koreans for two years. On his return home, Hall has to face unfathomable feelings of guilt and accusations that he had collaborated with the enemy. Across a range of such cases, Lifton saw veterans struggling for self-mastery as they found themselves caught between past and present selves. Like demobilized World War II soldiers, these veterans found returning home difficult, especially those who had been held in prison camps for long periods of time. But Lifton did not find radical variations between Western and Chinese subjects (most of whom had been well educated, and some of whom had attended revolutionary universities between 1948 and 1952, when "thought reform" was at its peak), only differing cultural and historical patterns that blurred the dividing line between education and indoctrination. Lifton encountered linguistic and cultural barriers in his work, but he concluded that his Chinese subjects displayed as wide a range of responses as his Western case studies, which complicated the assertion that brainwashing leads to a fixed psychological response and zombie-like behavior.

Although there are other arguments to suggest that Western prisoners of war in Korea behaved no differently from their peers in other wars, with their initial disorientation and blankness of response wearing off after repatriation, Lori Bogle and other critics counter this view by pointing to the fact that twenty-one Americans (as well as one British and over three hundred South Korean) prisoners decided to stay in Communist China after being released.[111] President Eisenhower dismissed this fact as an indication of inadequate preparation for the war and encouraged the US military to be more active in raising patriotism at home, as expressed in the 1955 Code of Conduct.[112] This did not just involve workshops and public broadcasts, but also talks from the likes of John Wayne and John Ford in Hollywood, suggesting that the war for hearts and minds would be conducted in the cultural sphere as well as in political life. Recent studies of the Central Intelligence Agency's sponsoring the Congress for Cultural Freedom in Europe to promote American ideas and culture during the Cold War need to be supplemented, then, by examinations of the role of the Department of Defense in promoting the Code of Conduct at home and using cultural channels that would not be traced directly back to the Pentagon.

One of Lifton's conclusions was that "the control of human communication" was central to the success of thought reform. This kind of "milieu control" can be brought about through coercion, Lifton believed, but at its most successful it convinces the subject that he or she is acting spontaneously rather than being directed by values that are alien to the self. Instead of allowing the individual to test reality against thoughts and beliefs, he or she becomes manipulated, controlled or suffocated by the environment. Most worryingly, especially if we consider the close links between therapy and religion that Philip Rieff described in *The Triumph of the Therapeutic*, it no longer becomes possible for the individual to distinguish false confessions from truth, or fantasy from reality. Although confession can be therapeutic in offering relief from guilt, it can also exacerbate deeper complexes and obliterate social realities, and in extreme cases the fragmented self is in danger of becoming a cipher, incapable of meaningful responses. Lifton's main concern was less to identify pockets of antiscientific zealotry (McCarthy's "blend of political religion and extreme opportunism," as he called it) or expressions of political reeducation (such as William F. Buckley's recommendation that alumni should decide on university syllabi), but to demonstrate that the institutionalization of psychoanalysis—"a combination of personal therapy, professional instruction, and organizational influence"—can itself lead to a form of milieu control or a quasi-religion.[113] Rather than resulting in personal freedom, then, psychoanalysis not only creates a culture of dependency but also has the potential to promote conformity.

Just as responses to the development of the atomic bomb led to profound questions about the social and moral role of science in the late 1940s and 1950s, so hints that biological and psychological warfare was being deployed in the Korean War led to similar concerns. It was the "deification" of science, the "expectation that science will supply a complete and absolutely accurate mechanistic theory of a closed and totally predicable universe," that worried Lifton, Oppenheimer, and other intellectuals during the Cold War.[114] In 1966 the Group for the Advancement of Psychiatry argued that the "budgets, organizations, and technology that can destroy mankind can also produce the most constructive achievements in world history," but the growing mistrust of the White House, US military, and government agencies during the early years of the Cold War suggested that science, medicine, psychiatry, and psychoanalysis were all caught up in the same ideological net.[115] At a time when Harold Lasswell was calling for "a proper balance between national security and individual freedom," the covert nature of top-secret mind-control projects was justified in the name of national defense, thus blurring the line between ethical medical experimentation and counter espionage.[116]

The main problem was not that science and medicine were enmeshed in Cold War hostilities, but that dangerous ethical issues arose that transgressed the Nuremberg Code and made US activities comparable to experiments carried out under fascism and communism that were profoundly anti-therapeutic. As the first section of this book has discussed, what was seen as a pinnacle of twentieth-century achievement only a few years earlier became mired in ideological problems during the early years of the Cold War. No longer was medical science the agent of hope that Assistant Secretary of State Butterworth announced in 1949; rather, it was dangerously close to becoming an agent of fear. This blurring of existential boundaries is something that Engelhardt and Lifton, among others, have identified. Lifton reminds the reader in *Thought Reform and the Psychology of Totalism* (1961) that the "god-pole" of science in its search for total control is not the opposite of its "devil-pole" in its potential for destruction; both might exist codependently, both "equally misleading and dangerous in their extremism."[117] Without checks and balances or an international agreement such as the 1947 Nuremberg Code or the World Medical Association's Declaration of Helsinki of 1964 to curb the ambitions of science, the world of ideas is left in a state of disequilibrium; medical research risks ideological co-option; and the individual—as Mailer argued in 1957—becomes a zero, a cipher "in some vast statistical operation in which . . . our death itself would be unknown, unhonored, and unremarked."[118]

PART TWO

Organization

1953–1961

4   *Organization Men*

INDIVIDUALISM VERSUS INCORPORATION

Science—The Endless Frontier, the influential report written in 1945 by President Franklin D. Roosevelt's science advisor, Vannevar Bush, recommended that "research in the natural sciences and medicine" should not simply be expanded "at the cost of the social sciences, humanities, and other studies so essential to national well-being."[1] The rise of the social sciences in the decade following this report challenged the privileged position of the physical sciences in the early years of the Cold War, but business and technology were the primary keepers of national well-being during the Eisenhower years, in what amounted to a top-down attempt to reconcile domestic prosperity with Cold War preparedness. Although President Dwight Eisenhower worried that too much federal control would jeopardize civil liberties and the privacy of ordinary citizens, he liked business leaders and claimed that "orderliness" is necessary to restrict "irresponsible human action."[2]

One such business leader was Charles E. Wilson. Dubbed the preeminent "American production man" by *Time* in 1951, Wilson was Eisenhower's secretary of defense from 1953 until 1957 and the public face of this business ethos in government.[3] Wilson is most famous for proclaiming in 1953 that he could not imagine a scenario in which what was good for the country would be in conflict with what was good for General Motors, whose president he had been from 1941 to 1953. This mention of his previous company is less significant than his coupling of the spirit of enterprise and a patriotic commitment to strengthen national values, which was in tune with the Cold War strategy to safeguard capitalist values in the face of socialist and communist competition. This model of increased domestic productivity might appear to be socially progressive, but Wilson's managerial philosophy could equally be seen as the extension of Cold War containment policies to the control of life in and beyond the workplace, particularly as he sought to restructure the Pentagon and Department of Defense along industrial lines. Wilson endorsed stable Cold War governance, but he resisted other policies, advising Eisenhower to rein in military spending, believing that "true security" derived from a healthy domestic economy, and speaking out against Senator Joseph McCarthy's rampant anticommunism.[4] Widespread concern that dissidents were working invisibly within American institutions (labor unions, the entertainment industry, and the government alike) lost its intensity in 1954, following McCarthy's failed televised attempt to indict members of the US Army, but broader factors reinforced domestic organization beyond the mid-1950s. "Organization" as an overarching concept, one could argue, was a joint strategy on the part of Eisenhower's "management administration" and big business to ameliorate the social problems explored in part 1 of this book and to stabilize the nation during the Cold War, without imposing the kind of state control practiced by the Soviets.

Perhaps the most important factor was the investment in technology by the government, military, and business, all of which shared, in some respects, the Soviet faith in rational science. Technology was the first line of defense against a communist invasion, as well as a safeguard of economic prosperity and a way for firms to shape consumer needs. Bush argued in *Science—The Endless Frontier* that technology should be designed in line with the skills and capabilities of workers, but just as important were new management and office structures geared to large workforces and increased productivity. Managerial proponents argued strongly for "superior management competence" to enable the nation to switch "back and forth between peacetime and defense production," based on robust organizational structures in which workers' functions were clearly defined and unnecessary activities eliminated.[5] Echoing the criticism of C. Wright Mills in 1951 that in a rationalized office structure the "employee group is transformed into a uniform mass," the management theorist Peter Drucker warned business leaders that workers should not be organized like machines, although he agreed that tracking behavioral patterns within the flow of production was strategically important for companies.[6] This emphasis on predictability—linked to the emerging field of cybernetics as a science of "information, communication, feedback, and systems"—helped managers to normalize behavioral variance against a golden mean of averageness.[7] Not all thinkers shared the "technocratic optimism" of cyberneticians Norbert Wiener and John von Neumann, but the emphasis on game theory and computer technology suggested that all human behavior could be mapped out as a rational pattern of motor neuron response, banishing irrationality in the brave new world of science and business.[8]

The Perils of Productivity

This chapter explores how this technocratic emphasis encroached on business, the workplace, and industrial and occupational healthcare. Chapter 3 demonstrated that the Cold War opened up a seam of distrust for authority—including the authority of organized medicine. Similarly, the paternalistic attitude of the business world served to promote both its own interests and the Eisenhower administration's priorities of stability and prosperity, but it also led to public dissatisfaction with the corporate world. Not only did this business attitude chime with Charles Wilson's 1953 statement about General Motors, but it also suggested that business saw itself as the caretaker of national values. A wave of social critics, including Mills, David Riesman, Erich Fromm, Paul Goodman, and William H. Whyte, criticized the organizational philosophy of large-scale businesses. At the same time that companies were beginning to take industrial and occupational health seriously, the emphasis on automatism and efficiency were arguably making employees more susceptible to illness. Business wanted a "productive" and "healthy" workforce (two adjectives that Eisenhower explicitly equated in his 1954 and 1955 State of the Union addresses), and there was a tacit awareness that health was a precarious condition in the 1950s. This is a central theme of part 2 of this book, which starts by focusing on the workplace in this chapter before discussing the organization of the 1950s home in chapters 5 and 6 to show the ways in which the categories of illness and health—particularly mental health—became regulated in everyday life.

The ideal type in the mid-1950s was part of the problem, at least according to Erich Fromm, who argued in *The Sane Society* (1955) that too strong an emphasis on averageness or normalcy could itself be pathological. And not only does overemphasis on mass productivity lead to alienation, but, as Fromm argued, it has a habit of transcending economic production and influences "the attitude of man to things, to people, and to himself."[9] In mass society, the process of abstractification becomes normalized: "The concrete reality of people and things to which we can relate with the reality of our own person, is replaced by abstractions, by ghosts that embody different quantities, but not different qualities."[10] In a version of the Marxist model of alienated labor, workers are apt to think about themselves as statistics or functions: a form of internal commodification that Fromm saw as deeply damaging to mental health.[11] The organization—both a metaphor for Eisenhower's administration and a synonym for "the firm"—can easily become an all-enveloping system, transforming the human worker into "the organization man" (a phrase immortalized in the title of Whyte's 1956 book), or giving rise to the abstract category of the "man in the gray flannel suit" (an image adorning the cover of Sloan Wilson's 1955 novel of that name was widely reproduced in advertisements and the popular press).

The focus of this chapter on business practices in the 1950s can be projected forward into the following decade, but it is important to note that the technocratic emphasis on scientific management did not survive the 1950s untarnished.[12] Indeed, critics associated with the new left—and other more radical thinkers—expanded Fromm's criticism and declared scientific management deeply anti-humanistic and potentially damaging to the health of workers and their families. Looking back from the mid-1960s, Abraham Maslow, for example, commented that normalcy is often presented as a "value-free" mode of description, but the danger is that averageness is often taken as "the best we can expect."[13] In such cases, "normalcy would be rather the kind of sickness or crippling or stunting that we share with everybody and therefore don't notice." Maslow argued that this existentially impoverished condition needs guidance and authority: "The experientially-empty person, lacking these directives from within, those voices of the real self, must turn to outer cues for guidance."[14] Echoing the Marxist humanism of Fromm, Maslow also reminds us of one of the most influential sociological studies of the postwar period, David Riesman's *The Lonely Crowd* (1950), and particularly the distinction Riesman made between "inner-directed" and "other-directed" personality types.[15]

Riesman shared with the economist John Kenneth Galbraith a belief that productivity had gone too far since the Great Depression. In *The Affluent Society* (1958), Galbraith saw benefits in the general improvement in standards of living and the "mountainous rise in wellbeing," but he worried about the degrading of public life, pollution, and the pernicious effect of advertising on an individual's aspirations—an advertising culture that President Eisenhower was to endorse in the Advertising Council's "Confidence in a Growing America" campaign of 1958, which the president believed could get the economy out of a temporary slump.[16] This suspicion of corporate culture led Riesman, in his preface to the 1969 edition of *The Lonely Crowd*, to agree with Galbraith that "public goods" had suffered in favor of "private goods," serving to downgrade intangibles such as "satisfaction in love and work."[17] It is this set of intangibles that Riesman had explored in the first edition of *The Lonely Crowd*. Riesman used a version of Fromm's character types to chart shifts in "social character," focusing on recent population trends that, to his mind, had given rise to "other-directed" people "sensitized to the expectations and preferences of others."[18]

Deploying a set of typologies that closely linked character types to social production, Riesman argued that "tradition-directed" individuals had been replaced by industrious "inner-directed" people during the Industrial Revolution. From the 1920s onward, they in turn were slowly succeeded by the "other-directed" social character, as production gave way to consumption. This might be read as a narrative of decline: the other-directed type was more liable to be influenced by outside forces and possessed weaker ego boundaries than the inner-directed character. But Riesman resisted nostalgia and warned against the tendency to "over-idealize inner-direction and to be over-critical of other-direction," seeing them as symptomatic of historical phases.[19] He did not argue that everyone in a particular period conformed to the prevailing character type, but he asserted that historically determined ideals shaped psychological horizons. The rise of private property was a factor in the emergence of the inner-directed type, but Riesman did not consider this an "essential condition," especially given that "ambitious, energetic, self-reliant men" could be identified under very different economic structures, such as those in Russia, Germany, and the United States.[20] Although Riesman's typology was influential, he was unsure how social change could be actively brought about, basing his treatise on the consequences of broad population shifts and the growth of the mass media.

The Lonely Crowd is often read as a thoroughgoing critique of postwar society that points to the rise of consumerism and mass culture for creating a national mood of anomie and lack of common purpose, even during a time of Cold War vigilance. Riesman was not concerned with health per se, or in constructing a "well-defined psychodynamic model," as Margaret Mead termed it, but he was interested in tracing general feelings of anomie to social production and population shifts. This was an attempt to pinpoint a mid-century condition and, in the words of Mead, to ensure "a future in which man will have both more power to control his destiny and more freedom within it."[21] Although Riesman did not add his voice to the two-cultures debate discussed in the introduction to this book, *The Lonely Crowd* pits humanistic forces against technology and tacitly associates health with personal autonomy.

Riesman might be seen to project the image of a northeastern male workforce onto the whole nation, but Todd Gitlin and Joseph Galbo have detected ambivalences in *The Lonely Crowd*.[22] These views echo the opinion of Arthur Brodbeck, who argued in 1961 that the book is not a jeremiad or a full-scale critique of industrial relations, but the theme of loneliness "haunts every page, like an insistent and sorrowful background music."[23] Wilfred McClay argues convincingly that other-directed types "have lost the fundamental core of consistency that makes for healthy individuation" and "risk ceding their inmost selves to social forces that care little for the integrity of the individual," but the fact that white-collar jobs provided opportunities for other-directed types to interact with other workers (rather than working with objects in industrialized workplaces) could be seen as a positive side of human-sector work or, perhaps, simply indicative of a growing service economy.[24] Nevertheless, Riesman argued that in the middle of the twentieth century, frustration at work—particularly in the white-collar sector—created a psychological need for consumables that could offer seductive escape routes. As I discuss below, marketing firms seized on this need for pleasure and the fantasy of sophistication to offset the tedium of city jobs—a trend that led Vance Packard to worry in *The Hidden Persuaders* (1957) about the increasing influence of advertising on consumer desires, particularly fantasies surrounding personal and family health.[25] Riesman did not condemn mass culture out of hand for encouraging passivity, as Theodor Adorno and Max Horkheimer had in the mid-1940s; rather than just another form of factory-line production, Riesman thought that the postwar culture industry possessed a degree of flexibility and catered more to individual tastes. This pandering to individuality tended to streamline and package individualism, however, and to link it closely to business logic. Thus, although mass culture could play a therapeutic role, it never moved very far from the standardization at the core of business organization. The problem—for Riesman and others, such as the broadcaster Ed Murrow—is that mass culture can often be a distraction, preventing consumers from understanding the capitalist structures that undergird its production.

The solution for Riesman was to encourage a more autonomous personality type, which was neither as inflexible as the inner-directed type of traditional labor nor as receptive as the other-directed type to the forces of consumer capitalism. Riesman's hope, as Galbo argues, was to encourage the public "to examine the potentially liberating aspects of the new mass culture" and not to sell short "human resilience against totalitarian control and media manipulation."[26] But the increased reliance on medicine and healthcare—from advice columns and the proliferation of pharmaceutical products to occupational health and more surgical procedures—made it less likely that individuals could work out health problems by themselves or with just a little medical help. The tensions between the individual as autonomous consumer, on the one hand, and someone dependent on medical authority, on the other hand, marked a major postwar fault line, suggesting that Riesman's inner-directed and other-directed types coexisted rather than representing two successive historical phases. Although his companion volume *Faces in the Crowd* (1952) provided empirical data that substantiated these social types, many novels and films of the 1950s portrayed double-facing characters, pulled between the demands of their environment and half-expressed anxieties about autonomy, work, and health.[27]

A Healthy Workforce?

The Lonely Crowd is often read as a portrait of a maladjusted nation, full of other-directed individuals who oil the wheels of capitalism but do so at great expense to their own well-being. As this chapter explores, criticism of the psychological demands of white-collar work and corporate life run throughout the 1950s, from responses to management philosophy through cultural representations, which I will discuss with particular reference to Rod Serling's television play *Patterns* (1955), Ernst Pawel's novel *From the Dark Tower* (1957), and Sloan Wilson's popular novel *The Man in the Gray Flannel Suit* (1955) and its 1956 Hollywood adaptation.

These accounts of the damaging effects of corporate life need to be offset, however, by a number of facts, most crucially that Presidents Truman and Eisenhower continued to invest in health services and that the National Institutes of Health increased its input into medical research significantly in the fifteen years following World War II, from $85,000 in 1945 to more than $155 million in 1959.[28] Together with a paternalistic attitude toward returning soldiers—which included the work of the Veterans Administration to secure suitable jobs and compensation for those who had been disabled in combat—industrial safety was high on the national agenda. There was a national conference about it in Washington, D.C., in 1948, followed by a major study on air pollution in 1949 and a conference on workers' compensation and rehabilitation in 1950. The emphasis over the previous fifty years had been on hygiene in heavy industry and on limiting the hours of the working day, particularly for women and children. By 1950 little research had been done on the relationship between physical and psychological stress, although company medical services were starting to make these links in relation to the stresses of war, and a 1954 study on *Suicide and Homicide* assessed how factors relating to workplace stress can lead to aggressive behavior, with sometimes fatal consequences.[29] Industrial hygiene focused mainly on preventive measures, first aid, safety codes, physical examinations, and, in some cases, health education. Where psychiatrists were used, it was to deal primarily with emotional conflicts between workers on behalf of the management, rather than to address occupational stress faced by individuals.

Throughout the 1950s, industrial research increasingly dealt with the varying concerns of the worker, shifting its attention from heavy industry to white-collar work. This marked a general swing not only from industry to business but also, using Riesman's terminology, from the inner-directed employee whose work involves "non-human objects" to other-directed employees who "think of work in terms of people—people seen as something more than the sum of their workmanlike skills and qualities."[30] The increasing emphasis on human relations in industry was reinforced in a report released by the Department of Labor, *How American Buying Habits Change* (1959), which focused on the "revolution which has transformed the [life of the] average American worker and his family from . . . a generally drab existence" into one of ease and security.[31] This change was facilitated by work that required less physical effort and fewer hours (the average non-agricultural working week was

40–41 hours in 1950, compared to 56 hours in 1900) and that came with more efficient equipment, higher salaries, and better opportunities. Business elites strongly supported government funding for scientific research via the National Science Foundation (formed in 1950), even though some industry leaders were worried about too much external interference—particularly those businesses that could afford their own research departments.[32]

The report promised that hard work could help individuals transcend their class status. Workers could look forward to equity in the workplace and a fairly affluent lifestyle—an assessment backed up by a 1950 consumer expenditure survey that revealed that earnings across various types of urban work had leveled out between 1935 and 1950.[33] The positive outlook for workers in the Department of Labor report is in line with the upward trajectory of Norman Vincent Peale's self-help narratives (discussed below), which linked the individual's well-being to promotion and status, but perhaps at the expense of cooperation with co-workers or a sense of shared responsibility and destiny. Although the report gives the unions credit for helping transform working practices, it characterizes most unions as shunning socialism and helping "to bring capitalist production to full fruition."[34]

The triumph of science model adopted by the report also applied to changes in the level and quality of healthcare, contrasting the health hazards of nineteenth-century factory work (dangerous machinery, poor sanitation, high accident rates, long working hours, low life expectancy) with significant increases in the numbers of doctors, nurses, and auxiliary medical personnel in the middle of the twentieth century. This was also true for medical services in industry, with on-site health protection estimated to be available to 40 percent of workers in 1947, providing them with emergency care, physical check-ups, diagnostic tests, counseling, and "industrial and mental hygiene programs."[35] The report credits unions with setting up fifty health centers by the late 1950s and praises some companies for introducing vaccines and providing vitamin pills for employees. Although the report identified health insurance as a problem in some regions (the highest medical expenditures were in the West) and detected variations among classes of worker (unskilled workers in the South spent the least on healthcare), the 1950 census revealed that health insurance figures for African American families had improved markedly since World War II, with half of them reporting that they had insurance.[36] These improvements led to a very positive summary in the report: the worker's "health problems are not his alone but the responsibility of the whole community working together. He knows that a vast army of scientific, educational, financial, and legislative experts is waging war against preventable maladies and against unnecessary suffering from unavoidable ills."[37] Although many reports of industrial ill health did not arise until decades later (an asbestos factory in Paterson, New Jersey, had seventeen healthy workers in 1954, but only two of them were still alive in 1974), the 1959 report raised concerns about work-based injury, sanitation (particularly nuclear contamination), and lack of health insurance for low-paid workers.[38] Of particular concern was the slow progress of research on and treatment of mental illness, which was seen as a significant drain on federal funds.

One frequently used term missing from the 1959 report is "human engineering." The fourth edition of *Industrial Psychology* (1958) linked the term to employee motivation, and Drucker referred to human engineering positively in 1959 in his conceptualization of production flow.[39] Associated with the principles of efficiency laid out by the efficiency expert Frederick Winslow Taylor and championed by owners of industrial production companies in the 1910s and 1920s, human engineering had been promoted by Hugo Münsterberg as beneficial to both employer and employee in reducing working time and helping to raise wages. Adopting a scientific managerial approach, Münsterberg's *Psychology and Industrial Efficiency* (1913) provided an intellectual rationale for "the managed life." Münsterberg recommended that "psychological engineers" pay serious attention to four groups of issues—selection and appointment; advertisement and display; fatigue, efficiency, and recreation; and "psychological demands for the arrangement of machines"—and he was positive that such attention would lead to "splendid betterments."[40]

Nearly half a century later, a team of European physicians, psychologists, and design engineers under the auspices of the European Productivity Agency examined the condition of the American workplace. Their report emphasized the dangers of "a forced and too rapid introduction" of human engineering, either because of the employment of "insufficiently qualified people" or through the militarization of the workplace, linking the growth of ergonomics to the use of military equipment in World War II.[41] Echoing Münsterberg's concern about worker fatigue, the European Productivity Agency report focused on long-term stress. The researchers were particularly concerned that human research was being carried out under the auspices of the military, and that the "capacities and limitations" of workers and equipment design were being skewed by military and government investment. The report offered a critical view of postwar workplace practice from a European perspective, recommending that more independent research should be conducted on the consequences of fatigue and the needs of older workers and women.

These concerns correspond with those expressed in a more balanced survey of industrial psychology carried out in 1948 by two Californian psychologists, Edwin Ghiselli and Clarence Brown. They applauded the reduction in the average number of working hours across the previous half-century, but they remained skeptical about the claim that shorter hours "provide the opportunity for a fuller life" or that "the work will come within the psychophysiological limits of the worker."[42] Their overriding concern was that human factors were often overlooked in favor of standardization, and that a crude mechanistic model was usually adopted instead of the view of the worker as a "thinking, feeling, and desiring organism."[43] Reacting against the frequent division between physical and mental work, the authors focused on "totalities of behavior," but they distinguished between jobs that emphasized "remembering, thinking, reasoning, judging" and those that required "speed and coordination of muscle groups."[44] The most important context for this study was the spate of labor strikes in 1945–1946 by coal miners, steelworkers, and railroad workers, particularly because Ghiselli and Brown identified employer-employee relations as the chief industrial problem, together with an overreliance on scientific models for managerial planning. The authors recommended independent investigations of working practices (focusing on fatigue, monotony, physical conditions, and shift work), a more nuanced approach to worker morale, and a better incentive system than the bonus model.

All these reports worried that Taylorist models were having negative effects on the worker's long-term health. The realization that working life was not solely mechanical led the International Labor Organization and the World Health Organization to draw up a common definition of "occupational health" in 1950 that focused on maintaining "the highest degree of physical, mental and social well-being of workers." This joint statement by the two organizations was designed to cover all conditions and grades of work, but occupational health was not fully codified until the end of the 1960s, with the formation of the Environmental Protection Agency in December 1970 and the signing of the Occupational Safety and Health Act by President Richard Nixon in the same month. However, even though the risks of using asbestos, for example, had been known since the mid-1930s, and an increasing number of lawsuits were lodged in the mid-1960s, the industrial manufacture of asbestos continued into the 1970s despite the efforts of the Environmental Protection Agency.[45]

Machine safety started to be taken seriously after a spate of accidents during World War II, and the increased number of jobs that involved working with chemicals and radioactive materials created the need for a set of coordinated guidelines. A number of states, notably New York and California, quickly produced safety guidelines for businesses, but the federal government was slow to respond. This was particularly true in respect to the psychological well-being of workers, even though doctors were calling for "planned coordination" between industry and the medical profession to strive for the "goal of true health maintenance for our employees."[46] This tallied with the August 1958 issue of the American Medical Association's journal *Archives of Industrial Health*, which was concerned with maintaining a healthy lifestyle to prevent sickness and absenteeism. The concern was stimulated by the belief that there was likely to be a personnel shortage in the 1960s; in fact, worries about the renewability of the workforce led Eisenhower to establish the Conservation of Human Resources Project in 1950. This paternalistic attitude toward the well-being of the worker could be seen to have humanitarian ends, but the journal issue argued that it is common sense to ensure that workers remain happy and healthy, so as to achieve greater productivity. Thus, occupational health became closely aligned with managerial practice rather than necessarily focusing on looking after the "true health maintenance" of workers and families.[47]

Given the increasing importance of psychologists during World War II, businesses became eager to employ them to design aptitude, personality, and achievement tests and to help with recruitment. Industry statistics showed that the number of big businesses using psychologists grew from 14 percent in 1939 to 50 percent in 1947 and 75 percent in 1952, with major companies such as IBM and General Motors employing them to improve the effectiveness of supervisors, office structures, and the design of consumer goods.[48] This brand of human factors psychology marked a shift from the machine emphasis of Taylorism, stressing the capabilities of the worker rather than processes or products. Despite the new emphasis on training and communication, many of the lessons applied to business in the late 1940s and 1950s had been learned during the war under the aegis of the War Manpower Commission, created by President Roosevelt in 1942. Although the commission's work was important for increased training and regulation of working hours, the relationship of these lessons to war suggests that firms gained from regimented control of workers, hiding behind the seemingly humane objective of employing psychologists to support the workforce. Postwar occupational health thus teetered on the fulcrum between genuine therapeutic concern for the worker and attempts to broaden the reach of managerial control.

Mental Health and the Organized Workplace

Perhaps the most important book to explore the relationship between national character and the postwar industrial boom was the social historian David Potter's *People of Plenty* (1954), which evaluated how an abundance of available goods had altered the aspirations of citizens following the Great Depression and wartime rationing. Based on a series of six lectures from 1950, Potter's book proposed that abundance was the new American frontier: economic prosperity had a direct effect on growing up, choosing leisure pursuits, and prospects of employment—not just promising more available goods, increased wealth, or better health, but shaping what Potter calls "the most intimate features of man's self."[49] The postwar culture of abundance provided "protection, care, shelter, and nourishment" to the young child, including increased reliance on technology (Potter gives the example of calibrating the temperature of milk in a baby's bottle) and the expectation of more individuated space (the child's own room).[50] Abundance raises a child's expectations, speeds up growth through better nutrition and healthcare advice, and reinforces the well-being of parents and children alike through the availability of material resources. However, although Potter was concerned about the ways in which advertisements exploited "materialistic drives and emulative anxieties," *People of Plenty* did not discuss what happens when optimism is deflated, when health gives way to sickness, or when work does not deliver satisfaction or the wages to allow the worker to keep in step with prosperity.[51]

Potter's book can be read as a corrective to postwar critics who were quick to castigate capitalism, business, and the anesthetizing effects of Cold War containment policy. But Potter was too optimistic in his depiction of the US national character, overlooking the potential drudgery of work and the significant gaps in the healthcare system that President Truman had tried to address in the late 1940s. In a series of articles from the mid-1950s onward—published in 1964 as *Abundance for What?*—Riesman filled in the details of Potter's picture of an abundant nation, bringing the Cold War into the frame and noting that many Americans "are coasting psychologically on the remaining gaps and deficiencies in the ever rising 'standard package' of consumer goods."[52] Riesman was very worried about the lack of public programs, believing that—despite Charles Wilson's attempt to scale down defense spending—the erosion of a public culture countered Wilson's vision of what was good for the nation. For Riesman, the 1950s marked an impoverished sense of the social good, and he believed that Cold War fears could not be quashed by consumer confidence. Potter's frontier of abundance brought the possibility of new vaccines, such as the polio vaccine in 1952, but below the surface were retroactive currents often ignored or sidelined in public proclamations about the nation's renewed prosperity. Medicine was central to the grand march of science celebrated by *Life* in 1950, but healthcare for mental illness had barely a toehold on the plentiful frontier outlined in *People of Plenty.*[53]

A fuller picture was provided by the National Health Assembly convened in Washington, D.C., in 1948 to assess the health of the nation. The resulting report, *America's Health*, recommended innovations in medical research and an increase in medical personnel (particularly psychiatrists), the development of hospitals (including the redeployment of veterans' hospitals as teaching institutions), and increased public education about nutrition. This report focused on international healthcare and cooperation, but it recommended a combination of public and private funds to develop the national infrastructure. One example of this philanthropic investment stream was funding from the Rockefeller Foundation, which established an International Health Board in 1913, inspired by the belief that "an applied science could unite a divided world" and that democracy and health are closely entwined.[54] The foundation sponsored research into the control of diseases (including yellow fever, hookworm, and malaria in the 1910s) and family healthcare (especially contraception and reproduction research in the 1930s through to the 1950s). However, although the foundation helped to establish departments of psychiatry at Harvard, Yale, Chicago, and Duke Universities in the early 1930s, psychiatric care remained a major concern, with a lack of expertise, insufficient personnel, and inadequate institutional support all contributing to "the shame of the states," as Albert Deutsch wrote in 1948.[55]

The creation of the National Institute of Mental Health in 1949 helped to shift the focus of the discussion away from debilitating mental illness (the subject of many studies in the 1940s) to promoting mental health in the workplace and the home. But it became increasingly apparent that, despite the growth in government-sponsored medical research, many Americans were suffering from everyday mental maladies and neuroses. In order to identify which groups of people were consulting doctors, the *American Journal of Psychiatry* published a report called "Who Goes to a Psychiatrist?" in May 1950. The article was based on a hundred patients who visited three psychiatrists in private practice. It claimed that the vast majority of the sample were people of "moderate means" (regular psychiatric consultations cost around $240 per year in 1950) and represented "a veritable cross-section of American life."[56] Claiming that "our patients were no more eccentric than those who would visit the office of any M.D.," the report shifted from specialized therapeutic techniques to a more diffuse set of treatments for conditions experienced by professionals, businessmen, laborers, students, housewives, office workers, and a few unemployed people.[57] The common complaint was a sense of nervousness, "internal tension, a feeling of depression, and a feeling of vague unreality," behind which lay "basic insecurity and [a sense of] uneasiness in relation to the environment."[58] We have already seen how such insecurities played out in the period after World War II and during the Cold War, but this uneasiness extended across such a broad cross-section of people that it was impossible to attribute it to particular circumstances (marital problems or impotence) or national conditions (mistrust of corporations, maltreatment by authorities, lack of work opportunities). As the next two chapters explore, significant patterns emerged in the 1950s that were associated with sexual confusion, familial expectations, and teenage anxiety, with alcohol, religion, and financial worries as minor factors.

The report's conclusions were linked to the diagnosis of these hundred patients: fifty-two of them were diagnosed as psychoneurotic, a category that included diagnoses of general anxiety, obsessive compulsive behavior, and hysterical reactions; twenty-six were functionally psychotic, with diagnoses including schizophrenia and manic depression; and twenty-two were "undiagnosed except by symptoms" such as alcoholism (four patients), barbiturate use (two), psychopathology (one), and homosexuality—which was then considered a pathology—(one). The psychiatrists advised fourteen patients to go to a sanatorium; sixteen of them received electro-shock therapy or insulin treatment; and the remaining seventy received psychotherapeutic treatment.[59]

This report makes interesting reading as a snapshot of who was seeking treatment at the beginning of the 1950s, but a follow-up letter to the editor of the *American Journal of Psychiatry* published later in 1950 pointed out that the data, although useful, were not detailed enough. The letter raised such issues as why more men than women saw psychiatrists; why there were more Catholics and Jews in the sample than the members of any other religious group; and why most patients were between twenty and fifty years of age.[60] Interestingly, the report makes no mention of race or region, two seemingly invisible factors at the beginning of the 1950s that—as chapter 7 discusses—became increasing prominent through the decade. Nor did either the report or the letter to the editor directly relate psychiatric issues to working life.

To assess these connections, it is worth briefly discussing the medical film *Feelings of Depression* (1950), prepared for the Canadian Department of National Health and Welfare by the Allan Memorial Institute at McGill University. Based on an actual case, the film relates the story of a reserved young man, John Murray, who is dependable and likeable but one of life's "bumblers." The film traces John's feelings of displacement to the day his mother brought home a baby brother, whose arrival threatened John's status within the family. His feelings of loneliness, particularly when his mother dies and his aunt comes to live with them, push him to act in a baby-like manner. The dispassionate voice-over is moralistic as well as clinical: "His attempt to win affection by imitating his younger brother ends in failure, as such attempts always do eventually. John must learn not to retreat in the face of his loneliness but to grow up." John's feelings of emptiness worsen when his father dies, forcing him to leave college for an office job, and they intensify when his younger brother announces that he is engaged to marry and has been given a promotion. John also gets married (without much emotional commitment), but his life starts to drift just as his brother finds recognition as a published author and becomes a father. As a result of both an unresolved conflict with his own father and feelings of sibling rivalry, John becomes "disturbed and angry with himself"—emotions that intensify when he loses his job after twelve years in the firm. This low point threatens to become a permanent condition, but the film ends with the possibility that John might recover his balance and sense of direction. We see him in the park interacting with children, and the narrator hints that, with psychiatry's "growing resources," he might experience "a fruitful release of his rich abilities and his long repressed capacity for enjoyment and warmth and happiness." Thus, *Feelings of Depression* is an example of a public health film in which the routine of office work and redundancy become elements in John's psychodrama, compounding his deep feelings of alienation and jealousy. The film does not seek to blame work, nor does it foreground the stresses of working life beyond the sense of expendability that John feels after working for a firm for twelve years and then being let go.

Another educational film made seven years later, *1104 Sutton Road* (1957) makes more explicit connections between work and well-being. Focusing on a typical suburban, lower-middle-class worker and newspaper-reading husband, the film uses the phrase "sometimes he doesn't seem to know his own mind" to pinpoint Adam Hathaway's general unease. A culture of efficiency at work "squeezes a little more out" of Hathaway every day, leading to fights with his wife over his level of pay and the demands of the household economy. The film deals with hierarchical roles in the workplace and status rivalry, when Butch, another worker, brags about his new automobile and makes a jibe at Hathaway's "old heap" of a car. The film's recommendation is that Hathaway should produce more to get what he wants and that the company should behave like a "mature adult" and "a good citizen" to alleviate his uneasy sense that his employer places productivity above human relations. Rather than focusing on luxurious houses and new cars, the film emphasizes the need for cooperation, affection, human understanding, and guidance in a well-balanced life.

These two films are not isolated cases. By the end of the decade, the Joint Commission on Mental Health and Illness published the results of a nationwide survey, *Americans View Their Mental Health*, which indicated that frustration at work was one of the chief precipitating factors in mental illness. This report identified male clerical workers and the wives of unskilled workers as among the most discontented working groups and noted, perhaps surprisingly, that many workers in less desirable jobs were either resigned to a lack of creativity or found emotional outlets elsewhere.[61] John Murray in *Feelings of Depression* does not seem to have any such outlet—his feelings of loneliness and inferiority lock him in a vicious circle, blocking activities that could relieve these pressures—whereas Adam Hathaway in *1104 Sutton Road* finds it difficult to identify the root cause of his unease, requiring the narrator to nudge him toward clearer awareness of his problems.

The section on work in *Americans View Their Mental Health* focuses on job satisfaction and difficulties in the workplace. The results suggest that self-worth is linked closely to the category and status of the job: for example, 42 percent of male professional workers expressed job satisfaction, compared to 13 percent of male unskilled workers. However, work-related problems were much higher among white-collar workers than in the other two categories, with lower-middle-class workers in clerical or sales jobs particularly likely to report such problems. The conclusion is that "white-collar categories are the only groups that are high in both dissatisfaction and the expression of problems . . . we might say that these white-collar categories maximize the frustration that derives from the nonfulfillment of high ego involvement and aspiration."[62] About 57 percent of clerical workers—10 percentage points higher than any other category—expressed a desire for another form of work. The dissatisfaction decreased with age: workers in the middle of the age range of twenty-one to thirty-four years suffered most in terms of dissatisfaction and work-related stress. Although *Feelings of Depression* does not dwell on the workplace, not only does John fit into this age range, but stories like his become a staple in many cinematic and literary representations of white-collar workers in the 1950s. In *Americans View Their Mental Health*, health in the workplace is equated to self-actualization, whereas feelings of maladjustment and inadequacy are closely linked to physical ailments such as insomnia, headaches, upset stomach, palpitations, and nervousness, as well as dependency on alcohol.

Such links between physical and psychological stress in the workplace were taken more and more seriously through the 1950s. In the second half of the decade, for example, *Archives of Industrial Health*, which focused primarily on work-related physical ailments, began to publish articles on stress and anxiety and on the role of the psychologist in the workplace, often from a management perspective. One such article, "The Measurement of Health" (1956), outlined three types of psychological examination that the employee is likely to undergo in an average firm: "prognostic," "present health," and "percentage" examinations (the latter helping to ascertain financial compensation for injury or disability).[63] Little mention is made of the manager's role in scrutinizing the firm's healthcare support, beyond the need to maintain periodic examinations to ensure that appropriate employees are recruited and that the workforce remains functionally fit.

During the 1950s, the Menninger Foundation also became very interested in work-related stress. Staff members of the foundation carried out an initial survey in 1954 and published a report in 1962 that drew on clinical experience and focused squarely on the individual rather than "the organization as an operating structure."[64] This report, titled *Men, Management, and Mental Health*, did not adopt an explicitly psychoanalytical approach, nor was it concerned with the psychological baggage that workers might bring to the workplace, where uncomfortable relationships with parents or siblings are likely to be projected onto dealings with managers and co-workers. The report's main aims were to establish the mental health implications of working for a large organization, but it also tried to counteract "the impersonalizing effects" of company mergers and growth and to encourage the manager "to examine his role and relationship of what he does to the mental health of his subordinates."[65]

The study focused on a large and diverse company, given the pseudonym of the Midland Utilities Company to ensure its workers' anonymity (the name reflects the famous studies that Robert Staughton Lynd and Helen Merrell Lynd conducted in the pseudonymous Middletown during the 1920s and 1930s). The firm had been established after World War I, had grown rapidly since 1945, and at the time of the study employed over two thousand people in various categories of work. It faced a potential change of direction due to the growth in its activity, with the middle managers detecting a widening gap between themselves and top managers, a "greater formalization of procedures," and less opportunity to offer the firm's customers personal service.[66] Within this milieu, the study hoped to assess to what extent a reasonable level of mental health was maintained—from factory floor workers up to middle managers. The investigators relied on a five-part definition of mental health: (1) treating others as individuals; (2) displaying flexibility under stress; (3) "obtaining gratification from a wide variety of sources"; (4) accepting personal skills and limitations; and (5) being both "active and productive."[67] This framework adapted Karl Menninger's notion of a psychological contract to explore the reciprocal relationships between managers and workers—which, the report noted, might be "affirmed, altered, or denied."[68] In the course of the interviews, particular concerns arose concerning various aspects of mental health, revolving around company relationships, interdependence, and changes of personnel and infrastructure.

The report argued that interdependence was vital in order to create a mutually supportive environment in which stress can be dealt with more easily. The investigators found counterexamples among female workers whose jobs were in similar categories: one group of workers extended their interdependence into their social lives, while the members of the other group displayed hostility toward their supervisor and a lack of support for each other. Whereas the first group received gratification from collegiality and recreation, the second group focused solely on their salaries—particularly workers whose personal relationships with their supervisor had broken down. The investigators detected a stronger sense of mental health among the first group, whereas anger, mistrust, and selfishness characterized the second. This was not wholly down to poor management, and the report did not seek to lay the blame entirely on supervisors and organizational structures that prohibited collegiality. But it recommended that the manager should be attentive to the psychological needs of his workers, anticipate conflict, and be constantly "aware of his own influence."[69] The study was also critical of increased automation, particularly when it affected the psychological contract between employer and employee. Younger workers seemed more willing to adapt to change, but the loss of established leaders left some workers feeling deserted or abandoned by familiar parental figures. The report emphasized the importance of flexibility to mental health, but it noted that workers are unlikely to sustain their motivation without support structures to enable them to develop in line with the company's priorities. Focusing throughout on the individual worker and his or her relationships, the report concluded with the assertion that if the goal of economic efficiency is promoted above human relations, then it not only jeopardizes mental health but is unlikely to lead to a flexible, sustainable, and interdependent environment.

Men, Management, and Mental Health was not the only such study in the 1950s. Psychoanalytical writings on the effects of work on mental health had begun earlier than the Menninger survey. For example, an article published in the Menninger Clinic's journal in 1951 compared the priorities of work and play. The author, Clarence Oberndorf— one of the first psychoanalysts in American private practice—compared the pleasure and gratification of play with the deferred satisfaction of work, which often is associated with "discomfort or deprivation."[70] Oberndorf noted that all workers hope that they will be rewarded "with something pleasurable," but "too much playfulness in the present" will lead to recklessness, while "too much concentration on work" leads to drudgery. He also noted that jobs in which the worker is directly involved in the end product carry libidinal satisfaction, whereas the role of an operative within a huge organization will often lead to daily drudgery. Not only is this lack of involvement likely to result in absenteeism or resignation, but it might well lead to psychopathological imbalance.

Countering this focus were other studies from the world of business that promoted the importance of a strong organization for the physical and psychological health of the worker. The well-organized workplace was often linked, at least tacitly, to a healthy mental attitude to working practice. One 1953 article, "Problems of Organization," written by Norbert Wiener, aligns a well-balanced workplace with the homeostasis of the individual: the worker is likely to malfunction or feel overloaded only if the environment induces inordinate stress. Unbalanced individuals, according to Wiener, need to be placed in "an environmental situation which is itself more or less automatically homeostatic and will tend to counter serious departures from equilibrium."[71] Other business advocates recognized the importance of worker participation for safeguarding equilibrium; an example is Alfred Marrow, president of the Harwood Manufacturing Corporation, which produced pajamas in its main plant in a small town in Virginia. Marrow recognized the value of a supportive union, incentive plans, and group involvement, all of which enabled workers to develop "genuine feelings of achievement, because they really help to form the company's decisions."[72]

Although balance and involvement suggest organic models of cohesion, *Men, Management, and Mental Health* implies that business practice in the 1950s was more often linked to mechanistic metaphors of automation. It was precisely this rhetoric of scientific management, information systems, and cybernetics that worried critics of business. Writing in the *Nation* in 1957, the Illinois sociologist Bernard Karsh linked automation to Taylorist notions of production flow, replacing "men's muscles," reducing "physical effort," and "eliminating human judgment in the administration or direction of the control of the machine." Karsh saw "business automation" as comparable to production-line industry, in which administrative and statistical decisions are made by machines outside the realm of human input. Although there is an element of science fiction here—reflected in the title, "Automation's Brave New World"— Karsh's analysis chimes with William Whyte's argument in *The Organization Man* that integrity for business is not measured in terms of the worker's skills or qualifications but what Karsh called the "organization and planning and the continuously smooth functioning of the operation," in which ever "greater value [is] placed on the operating unit as a whole."[73] In such an environment the individual is in danger of erasure, replaced by the operative or the unit of an organization. Even the American doctor was described, in 1967, as "an organization man—dependent upon society to provide the hospital for his workshop, dependent upon scientists and a whole host of specialists for assistance in the treatment of his patients, dependent upon an enormous and growing number of paramedical personnel for technical aid."[74] The high social status of doctors in the 1950s protected them against anonymity, but this description is not so dissimilar from Norman Mailer's apocalyptic warning to his fellow Americans in the Cold War, quoted at the end of the previous chapter, that they were in danger of becoming a cipher "in some vast statistical operation."[75]

Self-Help, Status, and Incorporation

Earlier in this chapter I suggested that self-help and business were compatible in the 1950s, but how exactly did discourses of self-reliance fit with the business orientation of Eisenhower administration and the twin emphasis of big business on management and technology? Although diversity, freedom, and the frontier of abundance (as Potter characterized it) were strong ideological weapons against communism, disenfranchised workers and those who had lost a stake in the social order could easily undermine organizational cohesion. This was a major reason why returning veterans were simultaneously honored and feared, particularly those with physical or psychological injuries. It was also a reason why so many articles appeared in the popular press in 1957–1958 on the topic of the erosion of masculinity, as traditional models of self-reliance were being replaced with conformity to the "gray flannel" model of white-collar work. The stereotype of the urban office worker making the daily commute from his northeastern suburb is one of the compelling abstractions of the mid-1950s, but these workers are often portrayed as uncomfortable participants, as if the autonomy that Riesman recommended had been sacrificed in favor of security. As Riesman noted, too much autonomy "threatens the whole shaky mode of adaptation" to postwar mass society.[76] The huge swing toward white-collar work in the late 1940s and the 1950s appears to confirm the prevalence of Riesman's other-directed character type, but that type sits uneasily next to such apostles of self-help as Norman Vincent Peale, who was one of the best-selling authors of the 1950s.

Peale is particularly important because he shifted from writing spiritual self-help books in the 1930s, which were aimed at raising the reader's morale during a time of economic hardship, to more assured books after the war that were geared to times of economic prosperity. The later works included *A Guide to Confident Living* (1948) and *The Power of Positive Thinking* (1952), probably his best-known work. According to Peale, fatigue, lassitude, nervousness, and lack of direction are debilitating conditions that can be overcome with the power of the mind and spirit. Echoing William James's recommendation early in the century that individuals should actively will themselves into a healthy life through the release of positive energies, Peale advocated a positive attitude to work and home that would nourish the spirit. His ideal American at

mid-century had an energetic but disciplined approach to life, but Peale tacitly promoted acquiescence toward the social and political status quo. To trust in God's will
offered comfort but also adherence to a metaphysical organizing structure that was
potentially at odds with self-reliance. In the words of Donald Meyer, Peale's philosophy induced "automatic behavior through the medium of an autohypnotized sub- or
unconscious," leaving the "superambient realm of authority" beyond reproach.[77] Not
only did a lack of specificity only thinly disguise Peale's right-wing leanings, but his
readers were not in a position to set rules or shape organizations: they had to work
within the structures presented to them from higher authorities in theology, business,
and government.

Peale introduces *The Power of Positive Thinking* as a book "written with deep concern for the pain, difficulty and struggle of human existence," teaching "the cultivation of the mind, not as an escape from life into protected quiescence, but as a power
center out of which comes driving energy for constructive personal and social living."[78] The force of his rhetoric lies behind the popularity of his self-help philosophy.
For example, the periodically amnesiac and depressed Will Barrett in Walker Percy's
1966 novel *The Last Gentleman* finds *A Guide to Confident Living* to be "a little volume of
maxims for businessmen" that makes him "feel good" with "its crisp and optimistic
suggestions" (see chapter 8).[79] However, it is never clear how the "inflow of power"
that Peale consistently promoted could drive "everything before it, casting out fear,
hate, sickness, weakness, moral defeat, scattering them as though they had never
touched you."[80] Despite his emphasis on "practical techniques" and a science of active
living "tested in the laboratory of spiritual existence," his success stories are wish-
fulfillment narratives rather than examples of hard-nosed realism.[81] In other words,
instead of focusing on medicinal remedies for lassitude or depression, Peale peddled a
"health formula" composed of "prayer, faith, and dynamic spiritual thinking."[82]

Meyer sees the 1954 *Guideposts* anthology *Faith Made Them Champions*—like
Guideposts itself, edited by Peale—as an example of the kind of genteel success story
toward which Peale was drawn. In many of the monthly issues of *Guideposts*, con-
tributors offered therapeutic homilies to help others with work anxieties, promoting
both individualism and fellowship among Peale's readers. Peale often drew on negative life choices, such as alcoholics in *The Power of Positive Thinking* who rehabilitated
themselves through strength of spirit, and in *The Tough-Minded Optimist* (1961) he recommended that his readers should live "without slavish dependence on pills" in favor
of "those basic resources of health and vitality which are to be found in right thinking
and the healing power of faith."[83] Illness for Peale vanishes when one adopts a positive
attitude to life, and in *Faith Made Them Champions* he reports that aggression, "dys-
pepsia, the taut nerves, the ulcer, the coronary and the angina" are eradicated in pursuit of noble goals.[84] This *Guideposts* publication includes extracts by the baseball star
Jackie Robinson and the decathlete Bob Mathias, who were forced to overcome racial
and medical hurdles (Robinson faced racial prejudice and Mathias battled anemia),
but these short sketches (or "daily devotions") provide examples of inner faith largely
uncomplicated by external factors. The absence of historical, social, and theological

detail characterized Peale's style of can-do Christianity, but it also left him open to attacks from the church for not defining what kind of God could inspire such activities. In *A Guide to Confident Living*, self-interest was easily reconcilable with belief in the supreme power of God, but divinity was an empty signifier to be filled with faith and trust in processes beyond human understanding.

At a time when other prominent theological writers such as Reinhold Niebuhr were emphasizing sin, the need for the nation to show international responsibility, and the historical ironies to which all nations are subject, Peale's books were comforting because they offered an insulated world of wish fulfillment. Deprivation, illness, war, and emotional conflict could hardly dent the supreme confidence that Peale hoped to inspire in his readers. On this score, George Stephenson, a Mississippi pastor, publicly criticized Peale for ignoring "hardships and tragedies," complaining that in *The Power of Positive Thinking* "these problems seem too easily solved, the success a bit too automatic and immediate, the answers a little too pat, and the underlying theology a shade too utilitarian."[85] This was followed by harsher criticism in 1954–1955, when Peale started to promote his ideas on radio and in popular newspaper and magazine columns; he was then criticized for ignoring the progressive role of the church and peddling middle-class homilies about betterment and success. In short, Peale's model of robust self-reliance could be interpreted as a chimera that disguised social acquiescence behind the sheen of individualism and an active lifestyle.

Although Peale's self-help narratives reconciled the needs of the individual to compliance in the workplace, it also left Riesman's other oriented personality type open to forms of manipulation that Peale did not even begin to address. For example, even though Peale was wary of pills, drug companies were targeting physicians to promote new performance-enhancing pharmaceuticals for exhausted workers. The use of narcotics to improve concentration and work performance go back to the 1920s, but physical efficiency tests carried out during World War II by one Missouri-based pharmaceutical company, Dios, suggested that Neurosine ("a combination of synergized bromides and therapeutic adjuvants") would increase work output by 21 percent.[86] Presented in scientific language, with no images except charts and tables, the Dios report measures work output in terms of horsepower per second, with the peak output achieved two hours after taking the medication. The therapeutic effects, so the report claims, are that Neurosine brings down the pulse rate of nervous individuals but does not affect the breathing rate. It can be used to treat hyperthyroidism, insomnia, epileptic convulsions, neuroses, menopause, and even alcoholism, suggesting that the drug is better than other barbiturates on the market because it increases physical efficiency while relieving nervous symptoms. No side effects are mentioned except for the warning that Neurosine should be avoided by those suffering from "impaired renal elimination." Based on the premise that unemployment can lead to "mental invalidism" and that "most nervous patients fare better when they keep on the job," the report recommended Neurosine to physicians working on the "home front" as an "important service in the all out fight against the Axis."[87] Neurosine was just one means of allaying work anxieties and bringing about a state of passivity in which tasks could be accomplished without distraction. Barely submerged tensions between activity and passivity run through Peale's writings and also find their way into industry reports that promoted loyalty and commitment to a firm while simultaneously constructing ideal types of occupational identity.

In her doctoral thesis on emasculation in the white-collar workplace, Erica Arthur considers the way in which reports such as the *Public Opinion Index for Industry* (1959) constructed "the inactive work of the white-collar employee through a language of heroic physicality," which simultaneously affirmed the worker's individuality (often overlooked or denied in blue-collar work) and reinforced the image of "a generic white-collar employee, largely detached from specific employment conditions."[88] The *Index* was particularly sensitive to the charges outlined by Riesman, Whyte, and Mills that the emphasis on human relations in business masked new forms of alienation, rebutting criticism of organizational management with a series of statements made by six hundred company presidents and managers. The *Index* also promoted a book written by the president of the DuPont Company, Crawford H. Greenewalt, *The Uncommon Man: The Individual in the Organization* (1959), which Greenewalt had developed from his McKinsey Foundation Lectures at Columbia University's Business School the previous year. Greenewalt provided a barbed reply to business skeptics such as Mills and Whyte by championing the "uncommon man" as a self-reliant, energetic, and imaginative high achiever. In this way, the book manages to reconcile individualism with the demands of organizations, cunningly cast in natural imagery: "the constellation rather than the star, the forest rather than the tree, the sea rather than the wave."[89] Rejecting the view of an organization as a "monster or automaton," Greenewalt links business structures with "the sovereignty of the market place," picturing companies as "living mechanisms made up of human beings," drawn from a "melting pot" of backgrounds with diverse talents, skills, and aspirations.[90] Arthur argues that through the power of his rhetoric ("the organization is nothing more than a slice of life") and ability to yoke mechanistic and organic imagery ("living mechanisms"), Greenewalt was able to make his version of "Jeffersonian individualism" transcend slavish conformity to company principles, and that "his contradictory affirmation melds degrees of conformity with just the requisite dose of individualism" required to ensure that the employee furthers the interests of the company.[91]

This view chimes with the tensions that Vance Packard explores in *The Status Seekers* (1959) between the myth of classlessness and the "significant hardening of the arteries of [the] social system" during the postwar years.[92] Packard detected that this "hardening" or "stratification" was particularly true in big corporations where "employees are usually expected to comport themselves in conformity with their rank," based on a military model of deference to superiors.[93] Applying the Taylorist principle of efficient flow to white-collar work, Packard saw that many workers could not understand how their roles fit into the larger process of the firm and found their activities "fragmentized and impersonalized," giving them no access to the decision makers—or "the power elite," as Mills called them in his 1956 book of that name.[94] Packard argued that white-collar work might provide a clean environment and offer financial rewards, but that office work in large corporations was developing along industrial lines and was arguably less skilled than manual work: "many white-collared office workers—billing clerks, key-punch operators—are actually machine attendants, manual workers in any honest nomenclature."[95] Given the rigid routine of many white-collar jobs and the expected conformity to company principles and dress codes, Packard observed that jostling for status was often carried out in leisure time. The divide was not between white collar and blue collar, but between the upper middle class and lower middle class, organized on a military model of officers and enlisted men, or what Packard calls "the diploma elite" with a college education and "the supporting classes."[96] The divide might never be breached, Packard argues, but the common lower middle-class fantasy of attaining the trappings and status of those with privileged educational backgrounds was often played out in the cultural sphere.

Although Peale argued that everyone can have a fulfilling and energetic lifestyle, the material realities of work suggested that this aspiration was often in the realm of fantasy rather than actuality. We will see in the next chapter how a high-school teacher in a significant mid-1950s film, *Bigger than Life*, acted out this kind of class fantasy, but this goal helps to explain why companies felt the need to inject the mythology of heroic individualism into otherwise mundane office environments. Pitted against the humdrum "man in the gray flannel suit" was the exceptional or "uncommon man" upheld by Greenewalt. This remasculinizing rhetoric is not so far from the emphasis on energy and achievement in Peale's spiritual self-help narratives, especially because, as Arthur detects, Greenewalt's arguments "are little more than defensive rhetorical strategies and *The Uncommon Man* is notable for the absence of any practical solutions to the problems it engages with."[97] Peale chose an apt title for *The Tough-Minded Optimist* (inspired by William James's distinction between the "tough-minded" and "tender-minded"), to encourage his readers to visualize themselves into a "strong mental pattern."[98] In contrast, Greenewalt's rhetoric of the tough uncommon man exposes what Arthur describes as the "concern over conformity in corporate employment."[99] The relationship between Peale and the business fantasy of *The Uncommon Man* is even closer when we note that US Steel spent $150,000 on subscriptions to Peale's *Guideposts* for its employees, and many other firms bought into his version of uncomplicated individualism, which could be easily reconciled with corporate enterprise.[100]

Peale presented himself as being at the service of the average aspiring middle-class citizen, but he was also "God's salesman" (to use the title of a 1993 study) in a benevolent and respectable guise.[101] Peale shared a tough-guy rhetoric with successful salesmen and businessmen (with whom he often spoke and socialized), and he found ways of dealing with hardship and illness on the same footing as entrepreneurialism did. In the words of the Peale scholar Carol George: "abundance was thus as much an aspect of the realizable wish as good health. The techniques Peale advocated for dealing with illness and pain—picturize, prayerize, actualize—were the same ones he applied to material rewards."[102] But Peale differed from Greenewalt in his supreme emphasis on self-reliance, whereas Greenewalt tried to reconcile the spirit of the marketplace and the "creative force unleashed by a free rein on individual effort."[103] Nonetheless, a public-relations attitude and the power of language to transcend the realities of working life characterize both Greenewalt's and Peale's work as mid-century versions of mind cures. Rather than ignoring the psychology of human relations, they sought to motivate readers and workers and simultaneously to advertise business through persuasive rhetoric. This is not quite the same brand of market-research "hidden persuaders" criticized by Packard in his 1957 book of that title. Instead, Greenewalt and Peale promoted a version of individualism that did not safeguard personal autonomy but rather upheld a version of laissez-faire capitalism, either to mask a life of white-collar drudgery or as an abstracted model of single-minded endeavor that furthers the needs of business. This view chimes with Whyte's argument that "no matter what name the process is called . . . the committee way simply can't be equated with the 'rugged' individualism that is supposed to be the business of business."[104] Although Peale seems to support a version of rugged individualism, his close links to business suggest that this is another form of incorporation in disguise. And although the realms of business and culture might seem worlds apart, by means of their rhetorical flourishes, imagery, and spin, "God's salesman" (Peale) and business evangelist (Greenewalt) entered the world of fiction.

White-Collar Fictions: Between Work and Home

A special issue of the *Nation* in 1957 "Automation's Brave New World," juxtaposes the lead article by the sociologist Bernard Karsh with a report on a business conference held at the Statler Hotel in Ithaca, New York, the previous week, at which twelve thousand "top organization men" had gathered to discuss the topic of "The Executive Pictured in Fiction."[105] The goal was to better understand fictional accounts of business, particularly negative representations, portrayed on television, such as Rod Serling's play *Patterns* (1955) and the television adaption of John Marquand's *Sincerely Willis Wade* (1956); and in fiction, from Cameron Hawley's novels *Executive Suite* (1952) and *Cash McCall* (1955) to Sloan Wilson's best-selling *The Man in the Gray Flannel Suit* (1955)—all three of which were made into Hollywood movies. These texts were part of a broader cultural moment that included the Gene Kelly musical *It's Always Fair Weather* (1955), which depicts a banking executive, Doug Hallerton (Dan Dailey), who ten years after his return from war has become an uptight, pill-swallowing gray-suited neurotic whose pending divorce and inability to see beyond his bourgeois lifestyle has made him lose touch with his former war buddies. The guest speaker at the 1957 Ithaca conference (via telephone) was Rod Serling, who was a year away from launching the popular CBS science-fiction serial *The Twilight Zone* but who had recently profited from the Kraft Television Theatre's live studio production of *Patterns*.

Written in 1954 and broadcast on NBC in January 1955, *Patterns* tells the story of a hard-nosed company boss, Walter Ramsey (Everett Sloane), who creates a series of tricky work situations for an older worker, Andy Sloane (Ed Begley). Sloane believes in human values, but he has developed a weak heart and a stomach ulcer through work pressures and is introduced as a "battered, dying, yet strangely resilient man."

Irritated by Sloane's old-fashioned attitude to business, Ramsey hires Fred Staples (Richard Kiley), an ambitious but naïve midwesterner, as a rival to Sloane. Distressed by the company's priorities and publicly criticized by Ramsey in front of the company board, Sloane dies suddenly from a heart attack. Staples is horrified by Ramsey's role in Sloane's death and he briefly becomes the story's voice of conscience, berating Ramsey for lacking compassion and threatening to leave the firm (he does so in an earlier draft).[106] But in the television play and the film version, Staples (played by Van Heflin in the film) is won over by Ramsey's doctrine of enterprise despite his scruples about Sloane's death (Sloane is renamed William Briggs in the film) and his pledge to remain the firm's conscience.[107]

The key to the success of the television production was that, despite his ruthlessness and manipulation, Ramsey cares about his company, its successes, and its employees. In his conference talk, Serling stated he did not write the play from a Marxist perspective, nor was he attacking big business per se. Rather, his intention was to write a tragic play to expose Ramsey's machinery of power and the overemphasis on efficiency that leads directly to Sloane's demise. Serling told the conference attendees that he wished to emphasize Greek tragedy and power over the specifics of business ethics, much as Arthur Miller's play *Death of a Salesman* did in 1949. Corporate America does not come off unscathed in *Patterns*, though: the opening credit

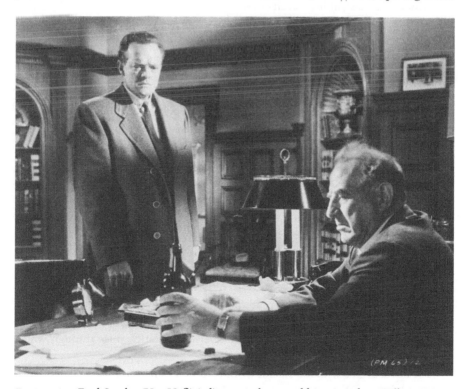

FIGURE 4.1   Fred Staples (Van Heflin) discovers that an older co-worker, William Briggs (Ed Begley), is close to a breakdown. *Patterns* (Fielder Cook, United Artists, 1956).

sequence of the United Artists film version visualizes the standardization of working life as a bank of monotonous office windows reminiscent of the alienating office imagery in King Vidor's film *The Crowd* (1928). In contrast, montages of deserted executive floors serve a similar, if less visually arresting, function in the television production of Patterns.

Also present at this conference was Ernst Pawel, a German émigré who had come to the United States in 1937 to escape Nazi persecution and whose 1957 novel *From the Dark Tower* caused greater consternation than Patterns among the business leaders. Criticized for oversimplifying the business world in his novel, Pawel replied that he saw dehumanization at the heart of the corporate enterprise. Referring directly to Whyte's *The Organization Man*, Pawel contrasted earlier heroic tycoons such as Rockefeller with the contemporary business leader: "The tycoon of today is almost anonymous—yet his power is enormous. There is a quality of inhumanity now. I believe that the basis and measure of everything is man—this used to be understood. Now it doesn't seem to be. . . . This feeling that is there seeps down even to the schools, to all of us, and it produces this quality of dehumanization—of blandness."[108] The *Nation* piece ends poetically, with an image of the Jewish émigré writer Pawel and Julius S. Glaser, president of the Glaser-Steers Corporation, sitting next to each other but each "alone with his private vision from the two dark towers" of literature and business, "so distant from each other."

As Pawel's comments suggest, *From the Dark Tower* takes a very bleak view of corporations, seeing them as "sound-proofed, air-conditioned beehive[s]" created along purely functional lines, in direct contrast to the manager's office in the dark tower, depicted as "a museum full of hand-carved antiques."[109] The novel tells the story of the Jewish American Abe Gogoff, who works for a life insurance firm in which most processes are automated (Pawel himself worked in public relations). In the Tower, decisions "are arrived at by committees—machinelike, impersonal, and therefore, infallible to the extent that no one is responsible for either failure or success . . . it takes the human element out of people. The human element is fallible and capricious; machines run much better without it."[110] Reflecting Ramsey's emphasis on machine-like processes in *Patterns*, the firm in *From the Dark Tower* is Kafkaesque in its totalizing organization, in which self-styled "underground men" like Abe must conform on the outside even if they continue to harbor their own thoughts.[111] This is in line with Whyte's optimistic view that individualism is possible in organizational life, either by developing countervailing attitudes to the company line or by scrambling the system by cheating on personality tests. Although there are dangers that outward conformity might swallow up inner radicalism, Abe gets by in a firm in which Jewish employees are rare. He also manages to retain his voice despite the "double talk" he encounters at work, emphasized in the first-person narrative voice through which Abe expresses unmediated opinions.[112]

The novel begins with the suicide of Bill Norden—an insurance executive, husband, and father—that reflects a trend in business fiction of the 1950s: the death of Andy Sloane in *Patterns* and of the CEO Avery Bullard in Cameron Hawley's management novel *Executive Suite* are both work-related, explicitly in the first case and implicitly in the second. The fact that Bill gasses himself in his car, cuts his wrists, and takes a bottle of pills suggests that he was very psychologically unstable, as if the excessive mode of death was an act of desperation rather than of release. Bill represents the link between home and work for Abe, while Miriam—Abe's wife—thinks of him as "the one man firmly rooted in two worlds—her own and that other, outside one, the world of business success and upper middle-class security."[113] The suicide casts a long shadow over the narrative, for it was Bill that encouraged Abe and Miriam to move to Long Island, turning the couple from "gypsies" into "suburbanites."[114] Bill's wife, Betty, is described as being shielded by "seven layers of ice," but her husband's suicide makes her needy and scared, and Miriam realizes that Betty wants something that the world of work seems to have forced out of her marital relationship.[115] A devotee of vitamin pills herself, Miriam had encouraged Bill to seek an analyst, whereas Abe sees in Bill's demise a weaker version of what he is trying to achieve: a successful partitioning of inner and outer worlds, "two separate lives at the same time." "It could be done," Abe muses, "given brains, courage, and cunning, it could be done. Bill had the brains and the courage, but there was in him no trace of cunning." Abe concludes that Bill had reached "the point of no return," from which he "was no longer able to extricate himself and drift back up into the light."[116]

Abe's attempt to lead a suburban life while retaining social awareness is depicted as courageous, pushing him to confront dissent, radicalism, and accusations of communism outside of work when he joins a neighborhood civil defense group. But given the choice later in the book between full incorporation into the firm or escape, Abe chooses the latter; by the end of *From the Dark Tower*, he has become a local newspaper editor in a remote town in the Rockies. The mountain view from his new home is "bleak at times and forbidding," but the rock is solid: "no one buried, no one trapped inside."[117] This existence differs from Potter's culture of abundance, reviving the memory of the nineteenth-century frontier before the West was closed. But the escape is incomplete for the Gogoffs. The mountain retreat is haunted by the image of an ever-expanding capitalist corporation that will someday "dwarf the mountain." The Tower has the potential to envelop even the mountain regions in time:

> Unless somebody does something about it. Unless everybody does something about it. Which is unlikely, considering the way people everywhere turn their backs on the mountain and look to the Tower for whatever it is they want to get out of life—a 5 per cent guaranteed mortgage, I suspect, and the happy assurance of a first-rate burial complete with scented, wormproof coffin.[118]

The mountainous West is more solid and authentic than the industrialized Northeast; the Gogoff family has a renewed sense of well-being and balance, and Abe starts writing again, "after ten years of apathy." But there is a question about whether the move is an act of good faith. Even though Abe thinks that the "poison" is "less virulent" in the West, the closing pages of the novel are haunted by the psychological baggage that travelers bring with them: "the same fears, frenzied values, and simple-minded faith in gadgets."[119]

Patterns and *From the Dark Tower* are two of the strongest cultural statements about the influence of postwar business on health and well-being, and they offer different outcomes: Staples sees the dangers of Ramsey's business philosophy but ultimately chooses incorporation, whereas Abe decides on autonomy and escapes to the West. More often than not, though, as discussed here and in the next chapter, a sense of unease or malaise runs through 1950s culture, connecting the spheres of home and work in ways that Abe tries to resist in Pawel's novel.

White-collar work was not new to fiction and film, but there was a noticeable peak in depictions in the mid-1950s linked to an interest in the sociology of suburbia. The rapid postwar rise of suburbs (twelve million Americans moved there between 1946 and 1958) made suburbia the typical habitat of the 1950s, with the suburbanite often standing for the average middle-class American. This mirrored an earlier trend in literary representations of white-collar work by stressing the normative patterns of suburban life, the "insistence on the ordinariness of such characters, whether to their credit or detriment, and on their subjection to habit and routine."[120] Although Riesman saw the emergence of the other-directed character type as closely linked to the rise of private property, he also saw the rigid organization of postwar suburbs (what he called a "massification of men") as leading not to more autonomy but as a direct extension of the white-collar workplace.[121] Levittown suburbs were a prime example of mass production, arising from the same logic of automatism as the companies for which many of suburbanites worked: an image captured in winter 1953 by a two-part feature in *Harper's* entitled "The Mass-Produced Suburbs."[122]

Despite, or because of, this conservative drift (Eisenhower was popular in the suburbs), the suburbanite was often treated with disdain, as Robert Wood observed in 1958—certainly by left-wing critics of business.[123] The gray-flannel-suited white-collar worker was often the husband and father of an identikit suburban family, satirized by John Keats in *The Crack in the Picture Window* (1956) as possessing the same "income, number of children, problems, habits, conversation, dress, possessions and perhaps even blood type" as his neighbors.[124] "John Drone," as Keats called him, lacked the self-reliance of his ancestors, was dependent on specialists for advice, and sets his sights on material security. The tendency to stereotype the "man in the gray flannel suit" was typical of the mid-1950s, particularly after the release of Sloan Wilson's novel and its film version, but in *The Organization Man* Whyte was careful not to homogenize suburban families; he saw "transient junior executives" living close by "mechanics, professors, lawyers, research scientists, travelling salesmen, [and] white-collar workers." Nevertheless, Whyte—like Wood—observed that friendship and neighborliness were often very thin; such propinquity is a "striking demonstration of how very deeply mass media and education have ironed out the regional and religious differences and prejudices that have separated people."[125]

Part of the problem is that Levittown was, as Whyte wrote in a 1953 *Fortune* article, a transient zone and "a second melting pot."[126] Such suburbs were linked closely to work through commuter-belt transportation systems, and, as Lynn Spigel notes, they became "terminals" for a "new traffic in media culture"—particularly television, but also advertising geared toward child rearing and consumerism.[127] Whereas Mills wrote in 1951 about the split between work and leisure, for Riesman, like Whyte, "the new assembled suburbs . . . are the consumption side of the managerial economy."[128] Suburbia often proved a trap for the likes of Sloan Wilson's protagonist, Tom Rath, who worries constantly about money and uses his ill-formed dreams of a wealthier, roomier, healthier life to fuel his erratic career choices. This bourgeois capitalist ethos meant that the spheres of work and home, although separated by a commute, were of a piece, and for more than one working man, the suburb represented "the big organization on his doorstep."[129]

The Man in the Gray Flannel Suit also dwells on the potential benefits of living a partitioned life, as Rath strives to divide the spheres of his life into manageable chunks, but during the course of the narrative these compartments clash with each other. Whereas Abe Gogoff is in his own way "an uncommon man" (to recall Greenewalt's phrase), Rath is an average type, emphasized by his clipped name (despite the muted emotion of his surname); the picture of him as "one of many men holding newspapers on their laps" during his commute from his Southport, Connecticut home; and his habit of thinking about himself as a series of statistics during a test that forms part of a job interview.[130]

Rath is not as suspicious of work as Abe is, nor does the novel seek to blame business for Rath's sense of unease as he tries to accommodate the desire of his wife, Betsy, to move to a bigger home and the need to earn more money by taking a risky position in a public-relations firm where, perhaps ironically, he is given the task of

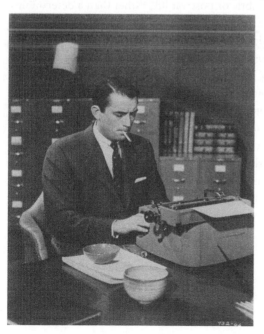

FIGURE 4.2   Tom Rath (Gregory Peck) struggles to tell his life story during a job interview. *The Man in the Gray Flannel Suit* (Nunnally Johnson, Twentieth Century–Fox, 1956).

promoting a mental health service. Whereas *Executive Suite* and *From the Dark Tower* open with actual deaths, *The Man in the Gray Flannel Suit* begins with a milder childhood illness, when the Raths' daughter contracts chicken pox. And whereas Pawel includes Cold War suspicions in *From the Dark Tower*, Rath is faced with unfinished business from World War II: he was a paratrooper in Italy and had an affair with an Italian woman who, unbeknown to him at the start of the narrative, has had his child. Themes of destruction (memories of the seventeen men he killed in Italy) and natality (the secret war baby) are interwoven through a novel in which work plays a significant role but does not overpower domestic stories, such as Tom and Betsy's relationship, the ghosts of Tom's parents, and traces of his wartime affair.

Work does not make Tom sick or lonely, but it does push him into an existence in which he must take risks to secure what he thinks is a living wage; and rather than a better income making him feel more secure, he is plagued by doubts and irritations. That said, Rath's new boss, Ralph Hopkins, adopts a paternalistic attitude toward him, and we see a human relationship taking primacy over the automated systems that dominate *From the Dark Tower* and lead to the demise of Andy Sloane in *Patterns*. In essence, though, Tom Rath's individualism is a limited and compromised one. He sees his life as a "vague unreality" (to recall a phrase from the 1950 *American Journal of Psychiatry* article), enticing him to dwell on fantasies rather than taking responsibility for his actions. The interlocking patterns of urban work and suburban life in *The Man in the Gray Flannel Suit* are hard to separate and too complex for us to identify a simple cause-and-effect sequence.

Born out of Wilson's experience as assistant director of the US National Citizens Commission for Public Schools, the novel offers an example of a more benign attitude toward business as part of the fabric of postwar life, rather than a determining factor in the health, well-being, and happiness of its employees and their families. In this way the novel suggests that domestic and working life can be reconciled, and that business in the 1950s was not just about a duped workforce suffering from new forms of alienation and monotony. Rath does not need to fight the organization, particularly as its president looks out for him, and he senses that things will work out, that democratic values will be upheld, and that the paternalistic structure has his best interests at heart. National politics are not given an explicit role in *The Man in the Gray Flannel Suit*, but, in this story set in 1955, Rath's boss, Ralph Hopkins, would have bought into Defense Secretary Charles Wilson's view that what is good for business is good for all Americans. And, just as business was struggling to come to terms with the health of its employees, so—as the next chapter discusses—domestic health was also in the spotlight in the 1950s.

In the Family Circle

THE SUBURBAN MEDICINE CABINET

In 1952 the Eisenhower-Nixon presidential ticket made the promise to "clean house," which was a well-chosen metaphor designed to exploit suspicions that the Truman administration contained hidden communists and other subversives. The two Republicans promoted themselves as family men, as evident in Richard Nixon's live television plea of September 1952 to spare the family dog, Checkers—a broadcast that served to deflect the charge that Nixon had received illegal gifts. The public had to wait eight years, until the 1960 Kennedy-Nixon presidential debate, to see what at the time was the defining moment of televised politics, but Dwight Eisenhower and Nixon were eager to use the mass media to project a homely image to complement Eisenhower's reputation as a heroic wartime general. Even Adlai Stevenson, the Democratic presidential candidate in 1952 and 1956, referred to what he called a "New America" of neighborliness in his second campaign, and the media was full of images of family harmony and "togetherness," to cite the tagline of an issue of McCall's.[1] Through popular TV shows such as The Adventures of Ozzie and Harriet, Leave It to Beaver, and Father Knows Best, the mass media affirmed the white middle-class family as the cornerstone of the Eisenhower years. Neo-Victorian values, the return to the domesticity for many wives and mothers, and the drive to raise children in the safety of the suburbs reinforced the ideology of the nuclear family.

Thus we switch focus in this chapter from work and business to the organization of the family home as the second pillar of a healthy nation in the mid-1950s. The normative ideology of the nuclear family did not arouse as much criticism as business practices—at least not until the early 1960s. As we will see in this chapter, though, the structures of suburban life prompted sociologists, psychologists, psychiatrists, writers, and filmmakers to ask far-reaching questions about family health and the place of medication and therapy in the American home. This discussion will enable me to explore cracks within the family circle in the next chapter.

The Medicalization of Family Life

Writing in the mid-1970s, the social theorist Christopher Lasch argued that marriage as a supreme symbol of a democratic nation reached a "crashing crescendo in the Age of Eisenhower."[2] Lasch was interested in exploring not just the basis of the orderly household, but also the ways in which family life was regulated during the Cold War. Lasch argued in Haven in a Heartless World (1977) that families were expected to aspire to an ideal of domestic order that could be achieved through a mixture of self-help and reliance on professional advice, expelling "the irregular, the unpredictable, the unmanageable" from the home.[3] Concern over the psychological damage to war veterans rarely encroached on this idealized model, with its strong and well-adjusted wage-earning husband and father, supported by a wife who could run an efficient household, tend to the nutritional needs of her husband and children, and provide emotional stability for each family member. A 1956 study of Crestwood Heights, a typical Canadian suburb (comparable to many postwar American suburbs), claimed that this idealized family life "bears much more resemblance to Christian ethics and to democratic practice than did the authoritarian pattern of those more traditionally religious families of Victorian days."[4] This view was supported by the 1950 Census, which revealed that 80 percent of American families fell into the nuclear category; only 10 percent were headed by a woman without a spouse, and unmarried adults living together were a small minority of households.[5]

An understanding of family health in the 1950s requires two contrasting perspectives. The first view focuses on medical advances and the development of vaccines that promised to rid American families of invasive diseases. Medical breakthroughs came thick and fast during the decade. For example, Jonas Salk's polio vaccine (developed in 1952 and released to the public three years later) promised to relieve parents of the fear that their children would suffer from a hitherto incurable disease; 1952 also saw the first pacemaker (replaced by a battery-powered pacemaker later in the decade); a year later a heart-lung machine was invented in Philadelphia; and the first successful kidney transplant took place in Boston in 1954. The rise of vaccines, antibiotics, antiseptics, and sanitary products were triumphs of 1950s medicine, leading the *Ladies' Home Journal* to proclaim that the twentieth century was the "Golden Age" of medical discovery. This faith in breakthrough developments was echoed in other popular magazines—such as *Redbook*, *McCall's*, and *Life*—with articles such as "Hormone Stops Disease" and "Polio Is Being Defeated," even though the text was not always as optimistic as the title.[6] Two decades later, the *Ladies' Home Journal* began its *Family Medical Guide* (1973) with the words: "The evolution of modern health care is an exciting story in itself; but even more exciting is the realization that today, for the first time in human history, continuing good health is an attainable goal for every American family."[7]

Challenging this triumphant narrative of the rise of modern medicine, the second view emphasizes the limits of medical knowledge and questions the effectiveness of healthcare. A major reason why President Truman tried to reform healthcare was that he believed the medical profession was failing the American people by prioritizing business and profits over medical responsibility. The limits of knowledge and ethical dilemmas periodically came to the fore in postwar medicine, revealing a more troubled decade for healthcare than is often documented. This was particularly the case from the late 1950s onward when, as Bert Hansen argues, "cracks of hesitation and skepticism" arose in the heroic narrative of medical advancement.[8] The rise in medical prescriptions in the 1950s does not confirm a healthy period but suggests an anxious or "tranquillized" decade (to use the poet Robert Lowell's phrase), in which a variety of alleviating substances were to be found in the middle-class medicine cabinet.[9] Alongside tonics, aspirin, laxatives, emetics, astringents, antiseptics, bandages, and a thermometer (all found in the typical New York home in 1936), the 1947 medicine cabinet was likely to contain sedatives and some form of barbiturate, which were replaced by the popular tranquilizer Miltown in 1955.[10] So widespread was the craze for tranquilizers in the mid-1950s that the Iowan humorist Harlan Miller satirized the reliance on pharmaceuticals in his regular column for *Ladies' Home Journal*:

> Our medicine cabinet seems to contain liquids, pills & capsules for almost every ailment & orifice of the human body. Here are two kinds of thermometers, & there are powders to be applied "as needed," & here are suppositories apparently intended to relieve a child's blockade. Here's a red liquid that smells awfully good. You could probably serve it as an after-dinner liquor. . . . In moments of scepticism or resignation I've thought that almost any mild ailment or distemper might be assuaged by reaching into the medicine cabinet, picking almost any non-poisonous bottle or box of pills at random, & swallowing a modest portion. But this method is not for those of little faith.[11]

Although Miller was fascinated by household medications, he recommended that each bottle should be carefully labeled: "Don't imagine I'm pretending I know anything about the pills & fluids even in my own medicine cabinet much less yours."[12] The Crestwood Heights study reinforces this view, asserting that "much zealous trust is place in the contents of the medicine cabinet."[13]

The public often received mixed messages. Self-help books stressed the importance of perseverance and faith (usually in business and religion), while popular columns and advertisements touted therapeutic techniques, medicinal remedies, and indispensable consumer products. By the end of the decade, three-quarters of doctors were prescribing Miltown on a regular basis, convinced by advertisements such as one released in 1950 by Wallace Laboratories, which claimed that 70–95 percent of nervous patients "recovered or improved" after taking Miltown, making it easier "to lead a normal family life and to carry on their usual work."[14] Miltown became a national craze. As Andrea Tone notes in *The Age of Anxiety* (2009), in 1956 one could buy diamond-encrusted pill boxes from Tiffany's; drink Miltown cocktails in Los Angeles; and laugh at Miltown jokes delivered by Bob Hope, Milton Berle, and Red Skelton; while the regular use of uppers (amphetamines) and downers (barbiturates) later featured in Jacqueline Susann's best-selling *Valley of the Dolls* (1966), in which prescription drug addiction blights the lives of three talented postwar women.[15] Populist self-help advocates such as Norman Vincent Peale continued to emphasize self-reliance and warned against prescription drugs, but the vogue for tranquilizers in the mid-1950s can be interpreted as a conservative response to postwar anxiety, smoothing over "fissures that, left unattended, threatened to widen into more serious chasms."[16]

Whether or not one lived the celebrity lifestyle of Norman Mailer, Tennessee Williams, or Lauren Bacall—all of whom took Miltown in the mid-1950s (along with many others, such as the screenwriter Rod Serling)—medicalization crept into home life, from hygiene and housekeeping to sleeping habits and sexual behavior. But little was known initially about the addictive properties of Miltown, leading to a growing unease that drug treatments for everything from heart disease to schizophrenia had not been thoroughly tested for side effects. Miracle cures and overenthusiastic medical claims were questioned as early as 1946 in a *Collier's* article, "The Case of the Missing Miracle," which detailed "a host of diseases and reactions we know absolutely nothing about" and claimed that "the successful sulfas, penicillins and streptomycins represent no more than a very limited beachhead in man's war against bacteria."[17] Caricatures of mothers "thinking they were protecting their children from disease" but actually serving "penicillin tablets, scattered like alphabet noodles or witch-doctor potions in their soup" implied that for every optimistic medical breakthrough there was in fact much that was still unknown.[18]

It is quite easy to polarize these perspectives: that robust social structures and technology were bedrocks of Cold War stability, or that pharmaceutical companies were out to hoodwink families with the promise of miracle cures. Useful correctives to this second view have been published, such as Dennis Worthen's *Pharmacy in World War II* (2004), but many critics from the mid-1960s onward viewed the drug companies as a key component of a corporate nation, with products trickling down to local drugstores and profits going straight back to big companies, a situation explored by the psychiatrist David Healy in a number of books, including *The Antidepressant Era* (1999) and *Pharmageddon* (2012).[19] A close examination of postwar domestic healthcare actually reveals a variegated picture, as quack salesmen offering tonics and cures jostled with warnings from the Food and Drug Administration (FDA) about the boundaries of legitimate medicine. Such an examination also highlights complex gender interactions within the home over medical knowledge, internal tensions within family units, and fissures between potentially incompatible ideals of self-reliance and togetherness. Combining the two perspectives helps us to move the discussion from the oscillation between reintegration and fragmentation discussed in part 1 of this book toward the view of organization and anxiety as the psychosocial poles of postwar American life. These poles are neatly summed up in *The Family: Its Function and Destiny* (1949), which brought together essays by Talcott Parsons, E. Franklin Frazier, Ruth Benedict, Erich Fromm, and Max Horkheimer. The volume's editor, Ruth Nanda Anshen, asserts that "human thoughts and human knowledge have never before been so abundant, so kaleidoscopic, so vast, and yet, at the same time, never so diffused, so inchoate, so directionless."[20]

It thus becomes clear that Eisenhower and Nixon's 1952 campaign slogan "let's clean house" and the candidates' emphasis on the stability of the nuclear family hid a plethora of social and ideological tensions. The intimacy of home life often permitted what Parsons called "a kind of freedom for the development of personal feelings and attachments" that was rare in public life.[21] But the 1950s family revealed the paradoxical forces of threat and stability that marked Cold War culture, leading Anshen to reflect on how "the moral ambivalence of our society has penetrated . . . the family and the home. The failure of society is reflected in the failure of parenthood, for it is within the family that the seeds of anxiety, fear and delinquency are sown."[22] Just as the concept of the sealed domestic sphere is embedded in the phrase "nuclear family," so the Cold War subtext of "nuclear" reveals a troubling ambivalence about the American home. The nuclear family was often seen as an ideal, but the term also meant that "home, since the advent of hydrogen bombs, ha[d] lost its older meaning as a place of refuge."[23] This ambivalence reflected the status of medical, psychiatric, and psychological research: medicine sometimes bolstered the nuclear family and at other times underlined its frailty.

Challenging the received wisdom that located pathology within the individual (the disease model), a growing postwar trend in the social sciences focused on family relationships (the environmental model), noting that pathology is likely to arise if the unit is destabilized. This led the psychologists Nathan Ackerman and Theodora Abel (along with the psychiatrist Murray Bowen) to pioneer family therapy as a flexible method for tackling familial problems. Their work was facilitated through the Ackerman Institute for Family Therapy, established in New York City in 1960 after the publication of Ackerman's *The Psychodynamics of Family Life* (1958). Deborah Weinstein notes that "instead of invoking a linear model of cause and effect to explain why some children developed schizophrenia or became juvenile delinquents . . . family therapists proposed to study the family as a dynamic system with interacting components, an underlying structure, cyclical patterns, and the capacity to self-regulate through feedback mechanisms."[24] After 1951, under the aegis of the Group for the Advancement of Psychiatry's Committee on the Family (a branch of the American Psychiatric Association), studies of families became fairly common, based on the belief that family health can be understood only through broad study of complex patterns of value and practice. We will see in chapter 6 that this emphasis on intrapersonal systems was an important shift in therapeutic practice in the 1960s, but it placed a weighty responsibility on parents—particularly mothers—to raise their children correctly.

Margaret Mead commented at the end of the 1940s that, although there were strong pressures to regularize family life, she glimpsed within each American home a "different picture."[25] These pressures were acute in the mid-1950s, reinforced through the mass media and advertising as well as by serious medical, psychological, and sociological studies. However, that should not lead us to overlook the home as a place in which these normalizing trends could be remolded or resisted. In order to explore differing conceptions of postwar family health, this chapter focuses on medical writing that circulated in the professional and popular spheres in the mid-1950s, in addition to representations of domestic medicine in educational films, child-care manuals, advice columns, film melodrama (Nicholas Ray's *Bigger Than Life*), domestic poetry (Robert Lowell and Phyllis McGinley), and suburban satire (Richard Yates's *Revolutionary Road*). It considers the promises of domestic healthcare, better nutrition, and domestic stability that were tempered by the expectations of, and strains within, family units. In particular, the chapter discusses the pressures on parents—especially mothers—and the growth of pediatrics and child psychology, in which Erik Erikson's developmental psychology and Benjamin Spock's advice to parents need to be juxtaposed with the Freudian currents running through popular culture and the different roles that dietary advice, pharmaceuticals, and surgery played in family life.

Family Health and Nationhood

The term "nuclear family" was used commonly by sociologists after 1947. The Yale anthropologist G. P. Murdock, for example, described the nuclear family as a "universal human social grouping" that "exists as a distinct and strongly functional group in every known society."[26] Such continuity was important during Eisenhower's two terms in the White House, as he and his policymakers sought to stabilize social structures in the face of communist threats. But earlier sociological studies, such as the two editions of Robert Staughton Lynd and Helen Merrell Lynd's *Middletown* (1929, 1937), show that the nuclear family had deeper demographic roots. For example, the Lynds noted that in the mid-1920s, 86 percent of the families in a regular town like Muncie, Indiana (the real "Middletown" that they wrote about), owned their own homes.[27] Perhaps, then, little had changed between the 1920s and 1950s. However, the connection made between nuclear weaponry and the tight-knit family was no accident, particularly as Eisenhower's administration saw the stable nuclear family as a line of ideological defense.

That was one reason why Eisenhower emphasized healthcare, with a particular focus on family health. In his 1953 plan to reorganize the federal government, he established the Department of Health, Education, and Welfare (HEW) to oversee further research into cancer, heart disease, diabetes, and polio; aiding the construction of more hospitals; promoting good sanitation; and ensuring the more equitable provision of healthcare—all measures that Truman had supported in the mid- to late 1940s. Fearing that the country was not properly caring for its veterans, Eisenhower was serious about improving provision for disabled Americans, especially troops badly wounded in World War II and the Korean War. But the creation of HEW was more a symbolic moment than a historic turn in US health reform; it was not until after 1958, for example, that health issues among the elderly were seriously addressed.

Arguably healthcare was not as high a priority as it should have been during Eisenhower's first two years in office, but the establishment of HEW was the fruition of his promise to clean the national house.[28] He quickly realized, as Harold Diehl put it, that "good health is essential for the national welfare and even national existence."[29] Soon after the republication of Diehl's 1942 War Department manual *Elements of Healthful Living*, Eisenhower delivered a speech on the "Health of the American People" to the House of Representatives in January 1954, stating: "Only as our citizens enjoy good physical and mental health can they win for themselves the satisfaction of a fully productive, useful life. . . . The health of our people is the very essence of our vitality, our strength, and our progress as a nation."[30] The president touched many bases in his speech: the need to develop better insurance plans, public health programs (including the proposal to improve health conditions among American Indian populations), mental health, the role of the World Health Organization, and problems of pollution. The following year, 1955, was a particularly important year for health reform. Congress passed the Mental Health Study Act with the goal of reevaluating "the human and economic problems of mental health," and the Joint Commission on Mental Illness and Health was formed. The commission's report, *Action for Mental Health*, pressed for reform, but it was not published until 1961.[31] And not until the 1960 presidential campaign did medical care appear high on the political agenda, a topic that the third part of this book examines in relation to reformist impulses and social obstacles, such as those faced by Oveta Culp Hobby (the first secretary of HEW, who legalized and set up distribution of Salk's polio vaccine) in the wake of the historic *Brown v. Board of Education* ruling.

However one assesses Eisenhower's record on health reform, it is clear that HEW was the president's attempt to ensure stability by means of better health and education provision. However, HEW only partially addressed concerns about the contemporary changes in family life. For example, many writers in the late 1940s worried that the typical family was shrinking in size, due to the shift toward metropolitan patterns of living and the choices women were making between motherhood and careers. In 1960 the cartoonist Herblock used "split-level" imagery to satirize the increasing divide between a wealthy businessman relaxing at home and a poor family huddled around a kitchen table, with only meager welfare offerings from HEW for comfort. More optimistically, the popular publications *Redbook* and *American Magazine* promoted stable family life in the emerging suburbs, as well as the "logical division of labor" between married partners, as Vance Packard and Clifford Adams termed it in 1946 (although Packard later revised his stereotypical view of working women), with the husband's workplace responsibility balanced by the wife's roles as homemaker and mother.[32] The suburbs could offer relief from urban congestion, affordable housing for veterans, and a safe environment in which to raise children, but the reality of suburban life was not as cozy as mass-market magazines would have it.

In fact, some popular publications in the late 1940s suggested that the family was in a precarious position. *Life* magazine, for example, published a feature article titled "The American Family in Trouble," based on the Harvard sociologist Carle Zimmerman's study *Family and Civilization* (1947). The article bemoaned the urbanization of American families because it promoted competitive individualism above team spirit: "The individual now looks outside his home for his interests. He is atomistic, an individualized fragment rather than part of a unified whole."[33] In upholding the view of Henry Luce, editor of *Life*, that the family should be an ideal model of harmony, the article is streaked with realism. It is particularly scathing about consumerist elements of the mass media and the irresponsible emphasis on romantic love that encourages impulsive choices.[34] Although the article does not directly address medical issues, it claims that, when families lose their self-sufficiency, interventions by welfare aides, counselors, and social workers are unlikely to bridge the cracks. This sense of despair was developed in the revised edition of *The Family: Its Function and Destiny*, which pictures the late 1950s family as having lost its "living center" and becoming a "heterogeneous mass of isolated pieces of reality."[35]

Celebrations of family life punctuated these concerns, including "How America Lives," a long-running study of the mid-century family in the *Ladies' Home Journal* that began in 1940. Although it was not as rigorous as the Lynds' Middletown project,

Split-Level Living

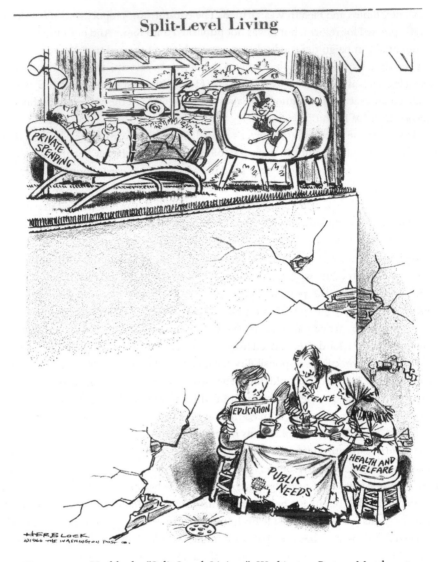

FIGURE 5.1   Herblock, "Split-Level Living," *Washington Post*, 9 March 1960.
© The Herb Block Foundation.

"How America Lives" charted diverse family patterns across regions, classes, population densities, costs of living, and family sizes. Using statistics from the Department of Commerce and National Resources Board, the magazine picked families "by formula" to study "the factors that combine to create a typical family within a given income, occupation and population bracket."[36] The *Ladies' Home Journal* focused on how the middle class (its primary readership) spent its income, but "How America Lives" also included some poor families living on welfare and a struggling black sharecropper family in Mississippi. Designed to affirm the typical family's resilience during the Great Depression and to embrace democracy in contrast to the rise of extremism in Central Europe, "How America Lives" provoked a stream of readers' letters that identified omissions in the families profiled. Other letter writers sensed a demeaning attitude to the Mississippi family ("How America Lives" mirrored *Middletown* in its marginalization of African American family life). The *Ladies' Home Journal* published a summary of readers' criticisms, but such negative comments did not detract from the picture of prosperous families or the conclusion that mothers "are really interested in providing the best possible health for their families, and do the best they can with what they have."[37]

Perhaps the most high-profile celebration of the family was *The Family of Man* exhibition, held at the Museum of Modern Art in 1955. Instead of simply focusing on the American nuclear family, the exhibition used over five hundred photographs (many by amateurs) from sixty-eight countries to portray the diverse forms and trajectories of family life. The photographs focus on a variety of kinship structures, rather than upholding an ideal family type as a building block for Western capitalism. Although the curator, Edward Steichen, argued that photography should operate at a distance from any particular "philosophy or ideology or system of aesthetics," *The Family of Man* can be read as an anticommunist exhibition, pitting diversity, freedom, and creativity against dogma. However, it is also a collective visual text that celebrates the longevity of the human family in the face of nuclear threats.[38] Images were grouped into categories that provided glimpses of birth, childhood, work, family, old age, death, with further images of children toward the end of the exhibition. Representations of illness are largely absent, with grief and loss depicted in a sequence covering the Great Depression, poverty in Asia, and a pair of haunting images from the Korean War. In the first, a distraught soldier from the US Signal Corps is tenderly comforted by another soldier; the second (from *Life*) portrays a group of female Korean prisoners of war confined behind barbed wire, their faces revealing a troubling mixture of bewilderment, anxiety, and rage.[39]

Just as the family becomes a generalized abstraction of togetherness in the exhibition, so illness is divorced from particular symptoms and conditions. The clearest depictions of family life are a series of images of nuclear and extended families from Italy, Japan, Botswana (then a British protectorate), and the United States, confirming that the existence of the family unit—connected by heredity, kinship, and emotional ties across three or four generations—bridges developed and primitive societies.[40] The images draw visual parallels between stages of the life cycle and differing cultural experiences, focusing particularly on birth and parenthood. They are accompanied by a range of humanist quotations from Shakespeare to Jefferson, and from Pueblo Indian philosophy to the United Nations Charter. However, perhaps because the exhibition included a number of images from *Life*, this central focus might be read as a form of subconscious cultural imperialism, or what Eric Sandeen terms "the projection of American values onto a newly subjugated world."[41] This imperialist interpretation is not wholly convincing, but Sandeen's reading does help to frame the exhibition within the Cold War emphasis on generalized and abstract notions of experience, sanctifying the family and speaking "earnestly to the middle class" as "representative citizens."[42]

This leaning toward abstraction was sometimes framed in terms of Cold War polarities—"the democratic mind" versus "the communist mind"—but it was also inscribed in the methodologies of the blossoming social sciences. Not all researchers followed this trend (as we will see in the next chapter), but the drive to identify a national character from statistics was common in the 1950s. One example is the Kelly Longitudinal Study of 1955, in which three hundred New England couples (all white, middle class, and Protestant) were questioned about family life, careers, marriages, and children. The historian Elaine Tyler May uses the Kelly Longitudinal Study in her book *Homeward Bound* (1988) as a snapshot of 1950s domesticity, in which "sexual containment" and "reproductive consensus" prevailed during the baby boom.[43] The findings of the study prompted the Commonwealth Fund to sponsor Earl Koos of Florida State University to examine the health of an average-size stable community in New York State, a "small-town America in microcosm."[44] Entitled *The Health of Regionville* (1954), Koos used more varied data than the Kelly Longitudinal Study and is therefore helpful for assessing the place of postwar medicine in family and community life. The town that Koos called Regionville contained one hospital and was home to five doctors, five dentists, a nurse, and a chiropractor, but its citizens had access to additional facilities in the region—including six other hospitals (each with 800 beds), fourteen doctors (each treating 1,200 patients), and other personnel including osteopaths, optometrists, and podiatrists. The project does not offer an anthropological study of Regionville, but it tracks how the town's residents reacted "to illness and to measures for maintaining health."[45]

Koos divided the 514 families that he studied into three broad classes, based on income and housing. Class I covered 10 percent of the sample (51 families) and was largely made up of nuclear families that included children and a white-collar father who owned a house and car and had reasonable savings. Class II constituted 65 percent (335 families) and included blue-collar and unskilled workers who earned wages (rather than salaries) and had modest houses, 70 percent of which were mortgaged, with only small savings. Class III (128 households) represented the final 25 percent, families in which fathers were often unemployed and that lived in rented accommodations, had second-hand cars in some cases, and rarely had any savings. Koos's interviews covered each of these family types, focusing on those who were likely to visit a doctor for a variety of symptoms, from loss of appetite and headaches to passing blood in their stools or finding a lump in their chest or breast. In most cases, members of class I were more likely to seek a doctor's advice, particularly when someone had severe symptoms, than members of class III. For example, in cases of excessive vaginal bleeding, 92 percent of class I, 83 percent of class II, and 54 percent of class III would seek medical attention. The figures in cases of finding an abdominal lump were 92 percent of class I, 65 percent of class II, and 34 percent of class III.[46] In summary, Koos found that class III respondents showed "a marked indifference to most symptoms."[47] He suggested a number of explanations: "the threshold over which one stepped in becoming 'ill' was a highly variable one"; the cost of treatment weighed heavier on class III members; and the "sense of urgency" varied for different family members, with working-age men in all three groups less likely to seek medical attention.[48]

Members of class I typically outstripped those of classes II and III in their use of medical facilities and knowledge of healthcare. Koos concluded that, despite the typicality of Regionville, each class had "its own symbols, customs, traditions, ideals, and aspirations, and its own behavior patterns" closely linked to financial and class status but also informed by education and the values of the whole community.[49] Avoiding a focus on the extremes—"the haves" (class I) and "the have nots" (class III), Koos spares a thought for those in class II who possess

> some of the knowledge, some of the aspirations, and much of the intent found in Class I, and little of the disregard shared in Class III. But having the watered-down perceptions of Class I without also having that group's ability to act upon them is of little help. , , , Class II families are confronted, then, with the important problem of how to meet needs which they recognize but which the total social environment fails to supply help in meeting.[50]

Without creating a moral category for class II or trivializing the position of class III, Koos touched on an important blind spot in the drive to generalize about the postwar middle-class experience that often left the lower middle class unrepresented or not clearly depicted.

Women and the Healthy Home

The ideal of the postwar family was enshrined by Vice President Nixon's emphasis on domesticity in what became known as his kitchen debate in Moscow in 1959 with Soviet Premier Nikita Khrushchev. As this high-profile event suggests, marriage and parenthood were commonly linked to responsible Cold War citizenship and family togetherness, reinforced via a range of media, from advertising and statistical surveys to the popular press and television sitcoms that promoted wholesome suburban lifestyles and neighborliness.[51] Suburban life compared favorably with urban living in the 1950s: suburbanites could enjoy longer lives with fewer infections, lower infant and maternal mortality rates, and less chronic disability. Mothers needed to be good managers of domestic hygiene, though, keeping their homes clean and sanitary. The 1956 Crestwood Heights study claimed that hygiene was not "won by casual conformity to health rules, but by meticulous, costly, and constant vigilance."[52] Mirroring the results of the Regionville study, relatively high income levels for suburban families meant that precautionary or preventive visits to the doctor, dentist, pediatrician, and gynecologist were frequent and "crisis hospitalization" rare.[53]

However, all was not well in suburbia, particularly for the supposedly "happy housewife," an idealized construction that was disparaged from 1963 onward by Betty Friedan and other feminists. A decade earlier, in a December 1949 article for *Harper's*, the popular poet Phyllis McGinley defended the suburbs from accusations that they mold a "stock character" that leads a life of "smug and prosperous medi-ocrity."[54] Instead, McGinley identifies in a New York commuter suburb, which she calls Spruce Manor (not dissimilar from her own Westchester County suburb, Larch-mont), a diverse community whose members have in common only the commitment to "pay off the mortgage and send healthy children to good colleges." Spruce Manor might be "architecturally insignificant," but, for McGinley, it is a "pretty town," full of life and vitality and containing "invigorating and stimulating" lifestyles.[55] Although McGinley was aware of the sometimes repetitive nature of suburban life, she did not think it monotonous or mediocre, delighting in its small joys, and ending with the Whitmanesque exclamation of her title: "Suburbia: Of Thee I Sing."

The literary critic Jo Gill reads McGinley's essay and her poems "Spring Comes to the Suburbs" (1947) and "June in the Suburbs" (1953) as celebrations of domesticity, but in other poems by McGinley, such as "A Malediction" and "Executive's Wife," the home becomes "a space in which all sorts of new conflicts and pressures come to a head"—for example, latent aggression or "competitive consumption and display."[56] Despite McGinley's affirmation of suburban life (it should be noted that Larchmont had developed in the early twentieth century, unlike the postwar Levittown sub-urbs), for other female poets such as Anne Sexton and Sylvia Plath (as well as Betty Friedan, who criticized McGinley for being soft on suburbia), the attractions of the home were often deceptive. Gill notes that, although the arrangement of the kitchen and living room revolved around women's expectations, the suburban home was a "profoundly ambivalent space" for many wives and mothers.[57] As such, the private home was rarely a refuge, connecting closely with "reproductive morality" and strict codes of propriety. Arlene Skolnick proposes that this return to "the Victorian cult of domesticity with its polarized sex roles and almost religious reverence for home and hearth" marked the mid-century as a period of amnesia on gender politics, with only 24 percent of mothers with children under the age of eighteen remaining in the workforce.[58] Skolnick argues that, given Cold War uncertainties, it was not the return to Victorian values that was surprising but its "exaggerated form," which enforced the kinds of limited domesticity criticized by filmmakers and writers ranging from Douglas Sirk to Sylvia Plath.[59]

Specific reasons for this can be located in four texts published in the 1940s that examined the relationship between psychological structures and gender roles. The first of these is Philip Wylie's *A Generation of Vipers* (1942), selected in 1950 by the American Library Association as one of the major works of nonfiction of the first half of the twentieth century, and reissued in paperback in 1955. Wylie's book blamed overbearing mothers for raising spoiled sons who were unlikely to ever break out of the family circle or express their autonomy. What came to be called momism was a possible cause of a number of unexplained neuropsychological cases arising in World War II. This view was legitimized in 1946 by the psychiatrist Edward Strecker's report *Their Mother's Sons*, which pointed to maternal overprotection—what Rebecca Jo Plant calls "pathological mothering"—as the root cause of immaturity among recruits.[60] Two years after the publication of Wylie's book, the Austrian psychoanalyst

Helene Deutsch (at that point in her early sixties and living in Boston) published the first volume of *The Psychology of Women*. Deutsch drew heavily on biology and anatomy to argue that women, particularly mothers, should be content with a passive and submissive role. She argued that penis envy in young girls is transformed later into "inward activity" and the desire to have babies, thus providing a normative account of the woman's role.[61] This view was supported by the sociologist Ferdinand Lundberg and the psychiatrist Marynia Farnham in *Modern Woman: The Lost Sex* (1947). Lundberg and Farnham were skeptical that women could maintain control in professional work or as the head of the domestic household; women's desire to work, in the authors' view, was part of an institutionalized "masculinity complex" that had given rise to a generation of neglected children—in contrast to Wylie's view of overbearing mothers smothering their offspring.[62]

Modern Woman was an influential text, as shown by the character of Liza Elliott (Ginger Rogers) in the film version of the Broadway musical *Lady in the Dark*. Elliott is a modern professional woman (a "synthetic Woman of Fashion," as Lundberg and Farnham called her), but she is reliant on psychoanalysis and reveals a "bundle of anxieties" in which competitiveness is entangled with a deep rooted father complex.[63] *Fight against Fears*, the 1951 book by the *New York Times* reporter Lucy Freeman about her encounter with psychoanalysis, provided further evidence that successful professional women were suffering from depression, anxiety, and somatic maladies (dizziness, acne, and sinusitis in Freeman's case) that had a psychological root cause.[64] Alongside such symptomatic accounts, Plant argues that domestic expectations were linked to the responsibility of women to "restore the mental health of American men by nurturing more" (the charge of momism was usually leveled at overbearing middle-age mothers, thereby safeguarding the nurturing role for young wives).[65] Wendy Kline, in her study *Building a Better Race* (2001), considers the many pressures that women faced: from wartime propaganda intent on replenishing lost lives, the desire for normalcy after the war, anxiety brought on by the Cold War, and the rise of postwar bureaucracy. Although it seems tempting to choose the 1950s as the century's most typical decade for family life, it was unique in the strength of its "pronatalist culture" and the emphasis in placed on the caring roles of housewife, mother, and helper.[66]

Despite *Life*'s celebration of the achievements of American women in its December 1956 issue, it is easy to paint a bleak picture, stereotyping 1950s women as hapless victims of advertisements that promoted the small joys of suburban lifestyles. The mid-century psychoanalytic interest in the archetypes and myths of womanhood might be seen as important for tracing recurring patterns of the "pure woman" and the "good and bad mother," but the frustrations and anxieties of domestic life were largely ignored until later in the decade, except in diluted form in consumer magazines and the odd advice manual such as *Health and Hygiene for the Modern Woman* (1957).[67] The decade's major sociological studies—*The Organization Man*, *The Lonely Crowd*, and *White Collar*—were largely silent on issues of gender, except for glimpses of the female consumer and the manipulative wife who settles for "small tactical gains" in the home.[68]

In reality, new domestic technologies and time-saving devices in the kitchen promised to release women from housework but often left them isolated and listless. The limitations of domesticity have since led feminist critics to disparage 1950s films and television shows for idealizing the home and offering "easy, optimistic conclusions" about any problems that the suburban mother and her family faced.[69] Media images of the perfect housewife and the Hollywood sex kitten pushed women to think about themselves in terms of unrealizable superlatives, particularly once the early sheen of marriage and the excitement of having babies had worn off. The clean, healthy home could offer protection from germs and disease, but it could also be a breeding ground for neuroses and mental health problems. Richard Yates's satirical novel *Revolutionary Road* (1961), for example, narrates the profound anxieties of April Wheeler, a Connecticut housewife, over her role as mother of two as she dreams of leaving suburbia for a new life in Europe. The fact that April's psychological turmoil leads her to make a life-threatening decision is a narrative twist that emphasizes the unhealthy nature of her suburban existence.[70]

Published a year before *Revolutionary Road*, *The Split-Level Trap*, a study by the psychiatrists Richard and Katherine Gordon and the journalist Max Gunther, also offers a dark picture of suburbia. The authors focus on the tensions and illnesses brought on by suburban living and they bemoan the fact that the tranquility of suburbanites is found "only fleetingly in pill bottles and a cocktail glass."[71] They point out that in their New Jersey survey, substantially more women than men became psychiatric patients between 1953 and 1958 (an average of 32 percent of "young wives" between the ages of eighteen and forty-four, compared to less than 18 percent of "young husbands"), while hospitalized cases of hypertension and duodenal ulcers were significantly higher in suburban than in rural areas.[72] The authors take as a representative case Alice Hager, a young southern woman who moves north when her husband is offered a promotion and a transfer to New York. Living in relative affluence in a New Jersey suburb, Alice nevertheless suffers from severe paranoia and an irrational fear of authorities. Contextual factors include the memory of her parents fighting over money, her father's alcoholism, and later her mother's death, but the main determinants relate to her suburban life: her husband's long working hours; her sons' increasingly naughty behavior; aggressive and competitive mothers in her suburb; and her feeling of being cut off from any sense of community, particularly when she is excluded from a women's club intent on preserving itself from infiltration by newcomers. Feeling hemmed in, Alice begins suffering from anxiety attacks and slowly starts to lose her grip on the outside world. She displays symptoms of dizziness and high blood pressure but receives little support from the family doctor. Suffering from paranoid despair, she experiences an emotional breakdown and crawls into a dark closet, "shivering in terror, waiting for them to come and get her."[73] The authors surmise that Alice's condition stems from her "socially disintegrated town," "a world of people in restless motion," and people who are "anxious to move on and up" and who are intolerant of any family "that stands still."[74]

The Split-Level Trap divides suburban stresses into three categories: "sensitizers," which lower individuals' defenses and make them susceptible to anxiety; "pressurizers," or stresses that continue throughout life; and "precipitators," which often push the sensitized, pressurized individual over the edge.[75] The authors argue that social psychiatry needs to consider an individual's case history closely to detect sensitizers and attend to the specific habitat in order to identify factors that can lead directly to severe psychological problems. The journey into the city and the office environment (despite its often alienating regularity) acted as a safety valve for many working men, but the monotony and homogeneity of suburbia were pressurizers, and the competitive spirit of keeping up with (or surpassing) the Joneses was a precipitator for many suburban women, including Betsy Rath in *The Man in the Gray Flannel Suit*. Although she does not suffer from mental illness, Betsy's suburban anxiety is palpable throughout Sloan Wilson's novel and is dramatized by Jennifer Jones's anxious demeanor in the 1956 film adaptation.[76]

The Split-Level Trap argued that child rearing was a precipitating factor for many women, supported by the case study of a young wife, Gina Conning, who suffers restlessness, anger, and a strange sexual drive a few weeks after giving birth to an unplanned child. The stresses of suburban competitiveness and the entrapment of pregnancy are also major factors in what proves to be April Wheeler's fatal breakdown

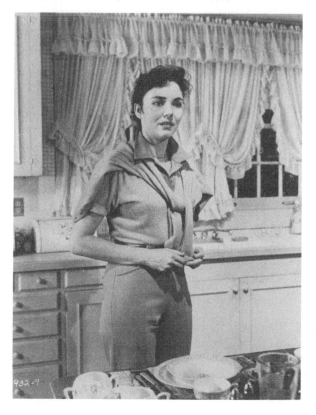

FIGURE 5.2 An anxious Betsy Rath (Jennifer Jones) in her suburban Connecticut kitchen. *The Man in the Gray Flannel Suit* (Nunnally Johnson, Twentieth Century–Fox, 1956).

in *Revolutionary Road*. April has become pregnant for the third time, and, in an attempt to carry out her dream of escaping to France with her family, she suggests to her husband, Frank, that she carry out a home abortion early in her pregnancy. Frank's response is to turn against her, wildly accusing her of penis envy, and recommending psychiatric treatment. His insensitive behavior and his later disclosure that he has had an affair with a co-worker are precipitating factors in April's breakdown, but the psychological horizon of her domestic troubles is very similar to the cases of entrapped housewives documented in *The Split-Level Trap*.

These case studies are revealing, but they unintentionally reinforce the experience of victimhood for many women in the 1950s. In contrast, the home could be a sanctuary and an area of real control, if the wage-earning husband handed over responsibility for the household budget and running the domestic economy to his wife. Although Wylie's category of momism was widely used and misused, his scorn—as Plant notes— was often directed at conservative, anticommunist, and patriotic women's groups that were at odds with an ideology of "pluralist democracy" and the experiences of many families.[77] This enables us to move away from the stereotypes of "momism" and "the lost sex" to suggest that many American women in the late 1940s and 1950s were agents of home economics and medical knowledge. The reluctance of many men to go to the family doctor or to interest themselves deeply in medical affairs was partly born out of the self-reliance of the war years; it was also partly because medical know-how was most widely available in women's magazines such as *Ladies' Home Journal*.

Although the housewife was often the intended target of advertising, tensions between commercial interests (tempting women to buy pharmaceuticals or hygiene products) and medical knowledge (often given a seal of approval by the American Medical Association) meant that mothers often had to work matters out for themselves, particularly if they were displaced from their wider family through a work-related move to the suburbs. Advertising campaigns in the interwar period suggested that health could be readily bought, but checks by the FDA on fraudulent advertising in the 1930s (particularly following the passage of the Food, Drug, and Cosmetic Act of 1938) and the American Medical Association's seal of approval scheme, were serious attempts to help parents to become responsible consumers. The FDA had no control over the therapeutic claims of drugs and could not "protect any consumer if he [or she] persists in believing what he [or she] sees in the press and hears over the radio and refuses to read the labels on the package," but it did help educate consumers to distinguish legitimate from bogus medicines. A good example of this value was the FDA campaign against Harry M. Hoxsey, who touted his "chemotherapeutic" cancer treatment as the only effective one on the market in the mid-1950s.[78] The effects of such advice

> [made it] possible for the skillful woman consumer to "buy" health for her family, but only by scrupulously uncovering deceptions that might transform her pantry or her medicine chest into a source of debility and death. For the modern wife and mother, becoming adept at sorting through this conflicting muddle became an increasingly important facet of running a modern home.[79]

According to this view, suburban sociability for many women not only meant coffee klatches and other social events but also provided an opportunity to share medical knowledge as well as gossip.

Although in some quarters there is still a nostalgic view of 1950s domesticity, since the mid-1960s it has been widely critiqued as an ideological framework linked closely to Cold War containment. In the 1990s, however, critics started to challenge the view that the postwar home was simply "a place of passive consumption with almost no relationship to productive forces in culture." Lynn Spigel, for example, has focused on "amateur arts" in the home and "alternative modes of production that go beyond the status of mere hobby."[80] In postwar fiction, though, it is hard to find such a positive account. *Revolutionary Road*, for example, opens with April Wheeler starring in a badly performed amateur theatrical production; her disappointment after the final curtain and Frank's inability to judge the emotional charge of the situation leads to the first of a series of intense marital arguments. Other amateur arts such as the paint-by-numbers craze in the mid-1950s barely make the status of art. Nevertheless, the presence of activities such as sewing, knitting, painting, and home decorating suggests a level of production that went under the radar of (mostly urban) cultural critics. Among these home arts was a practical knowledge about health care that returned agency to mothers and challenges the views that families simply deferred to their doctor's professional wisdom or that women were the unthinking victims of drug companies.

Medical knowledge was often linked to good housekeeping and nutrition. The feeling recurred throughout the decade that the government needed to act more decisively to control and reduce additives in food, but nutrition became part of middle-class life in the 1950s as a way of optimizing health.[81] The advertising of health products was parodied in a May 1952 episode of *I Love Lucy*, "Lucy Does a TV Commercial," in which Lucille Ball, while filming for a television advertisement, repeatedly demonstrates the medicinal properties of the tonic Vitameatavegamin—which, unbeknown to her, is 23 percent alcohol and ends up getting her blind drunk. Perhaps echoing the tagline that Vitameatavegamin tastes "just like candy," in a poem called "Positive Thinking," published in the January 1958 issue of *Ladies' Home Journal*, the female poet writes: "I lick my lips for castor oil, / Think vitamins are dandy, / Enjoy the sting of iodine, / Eat vegetables like candy."[82] The poet is concerned about the damage to the mother's own health (she is eager to take penicillin when offered), but the last couplet "I'm just a mother, martyred / To set a good example" indicates where her primary nutritional concerns lie.

Postwar studies of nutrition and healthy eating followed early-twentieth-century work such as *The Cost of Food* (1901) and *Dietary Computer* (1902), by the scientist Ellen Richards, and post–World War I studies of vitamins A and B intended to educate housewives about the importance of nutrients and vitamins in a balanced diet.[83] In 1949 Margaret Mead contrasted the young mother who follows her own mother by thrusting "the sugar-tit deeper into her child's mouth when it cries" to the "trim young housewife, clad in a charming apron," who measures out orange juice for her baby, perhaps hiding "shamefacedly from her own eyes the memory of what her mother did not do."[84] This picture of the modern woman in a scientific household led to the rapid growth of serious campaigns to market vitamins and minerals, especially those found in fresh fruit and vegetables, which helped to reduce the percentage of families with poor nutrition from one-third in 1935 to one-tenth in 1955.[85] National campaigns promoted the importance of vitamin C, which arrived on the market in the 1940s and could be taken to prevent scurvy and polio in young children and to maintain the health of skin, teeth, and gums.

Books such as *Nutrition for Health* (1951) were targeted directly at mothers. Published in McGraw-Hill's American Home and Family series, this work includes in each chapter a test of the reader's comprehension of key issues and memory of basic facts, such as the chemical elements found in the human body and the type of nutrient required in a particular case. The book emphasizes the "serious lag in getting these essential facts [about nutrition] to the general public" and an even greater lag "in convincing the individual that it is in his [or her] personal interest to improve his [or her] food habits in the light of modern scientific knowledge."[86] The book defers to specialists, but it also stresses self-help and careful parenting, encouraging mothers to apply their insights on sensible eating, calorie counting, and food preparation, made easier by improved methods of preserving and storing food in Tupperware—a brand name exclusively targeted at women.[87] However, the economic historian Clair Brown notes that 1950 was the high point for improvements in nutrition: the rise in frozen foods, snacks, sweets, partially prepared meals, and alcohol consumption led to "potentially harmful dietary choices" during the following two decades.[88]

Parenthood and Child Rearing

Lundberg and Farnham claimed in *Modern Woman: The Lost Sex* that having children could help improve strained modern relationships and shore up a crumbling home, but child-rearing techniques exhibited continuities with prewar parenting, despite the unusual spike in births between 1946 and 1957, a decline in infant and maternal mortality rates, and the increasing importance of television advertising targeted at young mothers. Rima Apple traces these continuities back to the early nineteenth century and to the first child-care manual (written by "an American matron," Mary Palmer Tyler, a mother of eight). In this 1811 work, *The Maternal Physician*, Tyler focused on hygiene and cleanliness, harnessing conservative beliefs to her personal experiences, enriched with "casual extracts from the most improved medical authorities."[89] Tyler set the tone for other writers to develop "scientific motherhood," as Lydia Maria Child did in *The Family Nurse* (1837), a text that linked "deference to medical authority and confident self-assertion," expressing the conviction that breast-feeding and attentiveness to her baby's body (including bathing and frequent changes of clothing) would help the mother become a skilled nurse and the child's "best physician."[90]

The science of child care continued to advance through the nineteenth century, and rather than mothers simply relying on instinct, they found sources of education in the growing discipline of home economics, in child-care manuals, and in magazine advice columns in publications like the *Ladies' Home Journal*, which emerged in the 1880s alongside *Babyhood* and *Good Housekeeping*, with its "Happiness and Health" column. Scientific expertise was encouraged by doctors and social reformers to improve parenting and relieve anxious mothers. For example, an immunization program began in the 1920s to control diseases such as diphtheria and found its greatest success in the polio vaccines administered in the second half of the 1950s.[91] Deference to medical wisdom, as Apple argues, had a paradoxical effect, making mothers "responsible for the health and welfare of their families" but denying them ultimate control.[92] Reliance on external authority was best symbolized by the mass release of the government-sponsored pamphlet *Infant Care*, first published in 1914 to educate the "average mother of the country," especially women in immigrant and rural communities. Its success was so great that by the 1940s twelve million copies had been sold, in a steady stream of editions that addressed the concerns of new generations of mothers. Not only did *Infant Care* provide parents with advice about bed-wetting, feeding, and bathing, but it steered lifestyle choices, recommending "suburban homes or those on the outskirts of cities or close to public parks," which could give children "the best chance for proper growth and development."[93]

This tendency to publish new manuals to reflect changing times was common among advice books and in the mainstream press, culminating in John Watson's *Psychological Care of Infant and Child* (1928), Dorothy Whipple's *Our American Babies: The Art of Baby Care* (1944), and the first edition of Benjamin Spock's *Dr. Spock's Baby and Child Care* (1946). Spock steered away from Watson's behaviorist approach to child care, attempting to combine Freudian psychoanalysis (in which Spock had been trained at Cornell University Medical School in the 1930s) with a common-sense advice manual that would appeal to a middle-class readership.[94] Quite often Spock found Freud's emphasis on infantile sexuality misleading; psychoanalysis certainly proved inadequate to the practicalities of toilet training and sterilizing bottles, leading Spock "cautiously" to blend pediatrics and psychiatry "as if the two forces might blow up if mixed improperly."[95] In its 507 bite-size sections and piecemeal use of Freud, Spock took a developmental approach to child care, focusing on the child's potential and the primacy of the mother's love rather than on the pessimistic Freudian view that neurosis is a constant companion from an early age. Spock stressed that he had used "diluted extrapolations of Freudian concepts," now masked in "friendly phrases and American colloquialisms," but his manual more obviously harks back to John Dewey's liberal and pragmatic emphasis on the child's capacity to learn.[96] Spock begins his book with the infant's earliest moments and moves through developmental stages to older children (and, in later editions, adolescents). It is as if he were trying to offer a stable counterpoint to the psychic fragmentation of World War II—the period during which he wrote this work, while serving as a psychiatrist in the US Navy Reserve Corps from 1944 to 1945.

There was one major difference between Spock's book and scientific motherhood. Although Spock offers a wealth of advice to mothers, he believes in the mother's instinct to do the right thing by her baby at the right moment, including breast-feeding—which he viewed as more natural than using a bottle. He even suggests that the mother should be wary of experts and that she needs to take a firm and confident approach. According to Spock, child rearing cannot be wholly controlled, even though some advisors would say that regulation of all aspects of the young child's life is paramount. In fact, the book seems to have it both ways in recommending combinations of planning and letting nature run its course; of science and instinct; and of Freudian insight, common sense, and folk wisdom. In many ways, though, the book fits neatly into the postwar moment, when the values of progressivism and the New Deal jostled with more conservative pressures to reorder society along lines of Victorian propriety. There is much in Spock's book that harks back to earlier popular advice for parents, but there were some novelties as well, including allowing children to suck thumbs or pacifiers, broaching the subject of masturbation (which Spock considered normal unless practiced excessively), and dealing with the darker fears of estrangement and loss that arise regularly in Freudian thought.[97]

Although Freudian ideas pepper *Dr. Spock's Baby and Child Care*, psychoanalytic currents featured more strongly in the work of the child psychologist René Spitz. A Hungarian who moved from Vienna to Paris and then to the United States in 1939, Spitz used Freudian ideas to explore anxiety in early life. Following many years of research on hospitalism—a condition in which infants wasted away while they were in a hospital—Spitz produced a series of educational films based on his work for the Psychoanalytic Research Project on the Problems of Infancy at the University of Colorado in the 1940s and 1950s. One of these films, *Anxiety: Its Phenomenology in the 1st Year of Life* (1949), looks at birth trauma when no anesthetics are used in childbirth (a practice adopted by those who thought that anesthetics could damage the fetal brain) and distress when the newborn baby is deprived of its mother's smiling face. This second theme is taken further in *Motherlove—The Baby's Greatest Need* (1951), which contrasts happy babies being breast-fed and playing with their mother to those who have lost their mothers and display "a severe mourning reaction" and the beginnings of "long-lasting psychiatric disturbances."[98] Spitz focused on the mother-child relationship and various potential problems in it, ranging from psychotoxic diseases caused by the "wrong kinds of relation" to emotional deficiency due to "inadequate emotional supplies."[99] According to Spitz, the baby's resultant hostility toward the mother is displayed variously through vomiting, breathing problems, and, later, playing with feces.

Spitz's work became important for understanding infant psychology and the emotional scars that can be carried into childhood and adult life, which other researchers such as the psychologist Harold Skeels had studied in relation to mental retardation in children who had been deprived of their mothers at an early age. By experimenting with different surrogate mothers, Skeels showed that early stimuli can dramatically improve a child's IQ and promote an integrated personality.[100] Spitz's film *Motherlove* offers no practical answers to the loss of the mother (it warns that "depriving the baby of love is as bad as depriving it of food"), and the absence of fathers in the film suggests that a loving mother is irreplaceable. Unlike Helene Deutsch, who stressed the primacy of the mother's "emotional warmth" but largely ignored external factors, Spitz focused in another film, *Shaping the Personality* (1953), on the complex elements—biological, psychological, and economic—that inform the mother-child relationship.[101] In *Shaping the Personality*, the mother is an anchor and source of nourishment, which is absent or distorted in the cases of unwanted and overstimulated babies (an example of the latter type has an "intellectually ambitious" mother). Nevertheless, the film neglects wider social and cultural factors such as education, age, ethnicity, family size, and social class.[102]

Spitz's view about the unique and powerful relationship between mother and child was reinforced by the British psychiatrist and pediatrician D. W. Winnicott who, like Skeels, had been working on the relationship between mothers and children since the mid-1930s. Following Melanie Klein's groundbreaking study *The Psychoanalysis of Children* (1932), Winnicott wrote on a wide range of topics including birth trauma, child neurosis, child care, good mothering, and transitional objects that play an important role in childhood—such as security blankets. Although Winnicott was not widely read in the United States in the 1940s and 1950s, his "primer of first relationships," *Mother and Child* (1957), shared with *Dr. Spock's Baby and Child Care* the use of plain language to address topics of infant feeding, digestion, crying, weaning, and childhood learning (as well as broader issues of having twins, adoption, and children's lying and stealing). Winnicott's target was mothers "who are ordinarily good at looking after their own babies," stressing that the initial year is a crucial foundation for a healthy adulthood.[103] *Mother and Child* differs from Spock's book in two regards: in stating that the medical professions need to be more proactive in providing support and information to young mothers; and in redressing the myths of maternal domination by stressing the importance of dependency in infancy and childhood.[104] Based on the empirical studies of Spitz (among others), Winnicott argued that the "good enough mother" learns to completely adapt to her infant after birth and then slowly concede less and less to her child's needs in line with the infant's "growing ability to recognize and accept reality."[105] Thus, he saw the spectrum of dependence and independence as central, linked closely to the infantile creation of a maternal illusion (the breast as part of the baby) and the gradual disillusioning of the child (through weaning and other forms of separation). Winnicott did not call on modern mothers to become psychologists, but he recommended that they understand (and perhaps even record) the behavior of their children as they expressed these energies through play, drawing, painting, and other opportunities to create.[106]

Erik Erikson was also very interested in the role of mothers in shaping the modalities of childhood and maturation, but—unlike Winnicott and Spitz—he looked beyond the primary bond of mother and child to the psychodynamics of family life and developments over the life cycle. Instead of seeing the baby's psychological evolution from complete dependency to increasing independence from the mother as a linear narrative, Erikson argued in *Childhood and Society* (1950) that the growing child moves between the poles of trust and mistrust, initiative and guilt, intimacy and isolation, modalities that are often carried into adult life. As an émigré intellectual,

Erikson saw this oscillation between polar opposites as a distinctively American trait, claiming that many Americans base their ego-identity on a combination of "dynamic polarities such as migratory and sedentary, individualistic and standardized, competitive and cooperative, pious and freethinking, responsible and cynical."[107] In the domestic sphere, these polarities give rise to a spatial structure (the world of play, the space of the home) and an evolutionary structure as the child moves through a series of developmental phases. Erikson saw certain blockages to these life-cycle phases, however: for example, he viewed momism as an unhelpful middle-class discourse that was retarding the nation's "dynamic potential."[108] Without taking an overtly hostile view toward "mom" as a maternal type, Erikson thought that momism was one of a "series of overcompensatory attempts at settling tentatively around some Main Street, fireplace, bank account, and make of car."[109] Some mothers might be drawn toward (or see the virtues in) adopting this role, but Erikson saw momism as another version of postwar standardization, denying mothers the potential to mold their own personalities to their family situation and to their own needs.

Parental Stress, Drugs, and Surgery

In her 1959 poem "Girl's-Eye View of Relatives," Phyllis McGinley portrays fathers from a girl's perspective as "dragon-seekers, bent on improbable rescues."[110] Winnicott's *Mother and Child* preserves a unique space for fathers as providers and protectors, but he detected "an especially vital bond between a father and his daughter," often manifested through the daughter's feeling of dreamy romantic attachment.[111] But rather than embodying the heroic soldier or the handsome film star, such as Cary Grant or Gregory Peck, the domesticated father in the 1950s was a more vulnerable type, an "uncertain hero," to use the term in a 1956 *Woman's Home Companion* article on beleaguered masculinity.[112] McGinley's juvenile persona goes on to say: "Scratch any father, you find / Someone chock-full of qualms and romantic terrors, / Believing change is a threat."[113] The anxiety that we saw in chapter 4 bubbling under the surface in work-related stress was also present in the suburban home, linked to romantic relationships and parenting but also to anxieties about children growing up and maturing sexually, as Deutsch explored in the mid-1940s.[114]

More recently, Stephen Cohan has argued in *Masked Men* (1997) that many representations of the 1950s home indicate that postwar men in general, not just fathers, found domestic life difficult to adjust to.[115] Cohan takes the 1959 poster of Hitchcock's film *North by Northwest*, showing an anxious-looking Cary Grant falling through space, as a symbol of fraying masculinity; this interpretation is furthered by a reprisal of the image in the title sequence of *Mad Men*, the hit AMC show whose protagonist, Don Draper, is haunted by an identity crisis of his own making and who lives a life that seems always on the edge of collapse. The Cary Grant image also is related to fears expressed in Wylie's *A Generation of Vipers* that the home could be a space of maternal suffocation for boys and grown men alike, while other fears linked to the ambiguous sexuality of emerging screen icons James Dean and Marlon Brando (although it wasn't public knowledge at the time, another icon, Rock Hudson, was homosexual). But this disorientation also found more intimate expression in the confessional poems of Robert Lowell, who saw illness and neurosis as facets of the enclosed hell of selfhood. Following his breakthrough collection *Life Studies* (1959)—in which he explored marital tensions in "Man and Wife" and a disordered psyche in "On a Mad Negro Soldier Confined at Munich"—he wrote in a later poem, "Eye and Tooth" (1964), about an optical infection that turned his eye "sunset red" and pushed him toward disturbing childhood memories.[116] In the poem, he thinks back on two moments: the extraction of his first tooth using a door handle, and the first time he caught a glimpse of a woman's naked body, through the bathroom keyhole. Now, trapped at home and looking "darkly / through an unwashed goldfish globe," the poet confronts his physicality and uneasy sexuality; finding no remedy to ease his optical pain, he concludes: "I am tired. Everyone's tired of my turmoil."

According to Cohan and other gender historians, masculinity was in turmoil in the postwar home. Not only was there the fear that domesticity could reduce the size and significance of men (as dramatized in *The Incredible Shrinking Man*, discussed in chapter 3), but there was also the fact that the family home became both the reward for, and the curse of, salaried work. This turmoil did not often find full expression until the late 1950s but, as chapter 4 discussed, it led to mostly inexpressible anxieties. For example, the epitome of the domesticated breadwinner, Tom Rath in *The Man in the Gray Flannel Suit*, is uptight in his profession and often uncomfortable at home.[117] In many 1950s stories, representatives of the managerial class share in the national story, usually linked to service in World War II, as is the case for both Tom Rath and Frank Wheeler in *Revolutionary Road*. However, as the article on the "uncertain hero" describes, "certain deep and perfectly normal masculine drives that were 'permitted' during a war . . . are not permitted in a suburban back yard." This 1956 article contrasts the "green, happy back yard" to the more primitive drives of violence, polygamy, and rebellion that, according to the article, need to be tamed, even though "if they are always and completely inhibited—the man in the gray flannel suit will stop being a man."[118] Although a wartime affair returns to haunt Tom Rath, his white-collar suburban life cannot accommodate the extreme forms of behavior permitted during war.

When McGinley in "Girl's-Eye View of Relatives" says that "change is a threat" to most fathers, she refers partly to an inability to relate to growing children (this inability can be glimpsed in *The Best Years of Our Lives*, in which Al Stephenson has no way of building a bridge between his wartime world and that of his growing children). But it also suggests that a life of uneasy conformity is often better than probing too deeply into the organized relationship between work and home. This partitioned life might have been preferable to the suburban entrapment of the typical housewife, but it also fueled largely unexpressed anxieties about masculinity and fatherhood. Tom Rath sees his Connecticut home (purchased in 1946 after his discharge from the US Army) as "a trap"; Tom and Betsy "no more enjoyed refurbishing it than a prisoner would delight in shining up the bars of his cell."[119] Unhappy with their "small" and "ugly" home ("almost precisely like the houses on all sides of it") they neglect to decorate it or to tend to the "weed-filled garden." When, in a rare act of untrammeled emotion at the start of the novel, Tom throws a vase against the wall, the resulting crack in the "shape of a question mark" seems to say something significant about their predicament, but Tom and Betsy just think that the crack is "annoying."[120] William Whyte noted in 1953 that many suburbanites "are fully aware of the all-pervading power of the environment over them," but they also "have no sense of Plight; this, they seem to say, is the way things are, and the trick is not to fight it but to understand it."[121] Tom and Betsy's question-mark-shaped crack suggests that such understanding, for them, can only be tacit or unconscious.

As we saw in the previous chapter, Tom's career path leads him to a public-relations job geared to promoting mental health. Although this might seem a surprising choice, given that he is not adept at analyzing his own motivations, it is related to Whyte's sense that the "lay curiosity about psychology, psychiatry, and sociology" meant that the relationship among identity, health, and happiness was closely linked to the home.[122] More self-conscious than Tom Rath, but equally as blind, Frank Wheeler in *Revolutionary Road* considers himself an expert on the sociology and psychology of suburbia, but he fails as a father: he nearly gives his son a fatal blow with a spade while gardening, and he struggles to fulfill his basic paternal functions. This persistent view of the husband as disengaged from responsible parenting is parodied in another 1958 poem, "Housebroke," published in *Ladies' Home Journal*: "A man is tamed for domestic life / When, lifting his feet to allow his wife / To sweep beneath 'em, he merely grunts, / Not losing his place in the paper once."[123] This simple poem (which appears on the same page as a serious article on Cold War morality) explores the fear that men were going soft in the home and are only able to "grunt" rather than to articulate their role (this discomfort is signaled by the first rhyming couplet, jarring with the off rhyme in the second).[124] There are no children in "Housebroke," but it echoed Whyte's interpretation of suburban lifestyles as matriarchal—or even what might be called "filiarchal," in the sense that children set "the basic design; their friendships are translated into the mother's friendships, and these, in turn, to the family's. Fathers just tag along."[125]

This sense of displacement and dissatisfaction was a contributing factor to the widespread incidence of heart disease in working men between the ages of thirty-five and sixty-four (including President Eisenhower)—which, along with cancer, led to much higher mortality rates among men than women in the late 1950s. The "stresses of modern living" were a major factor (to use a phrase from a meeting of the New York Heart Association in 1950), and the search for clinical cures intensified in the late 1940s and 1950s.[126] Cortisone, which had its first trials in Europe in 1948–1949 and was just as experimental as Miltown, was another wonder drug that promised to cure many conditions by mid-decade, including asthma, hay fever, gout, poison ivy, ulcerative colitis, rheumatic fever, leukemia, and periarteritis nodosa. This last condition, involving inflammation of the arteries, was often fatal, but cortisone treatment was thought to arrest or even reverse the condition. The problem, as revealed in a September 1955 article by Berton Roueché in his "Annals of Medicine" column in the *New Yorker*, was how to calibrate the required dosage or predict the complex side effects. Written during the boom years for tranquilizers, Roueché's "Ten Feet Tall" was a medical detective story focusing on the case of Robert Laurence, a high-school teacher suffering from periarteritis nodosa. The article describes the patient's "spectacularly brilliant" reaction to the cortisone prescription, but it also emphasizes that these effects "are seldom more than palliative and almost never permanent."[127]

The main problem with wonder drugs was the lack of clarity about their alleviative properties. Side effects ranged from the commonplace (nausea and headaches) to hormonal imbalance (leading to weight gain, diabetes, and unusual amounts of facial hair) and "awesomely new" effects, including "lowered resistance to infection . . . paranoia, schizophrenia, and manic-depressive psychosis."[128] Cortisone was an interesting test case for exploring the interface between physical and mental illness: this drug, administered for a physical complaint gave rise to a wide array of extreme psychological symptoms that followed the patient's initial dramatic recovery. At first Laurence feels as "bright as a button—capable of anything," but this new openness leads to increased appetite, irresponsible spending, loquaciousness, wild philosophizing, feelings of omnipotence, and dramatic mood swings—so much so that his wife, Nora, exclaims: "This wasn't Bob. There was no resemblance whatever. This was a man I'd never seen before."[129]

The article alternates between the husband's and wife's perspectives, but the story is told largely from Nora's viewpoint, as if Robert's grandiose new world can be captured only through an external description of his erratic behavior. Not only is he more emotionally open, talkative, and hungry than before, but he becomes more vulnerable to consumerist impulses, attracted to new clothes in bright colors for his wife, a workaday gray flannel suit for himself, and an expensive new car that he would not ordinarily have considered buying. In *Bigger Than Life*, Nicholas Ray's 1956 film version of Roueché's article, we see the husband, now called Ed Avery (stressing his average status), buy his wife, Lou, a bright orange dress, and he possesses much more energy than before his illness, as is evident when he plays ball in the living room with his son. Ray's film emphasizes the social dimension of the drug, particularly as Ed's first attack occurs just after he recognizes the blandness of his suburban life. Once he starts to take cortisone, he becomes a restless consumer open to a new world of possibility, but he also veers dangerously toward paranoiac megalomania: we see him switch from being a receptive, liberal teacher to a rigid dogmatist, preaching to parents about their "moral midget" children and narcissistically gazing at himself in the bathroom mirror as he toys with a more aristocratic appearance. But whereas Robert Laurence has an "alpine impression of himself" and sees himself as a revolutionary educationalist, this is undercut in *Bigger Than Life* by Ed Avery's primitive emotions and actions, emphasized by a threatening simian shadow (an illusion skillfully created by a limited light source) that looms over his son as Ed cruelly forces him to do his homework.[130]

Neither the film nor the article blames pharmaceutical companies outright (perhaps unaware of the government-funded Psychopharmacology Service Center, which was established in 1956 to test psychiatric drugs), but both point a finger squarely at the medical profession. During medical tests we see Ed (played by James Mason) positioned behind a crude X-ray machine that reveals the hollowness of his body, and an even cruder graph is superimposed over Ed's anguished and contorted face as the doctors attempt to calibrate the right dosage. Not only does this make the patient into a human guinea pig, but it poses questions of medical negligence when Ed is sent home as soon as he responds positively. The film explores the social reasons for Ed's condition: he holds down a blue-collar second job as a telephonist for a taxi firm (he works in a bookstore in "Ten Feet Tall"), but he hides this fact from his wife because she would consider the job beneath him. The main focus is on Ed's manipulative behavior as he becomes increasingly reliant on cortisone. In a fall from grace from his previous status as a "good enough" teacher, father, and husband, Ed begins to lie and scheme—even becoming a criminal figure when he poses as a doctor at a drugstore to procure more cortisone, after he has taken his dosage too quickly. These elements (and others such as Lou's unwillingness to work) are extrapolated from Roueché's article and emphasize the social and medical implications of the drug, as well as the psychodrama between husband, wife, and son as they struggle with its side effects.

The film critic Barbara Klinger sees Ray's style as "excessively symptomatic," but, rather than fitting it into a tightly defined genre of the family melodrama, exemplified by films directed by Douglas Sirk and Vincente Minnelli, Klinger reads *Bigger Than Life* as "ingeniously transgressive of the repressive Eisenhower era and its vision of the complacent nuclear family."[131] Ray achieves this through cinematographic techniques (the use of deep focus, Cinemascope, and a heightened color palette), and by skillfully deploying the mise-en-scène of the suburban home to dramatize the family psychodrama. Sometimes the space between characters is emphasized (when Ed arrives home after school, his son, Bobby, appears as a distant figure at the other end of the living room), and at other times the house seems claustrophobic, as the characters hem each other in. It is not always clear whether Ed is locked within an inescapable condition or whether Lou and Bobby are locked out of his world, but it is evident that the illness consumes them all.[132] Ed sees the forces of suburban containment more clearly when he is taking the drug, but his mood swings and egotism cause wild exaggerations in his perception. The scene toward the end—in which Ed and the school football coach, Wally Gibbs (Walter Matthau), fight on the stairs as Lou and Bobby cower in the darkness and the television blares out fairground music—shows a suburban home falling apart in the face of dangerous and uncontrollable forces.

Despite its scathing attack on medical responsibility, the ending of *Bigger Than Life* is upbeat, depicting the reunion of the family around Ed Avery's hospital bed, with the implications that the correct dose of cortisone can be calibrated and the curse of suburban living can be tempered by a new spirit of togetherness. However, the ending seems artificial and potentially ironic; like many critics discussed in this chapter, Ray felt that everyone clearly suffered from anxiety in the domestic "disturbia" of the Cold War, as *The Split-Level Trap* called it, and that neat resolutions of Hollywood films grated with increasingly complex life stories.[133] The domestic destruction

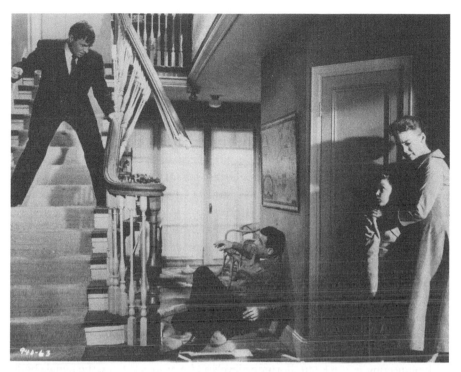

FIGURE 5.3   A psychotic Ed Avery (James Mason) destroys his suburban house and his family during a fight with Wally Gibbs (Walter Matthau). *Bigger Than Life* (Nicholas Ray, Twentieth Century–Fox, 1956).

of *Bigger Than Life* is only a couple of steps beyond Betsy Rath's proclamation early in *The Man in the Gray Flannel Suit* that "all I want is a decent house, without a damn-fool crack in the wall like a question mark, and without everything coming apart."[134]

Bigger Than Life was the most direct cinematic attempt in the 1950s to expose the negligence of the medical profession and the increased use of prescription drugs in everyday life. Malpractice among psychiatrists was not fully studied until the early 1960s, after three court cases between 1959 and 1961—including one in 1959 involving a patient who had become addicted to the narcotic painkiller Demerol after it had been prescribed to him by his doctor (Demerol was criticized for its addictive properties in *Valley of the Dolls*).[135] The year that *Bigger Than Life* was released was one of the peak years for tranquilizer use. An HEW report of 1956 noted the widespread use of tranquilizers for vascular complaints, psychiatric problems, and insomnia; it was believed that the drugs could control aggression and blood pressure and reduce the amount of electroshock and insulin treatment needed in institutions. But the study noted that although drugs such as chlorpromazine and reserpine (both introduced in 1953) "are a potential force for much good and can open a new era in psychiatry," a lack of sound data about the long-term effects of the drugs and reports of medical complications in patients suggested that they are "a potential source of danger."[136]

The HEW report was balanced in its discussion of the features of tranquilizers. There were three broadly positive ones: the drugs were relatively inexpensive; they had the potential to reduce the number of people admitted to hospitals, particularly mental hospitals; and they enabled general practitioners to treat mild depressive symptoms in outpatients. But there were also three drawbacks, which were arguably more profound: there was a temptation to use the cheap drugs; detailed studies were needed to explore the effects on a variety of patients (in terms of age, sex, race, and medical condition) and the particular therapeutic techniques deployed; and not enough was known about the toxic side effects of psychotropic drugs, including hypotension, parkinsonism, and psychosis, as dramatized in *Bigger Than Life*. The report concluded with a note of caution, stressing that follow-up tests were needed before the safety of such drugs could be assured.[137]

Nevertheless, the administering of tranquilizers such as Pacatal became commonplace, especially for women suffering from depression and anxiety.[138] Often neuroses revolved around the dual roles of mother and housewife; better day care for children or the readjustment of the parental roles might well have had a more positive and lasting effect than tranquilizers. The fact that there were so few practicing female doctors and psychiatrists (the 1960s saw a 20 percent rise in the number of female obstetricians and gynecologists) meant that diagnoses rarely tackled root causes, and medical treatment of "women's problems" often lacked sensitivity. Even with pioneering research into hormone levels and menstrual cycles, the female body was one of the least understood domains of medical science. For those drawn to psychoanalysis, Freud's male-centered view of psychic development left little room to explore female sexuality on its own terms, and for those taking a biologistic perspective, it was difficult to sever the link between "premenstrual physiology" and the exaggeration of "minor neurotic traits," as a 1963 symposium on "The Potential of Women" put it.[139] The Kinsey report of 1953 (discussed in chapter 6) improved public understanding of female sexuality, but a veil of ignorance hung over the decade, prompting the poet Adrienne Rich to write in anger in the mid-1970s that "I know no woman . . . for whom her body is not a fundamental problem."[140]

The obfuscation of women's health issues in the 1950s led to a number of investigations late in the decade. A two-part article, "Cruelty in Maternity Wards," published in 1958 in the *Ladies' Home Journal*, exposed what it described as torturous practices in hospitals, where the needs of young mothers-to-be were frequently neglected, doctors did not speak to their patients, and births were induced to suit the doctor's convenience.[141] The article, which received more letters than any previous article in the *Journal*, described "growing hostility" among mothers toward doctors, born out of a "gulf of ignorance, hostility, and just plain misunderstanding." While clearly supporting the mother's plight, the article (like the HEW report on tranquilizers) took a balanced perspective, calling for an "honest public discussion of the contentions of both sides."[142]

One area where American doctors fared better than their European counterparts was to the prescribing of thalidomide to pregnant women as a relief from morning sickness and insomnia. Manufactured by a Swiss company, thalidomide was widely prescribed in Western and Northern Europe between 1958 and 1962, and in Canada for eleven months from 1961 to 1962. However, thalidomide did not win federal approval in the United States, and as a result relatively few American babies were born with related congenital problems, including cleft palates, blindness, partial facial palsy, tumors, and limb deficiency. It did affect some mothers, though, who had purchased the drug abroad or by mail order.[143] Reports on the effects of thalidomide did not emerge until the 1960s, including a 1964 Montreal survey that focused on mother-child relationships and the fear that thalidomide children would be rejected by their parents, so extreme were the deformities and the mother's acute sense of conflict and isolation. The report noted that 75 percent of mothers were unable to discuss the matter with their husbands.[144]

Nonetheless, US medical practice did have a crueler side, which contributed to the sense of worthlessness among many women patients when diagnosed with hysteria or while undergoing surgery for conditions related to their sexuality. Evidence points to the experimentation with cobalt radiotherapy for breast cancer in the mid 1950s and a number of unnecessary hysterectomies were performed in that decade on women, particularly between the ages of fifty and sixty-four. The physician James Doyle detailed the erratic nature of ovarian surgery and mastectomy operations in the *Journal of the American Medical Association* in 1953, but the practice continued in the guise of aggressive "superradical surgery."[145] Barron Lerner points to the supreme authority of postwar surgeons, particularly when it came to palliative irradiation of ovaries or radical breast surgery, which often disfigured the patient and left permanent defects in the ribcage. Lerner's book *The Breast Cancer Wars* (2001) also notes the "mechanistic, reductionistic language" used by surgeons, including phrases like an "All-American operation" in which the task of fashioning a better nation is transferred from the patient-citizen to the skilled hands of the surgeon.[146]

Although sometimes quick to perform surgery, the medical profession at other times refused to intervene. The criminalization of abortion, in particular, meant that women had to seek unsafe measures outside of official healthcare. In 1962 one Arizonan woman, Sherri Finkbine, decided to seek the abortion of what would be her fifth child after she discovered that the tranquilizers she had been taking contained thalidomide, but she was forced to travel to Sweden after the administrators in her local hospital in Phoenix turned down her request for an abortion.[147] Abortions were only legal if the mother's life was in jeopardy, and as a result backstreet abortions and self-inducements were widely practiced despite their severe risks. In the mid-1950s, Alfred Kinsey estimated that 22 percent of women up to forty-five years of age had had at least one induced abortion, which a later study described as "a less shameful and frightening way to solve their problems than visiting a criminal abortionist," despite the dangers of self-harm, purgative drugs, poisons, and attempts at laceration.[148] Direct references to abortion are rare in 1950s fiction, but in *Revolutionary Road* Richard Yates tackles this taboo subject through the character of April Wheeler (as did Rona Jaffe in a less graphic way in her best-selling 1958 novel *The Best of Everything,* and Jacqueline Susann in *Valley of the Dolls*). In a desperate attempt to free herself from another unplanned pregnancy, April attempts a home abortion with a syringe, even though she knows it is too far into the pregnancy to be carried out with any degree of safety. April's calm, meticulous, and hygienic preparation does not prevent this home abortion from being fatal, and similar cases admitted to hospitals in the 1950s and early 1960s resulted in severe complications. When women did have illegal abortions, they were faced with equally unsafe methods or, as Joan Didion described in her novel *Play It As It Lays*, no information or counseling. "This is just induced menstruation," Didion's character Maria Wyeth is told, "nothing to have any emotional difficulties about."[149]

The lack of information about abortion—and the secrecy involved in two Planned Parenthood Federation of America conferences on abortion in 1955 and 1958—was a major problem, leading the conference organizer and sex education advocate Mary Calderone to call for more public information about abortion and for the physiology of pregnancy to be taught in schools.[150] Planned Parenthood lobbied for a relaxation of abortion laws following the 1955 conference and helped generate a body of information that slowly percolated outward, but the American Medical Association did not overturn its embargo on doctors' distributing birth control information until 1964, and not until the late 1960s did women's groups find that they could usefully mobilize around sexual health (see the conclusion of this book for further discussion of this point).[151] Although we might look to cinematic and TV portrayals of mental and physical health in the 1950s as alternative channels for public information, the almost complete absence of narratives dealing explicitly with abortion served to mystify the practice further. There are some hints about it—for example, in Alfred Hitchcock's 1940 film version of Daphne Du Maurier's *Rebecca*—and abortion is euphemistically discussed in the Hollywood version of *The Best of Everything* (1959), but even in the 1955 film *I Am a Camera*, set fairly remotely in 1920s Berlin, the Hays Code demanded that abortion should be turned into a case of false pregnancy.

The main problem was that idealized images of the nuclear family reinforced by the mass media and government involved profound silence on some topics, in spite of a growing realization that medicine did not have all the answers about sickness and ill health. Indeed, as "Ten Feet Tall" and the article on maternity wards in the *Ladies' Home Journal* demonstrate, after 1956 there was a wave of mistrust in medical authority and the suspicion that the uneven provision of healthcare was undermining the collective health of the nation. One could ward off minor complaints by having a well-stocked medicine cabinet, but far-reaching and sensitive support from medical quarters was frequently in short supply, or available only to the wealthy.

Although social mobility and lifestyle aspirations characterized the 1950s, the emphasis on the "average case" implied that health and illness were often dominated by normative categories, bringing medical disapproval, moral penalties, and social stigma to those who deviated far from the norm. As this chapter has explored, Freudian discourse and advice on child rearing in the late 1940s and 1950s was punctuated by profound silences on certain matters: the side effects of psychotropic drugs, the relationship between physiology and female sexuality, and advice on family planning and abortion. For this reason, looking back at 1955 from the perspective of the early 1960s (by which time information was available about psychiatrists willing to recommend therapeutic abortions on mental health grounds), Richard Yates resists giving April Wheeler her own narrative voice in *Revolutionary Road* until the final part of the story, when April's fate seems already sealed.[152] April's anxieties were shared by many married women, who felt constrained by narrow gender roles, limited cultural outlets, and mixed messages in the media about mother love, momism, and careerism, making it difficult for them to tell their own stories. However, as we will see in the next chapter, opportunities for self-expression as a marker of health did exist in second half of the 1950s.

6 *Outside the Circle*

GROWING PAINS, DELINQUENCY,
AND SEXUALITY

On 24 September 1955, at the age of sixty-four, President Dwight Eisenhower suffered a massive heart attack during a vacation in Denver. For a president contemplating a second term in office, this was more than just a return of the "mystery illness" he had experienced in 1949 before entering the political arena.[1] The fact that Eisenhower did run again in 1956, once more with Richard Nixon as his running mate, was a credit to his fortitude. To conceal the president's precarious health from the public, the Republican campaign team cleverly used television broadcasts and a number of strategic photo opportunities as an alternative to a grueling campaign in person.[2] But the victorious Eisenhower was frequently ill during his second term, undergoing surgery for Crohn's disease in 1956 and suffering a stroke in November 1957.[3] Although Eisenhower was serious about his health and continued to play golf, in 1957, the year that the US birthrate peaked, an ailing president offered a reminder to the nation of the frailty of old age.

Eisenhower's failing health provoked interest in the Twenty-fifth Amendment to the Constitution, which states that the vice president will take over in case of the president's "Death, Resignation, or Inability to discharge the Powers and Duties" of the office.[4] Not only did Eisenhower's illness raise the prospect of a physically weak leader, but a growing mistrust between Eisenhower and Nixon led to an uneasy alliance between the two men (there was some debate as to whether Nixon would be Eisenhower's running mate in 1956, and Eisenhower avoided endorsing Nixon as his preferred successor in 1960).[5] Aside from the speculation that Nixon was a paranoid narcissist with a borderline personality disorder, the combination of Eisenhower's frail physical health and the rumor that Nixon needed psychiatric treatment (as a 1955 journalist claimed) offers a more complex story of the late 1950s, which counters the heroic narrative of the grand march of medicine.[6]

Senator Joseph McCarthy's self-aggrandizing anticommunist claims faded from public view after he was discredited in the televised Army-McCarthy hearings in the spring of 1954. But just as Cold War suspicions lingered into the later years of the decade, even after McCarthy's death from alcohol-related hepatitis in 1957, so discourses of illness persisted through Eisenhower's second term, when speculation about the president's and vice president's health deepened the cracks that were emerging in the organized society of the mid-1950s. Although there are comforts in adopting an organized role (the happy worker or the giving mother), the more diffuse conceptions of health that circulated in the second half of the decade gave way to a different therapeutic strain—a topic that runs through part 3 of this book.

Before we get there, though, this chapter focuses on many Americans' growing unease with authority and institutional practice. Mid-decade films such as *Rebel without a Cause* (1955) and *The Blackboard Jungle* (1956) showed teenagers rebelling against authority figures, and more explicit struggles to assert sexualized identities appeared in other films, such as the MGM version of Robert Anderson's play *Tea and Sympathy* (1956), and Allen Ginsberg's free-verse poetry.[7] The chapter discusses these examples in the context of widely read studies by Benjamin Spock, Erik Erikson, Bruno Bettelheim, Robert Lindner, and Alfred Kinsey, which help to trace the life cycle—a term developed by Erikson—from childhood through adolescence and into young adulthood. This trajectory is useful for assessing the significance of health and illness in the late 1950s, and it provides a glimpse of a therapeutic revolution very different from that of the early part of the decade, driven by emerging ideas and new social movements.

Beyond the Cold War Consensus

Despite the work of the Department of Health, Education, and Welfare (HEW) and the availability of Jonas Salk's polio vaccine by 1955, statistical trends indicated that the nation was not getting any healthier. President-Elect John F. Kennedy's article "The Soft American," published in *Sports Illustrated* in December 1960, for example, noted that 51 percent of freshmen at Yale University passed a fitness test in 1950, but the rate had fallen to 43 percent in 1956 and to 38 percent in 1960.[8] Kennedy argued that Europeans were outpacing Americans in physical fitness, and he hinted at a broader Cold War concern: that foreign forces were threatening the physical and mental well-being of the United States. In his 1958 *Masters of Deceit*, J. Edgar Hoover went much further in arguing that communism was a disease that required containment and quarantine to prevent it from spreading; Hoover believed that it was the Communist Party's "objective to drive a wedge . . . into as many minds as possible [by means] of thought control."[9] Liberals such as Hubert Humphrey and Adlai Stevenson bought into these medicalized discourses by likening communism to "a political cancer" (Humphrey) and fearing that its effects were worse than "cancer, tuberculosis and heart disease combined" (Stevenson).[10] Entanglements between illness and communism also arose in right-wing protests against the fluoridization of drinking water, resulting from fears that this was an insidious form of mass medication rather than an aid to dental hygiene.[11] These entanglements are best illustrated, however, by the backlash to the seemingly innocuous Alaska Mental Health Enabling Act of July 1956. The bill was intended to ensure that Alaska, soon to be the forty-ninth state in the Union, had its own healthcare facilities, which would mean that Alaskan patients would no longer have to travel to Portland, Oregon, to be treated. But the conservative and anticommunist American Public Relations Forum and L. Ron Hubbard's recently formed Church of Scientology thought that this was an attempt to form Siberian-style United Nations camps in the Alaskan wastes as a means to practice mind control on American citizens.[12]

For liberals, such entanglements often focused on the questionable political integrity and mental stability of Vice President Nixon, whom Arthur Schlesinger Jr. had dubbed a "streamlined McCarthy" as early as 1950.[13] Vance Packard used Nixon as an example of "a new breed of American politician," the incarnation of the "hidden persuader" who favored Madison Avenue sales techniques over plain speaking.[14] The brooding image of "Tricky Dick" was parodied and pilloried by Democrats, journalists, and cartoonists throughout the 1950s. For example, in a January 1960 *Washington Post* cartoon, "Mirror, mirror, on the wall . . . ," Herblock portrayed Nixon as the wicked witch from *Snow White and the Seven Dwarfs*, complete with cauldron, syringe, and poison as he prepares himself for the presidency. Glimmers of duplicity, corruption, thuggishness, and intolerance fueled negative perceptions of Nixon and heightened liberal fears that his would be the finger on the nuclear button, and, during the 1956 election campaign, Adlai Stevenson referred to Nixon as the "guardian of the hydrogen bomb."[15]

That campaign was business as usual, with Stevenson again losing to the Eisenhower-Nixon ticket, but there was enough unease among some voters to suggest that Eisenhower's organized society was not as stable as he hoped. Along with liberals who wanted to see more progressive action in Washington, Herblock satirized Eisenhower as the captain of a rudderless boat in a 1956 cartoon titled "Ever Thinking of Starting the Motor?," in which healthcare disappears into the scribble at the bottom of the president's sail, underneath trade, foreign aid, schools, and civil rights. Cultural schisms also became more widespread in the second half of the decade. The emphasis on typicality, homogeneity, and averageness that lay behind public-relations spin and business speak, for example, only partially masked growing divisions and disharmonies at work and home, which increased as a result of the worldwide economic slump of 1958 and rising unemployment levels. Advertising campaigns continued to promote suburbia as the ideal location for middle-class nuclear families, but social critics were observing that behind the white picket fences lay a host of sociological and psychological problems.

The discussion of *Bigger Than Life* in the previous chapter suggests that unrest and illness were felt by husbands, wives, and children alike, often resulting from the conflicting demands of work and home. To be sick in the 1950s, especially for any length of time or with any degree of severity, was often to lose a stake in the privileged order: it meant being treated differently, sidelined, or watched. Cold War fears hit another peak with the launch of the Soviet satellite *Sputnik* in 1957, and discourses of illness often overlapped with forms of dissidence that threatened the Cold War ideal of a consensual and unified nation. Jacqueline Foertsch notes that the year *Sputnik* was launched, the Polish émigré Albert Sabin was preparing an oral form of polio vaccine for national distribution (after testing it on citizens of Eastern bloc countries), thereby challenging Jonas Salk's heroic stature as medical pioneer and adding a "polio gap" to the "missile gap."[16] Other evidence points to links between *Sputnik* and the rise of hyperactivity among schoolboys. Ritalin had been available since 1955 to treat behavioral disorders among children, but hyperactivity was first given a name in 1957

"Ever Think Of Starting The Motor?"

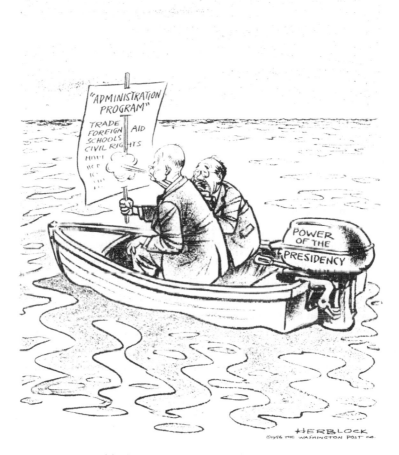

FIGURE 6.1   Herblock, "Ever Think of Starting the Motor?," *Washington Post*, 16 July 1956. © The Herb Block Foundation.

("hyperkenetic impulse disorder") and was arguably exacerbated the following year by the National Defense Education Act, when talented young boys were identified as the scientific brains of the future in an effort to combat Soviet prestige in the fields of science and technology.[17]

As we have seen, the workplace and the home were the privileged spaces of the organized society. Domestic containment in the home was often linked closely to the logic of the workforce, where illness could be accommodated as long as there was a good likelihood of recovery. The previous chapter also demonstrated the ways in which the workplace and home frequently became constraining topographies, often heightening anxiety or suffocation rather than facilitating the good physical health and healthy-mindedness that gurus such as Norman Vincent Peale advocated. However, as I discuss here, the middle-class norms that were reinforced in the white-collar workplace and the ideal suburban home often revealed liminal spaces within seemingly safe topographies. This can be seen in the cinematic interest of Douglas Sirk, Nicholas Ray, and Alfred Hitchcock in boundaries (windows, doors, and corridors) that opened up contained domestic spaces to neuroses and illnesses. Cracks within public spaces can also be detected in the ways in which "the ground rules of social interaction" that safeguarded "equilibrium" and "balance," as Erving Goffman put it in 1955, were increasingly challenged by different experiences and divergent voices later in the decade, exposing a more complex network of bodies, minds, and ideas than those legitimized by Eisenhower's organized society.[18]

The shift toward a quantitative notion of normality had begun to take hold in the late nineteenth century, but it was most closely linked to children's education in the 1910s and 1920s. The Child Health Organization and, after 1923, the American Child Health Association were responsible for a wave of post–World War I educational propaganda that linked psychological, educational, and intelligence testing to standard height and weight measurements, and the rapidly developing social sciences during World War II and the Cold War reinforced the use of "the normal" and "the average" as quantifiable terms.[19] But the myth of normality met criticism from C. Wright Mills, Paul Goodman, and others who questioned how rigidly this model could be applied, particularly to health and illness. A 1952 report by the Michigan Department of Mental Health, for example, revealed that 20 percent of the children in a regular school in Battle Creek, Michigan, had mental health problems: 2 percent were "seriously disturbed and in need of clinical treatment," while 17 percent were "maladjusted but only to a degree treatable in school facilities."[20] And in 1958, a *Ladies' Home Journal* article titled "How Neurotic Are You?" juxtaposed "normal people" ("those who grow up to focus their energies on main problems") with neurotics (who "dissipate much of [their] energy in emotional conflicts").[21] The article argued that "the neurotic process" is actually central to human development but is more often displayed by particular "types," including bachelors, spinsters, people with low IQs, and women prone to emotional stress. The piece links normality to good citizenship among married couples, parents, and college graduates, but it also suggests that neurosis lies on a continuum, lacks rigid boundaries, and is a condition to which anyone could be susceptible.

Although some exponents of popular psychology and sociology questioned the polarities of health and sickness, the most influential postwar psychiatric text—the first edition of the *Diagnostic and Statistical Manual of Mental Disorders* (1952), which came to be known as *DSM-I*—helped to institutionalize a rigid definition of normality and (perhaps unintentionally) stigmatized any behavior outside tightly controlled norms. *DSM-I* was established to overcome the confusion of psychiatric categories during World War II, particularly in the US Army—which decided to depart from the 1933 framework, *Standard Classified Nomenclature of Disease*, in an attempt "to express present day concepts of mental disturbance."[22] Psychiatric terms proliferated in the 1940s to such a degree that the chair of the American Psychiatric Association's Committee on Nomenclature and Statistics, George Raines, acknowledged that by 1948 the profession had reached a "point of confusion" similar to that of the 1920s.[23] However, this did not mean that the remedy, *DSM-I*, was immune to historical forces: the fear that deviancy might lead to social disorganization in the early 1950s crept into taxonomies, especially in relation to personality disorders, schizophrenia, "sexual deviation," and addiction. Although *DSM-I* was intended to improve diagnosis (the National Institute of Mental Health was to oversee treatment guidelines), it served to reinforce rigid medical categories that left little room for a broad spectrum of experience. The backlash against the work did not begin until its second edition was published in 1968, when homosexuality was again included as a mental disorder, but there were tensions between psychiatric nomenclature and other psychological and sociological models throughout the 1950s and early 1960s.

DSM-I tended to elide descriptive and evaluative categories and blurred social and biological conditions, but John Spurlock argues that tensions between psychiatry and developmental psychology after World War II revealed a broadly contested terrain that challenged binary categories.[24] These strains were closely linked to collective experiences and identity positions that did not have a privileged place in the social order, particularly two topics where sociology and medicine overlapped: homosexuality and juvenile delinquency.

DSM-I viewed homosexuality as a personality disturbance in conflict with dominant modes of sexual orientation. This belief was underlined by a number of social trends, among them J. Edgar Hoover's campaign to root out homosexual "sex offenders" in the late 1930s; the belief in the US Army and Navy during World War II that homosexuality was a "constitutional psychopathic state"; and federal mechanisms to disqualify homosexuals from serving via the Selective Service System (despite Harry Stack Sullivan's argument that sexual orientation should not affect a soldier's fitness to serve).[25] However, the postwar years also gave rise to tensions between practitioners who viewed homosexuality as the "malfunction of the endocrine glands" and those who saw it as a developmental phase through which many teenagers pass; according to this view, because adolescent groups tended to be homosocial, transitional friendships were seen as an important part of growing up.[26] Until the early 1960s, homosexuality in adulthood was widely deemed to be pathological, but homosexual leanings in adolescence could be "normal, transitory, and harmless," sometimes leading to fleeting homoerotic attachments—particularly among young soldiers stationed together for long periods.[27]

These tensions between psychiatry and developmental psychology suggest that "the normal" versus "the pathological" is actually too simplistic a model to describe the psychosocial terrain of the 1950s, particularly when we consider such impassioned attacks on averageness as the following quotation from 1949: "The 'average man' would be a sensationally horrible freak of nature if ever he should be created. He would be a more vague and inhuman shape than the most unrecognizable composite photograph, fuzzy in outline and possessed of more features than anyone ought to have."[28] This Frankensteinian depiction of the "average man," written in response to Alfred Kinsey's *Sexual Behavior in the Human Male* (1948), was a passionate defense of uniqueness and variety in the inner lives of Americans and suggests that the impulse to classify was only one trajectory within the social sciences. Critics since the late 1960s have regularly expressed concern that the institutional weight of *DSM* helped to normalize "the conservative view of homosexuality as pathology," rigidify clinical categories, and standardize what others saw as part of a developmental curve.[29] This criticism can be traced back to the late 1950s, when psychological testing—such as the series of Rorschach and Thematic Apperception tests carried out by psychologist Evelyn Hooker in 1957—helped to challenge this binary model. In her groundbreaking paper "The Adjustment of the Male Overt Homosexual," Hooker reported that clinicians could not readily identify a specific sexual orientation when they came to analyze images drawn by a sample of sixty nonclinical heterosexual and homosexual subjects.[30] Hooker's challenge to the Cold War view of personality as fixed, or the "enduring patterns of perceiving, relating to, and thinking about the environment and oneself" (to use *DSM*'s words) contributed to disagreements among psychiatrists and psychologists about adolescent behavior and sexual practice.[31]

The previous two chapters focused on work and home as the major modalities that defined national identity in the 1950s. In contrast, this chapter considers forces and discourses that put psychosocial organization under strain, particularly those linked to growing up and sexual orientation. This is less to suggest that the liberal therapeutic revolution of the 1960s (in which the youth, women's, and gay movements figured prominently) was on its way in the second half of the 1950s than it is to argue that challenges to medical normalization were close to the surface. Rather than being a consensual decade, the 1950s saw stability and instability, as well as normality and dissidence, exist in uneasy tension. These psychosocial tensions can be detected in the clinical literature, but they are most clearly in evidence in the cultural sphere. Fiction and film are the most helpful cultural forms here because they place these tensions within a narrative framework, tracing cause-and-effect sequences, the consequences of medical treatment and intervention, and the symbolic meanings of illness experiences. However, the more intimate cultural forms of poetry and personal letters (illustrated below in the discussion of Ginsberg's 1957 poem "Kaddish" and his journals) offer glimpses beneath the veneer of social and medical practices. So too does the popular press, which gave voice to a spectrum of opinions rather than agreeing on an official line. To recall the opening discussion of this chapter, Eisenhower's frail physical health and liberal concerns about Nixon's fitness for high office percolated through the later 1950s. In the same period, as the following sections demonstrate, we can clearly see that psychologists and cultural practitioners contributed to and intervened in medical debates.

Childhood and Growing Pains

When it was first published in 1946, Dr. Spock's *Baby and Child Care* placed children at the center of the postwar home. A regulated diet, a well-stocked medicine cabinet, and a clean house were seen as necessities to ward off childhood diseases like rheumatic fever and pneumonia. Two biological parents were also deemed essential to create a nurturing environment for their offspring, especially during the tricky ages of three to six.[32] Promotional campaigns for healthy suburban living reinforced the idealized middle-class family, and many doctors and child psychiatrists concurred, advocating a clean and caring environment as a central ingredient of a healthy childhood, together with good nutrition and immunization programs such as polio in the mid-1950s and measles in the early 1960s. Following a burst of research at the turn of the century into causes of infant mortality, deaths to babies and children dropped by 78 percent between 1910 and 1956; these declines were greater in areas that did not suffer from sanitation problems or overcrowding. But the downward trend in infant mortality slowed between 1950 and 1965, dropping just over 1 percent (before speeding up after 1965). In those years, deaths from pneumonia and influenza were at the same level as congenital abnormalities and a little behind premature births.[33]

A combination of scientific know-how and emotional engagement was essential for good child care, but Spock thought one could go too far with careful parenting, arguing that a parent who shows too much concern may affect a child adversely. He was more of a pragmatist than a champion of the family as filiarchy, though some critics have read *Baby and Child Care* as a text promoting "moderate permissiveness in childrearing techniques."[34] Spock realized that the family should not be rigidly organized but structured and flexible, allowing for different types of bonds and experiences—at least he certainly did by 1962, when he published *Problems for Parents*, a collection of his articles from *Ladies' Home Journal* that redress the child-centered view of *Baby and Child Care* by focusing on "quarrels [between parents], guilt about favoritism, resentment at interfering grandparents and difficult neighbors, doubts about comics, films, and television, the difficult of talking about death and sex, the frustrations of the housebound mother."[35]

Nevertheless, although many parents in the 1950s were wary about the negative effects of overmothering, the typical middle-class mother and father fulfilled tightly defined roles while accepting their children's individuality, as Christine Beasley advised in *Democracy in the Home* (1954). The promise that vaccines and antibiotics could banish perilous childhood illnesses and viruses meant that American homes were much safer than in the past, but many advocates of good parenting felt that family members had to abide by certain behavioral rules to maintain balance. Fears that the growing child could easily be thrown off track by an absent parent, inappropriate parental behavior, or bad habits picked up at school or on the street meant that the second half of the 1950s was more of a battleground than a safe haven for growing up, particularly with the acceleration of mass culture geared toward children and teenagers.

This normative model of family life, however, was at odds with the trajectory of developmental psychology, which focused on the maturing ego. In this respect, Erik Erikson and D. W. Winnicott recommended that parents should gradually increase their distance from the child as he or she matured, a view codified in Erikson's concept of the life cycle in *Identity and the Life Cycle* (1959), which posited a developmental learning curve through which the child moved en route to adulthood. Erikson's model offered an organic alternative to the mechanistic metaphors that dominated Cold War discourse, but he also suggested that maturation occurred through a gradual epigenetic process in which distinct character traits came to the fore at particular points in the life cycle. This smooth process of maturation might imply that Erikson, like Spock, was not interested in the jolts and sharp transitions of growing up, but Erikson detected that the movement from one phase to the next was through a series of experiential crises. He later called the moment of crisis "a crucial period of increased vulnerability and heightened potential," which might lead to "generational strength" but might also lead to "maladjustment" toward the family group or wider social milieu.[36] Erikson saw the life cycle as a dialectic in which two opposing polarities give rise to a particular ego quality: in early childhood the dialectic of "autonomy versus shame" gives rise to "will"; at play age, initiative and guilt give rise to "purpose"; industry and inferiority at school age contribute to "competence"; and so on through a series of eight stages, which taper off after adolescence.[37] It is easy to be critical of the universalism of these eight phases and the implication that the thresholds between stages are actually attainment goals, but Erikson's central focus was on ego development rather than the Freudian tensions between conscious life and the repressed unconscious. This developmental process starts in infancy, as the young child begins to understand the difference between "I" and "you"; toward its end are adolescents who define their egos through clothing, behavior, speech patterns, relationships, and social rituals.[38]

What happens if a child or adolescent is unable to resolve polarities at a particular stage of development is unclear in Erikson's schema. He was, however, as interested in the inhibiting factors in the development of a stable identity as he was intrigued by the self's adaptability. This might again suggest a normative model of development, in which opposing forces combine automatically to give rise to the next, more mature stage. In his defense, though, Erikson was sensitive to specific life stories and particularly interested in dislocation, migration (reflecting his own journey from Sweden to the United States in 1933), alternative cultures, and other conditions in which the individual's locality is disturbed. Erikson's memorable mantra "Change, Chance, Choice" might suggest a pioneering, optimistic spirit, but it also implies that certain aspects are beyond individual or group control and that unsettling experiences will often challenge ego development.[39] Crisis and adaptability are equally important for Erikson's life-cycle model; crises sometimes manifest themselves physically (for example, the frailty of posture in early childhood or bodily confusion in adolescence) and sometimes on a psychic level (such as the inability to distinguish reality from wish fulfillment or the breaking off a juvenile romantic attachment to a parent).

Erikson believed that activity was the key to health. However, this did not necessarily mean physical activity (although he probably worried about the passivity induced by the prominent place of the television in the 1950s home), as children can "actively stay put" and "actively hide" through shared experiences or play. Erikson argued that "patienthood" is usually "a condition of inactivation" brought on by invasive forces.[40] On this point he concurred with Spock in his belief that creativity and activity were essential ingredients of health—a view that led Spock to come down on the side of television as "the greatest educational force that has appeared since schools were established and printing was invented."[41] Although Spock noted that children often grow up with very different temperaments from their parents, both he and Erikson were concerned about negative patterning during the Cold War, which could undermine healthy ego growth, create feelings of disorientation, or lead to "a failure of nerve."[42] In his work at the University of California at Berkeley and, beginning in the early 1950s, at the Austen Riggs Center, in Stockbridge, Massachusetts, Erikson encouraged his young patients to create pathways for the emergence of their future selves. However, he realized that sometimes biology, kinship, and social forces are too immense to simply be overcome by force of will.

Erikson was drawn to romantic conceptions of an active and expressive self, but he did not use the terms "innocence" and "experience" to characterize childhood and adulthood. This was at odds with advertising and television programs, both of which tended to idealize childhood innocence and brush over the pains of growing up. Other trends, though, suggested that growing pains were more intense for the postwar generation than for preceding ones. This was recognized at the Midcentury White House Conference on Children and Youth held in December 1950, at which participants agreed that the passage from childhood to adulthood was not easy, particularly for those brought up in deprived environments or living with disabilities. Conference themes included the importance of a healthy personality, self-respect, and responsible parenting, but the delegates also recognized the need for local education boards to "accept full responsibility for providing adequately for the education of children with physical and mental handicaps," particularly as three-quarters of counties lacked adequate provision of special care.[43]

The conference took a much broader view of the child's world than Erikson did in his rather abstract epigenetic model. Some delegates—such as Spencer Crookes, director of the Child Welfare League of America—noted that child welfare and adoption policies had improved since the war. But Crookes stated: "I do not see how the conference can avoid the question of what war, even cold war, is doing to children and to family life."[44] These comments were reflected in President Harry Truman's speech to the delegates, in which he noted that "we cannot insulate our children from the uncertainties of the world" and asked parents to be vigilant in facing the "moral and spiritual dangers that flow from communism."[45] Truman emphasized a mixture of self-reliance and a safe home, but rather than simply reinforcing healthy personality, the conference had, in Ann Hulbert's view, a secondary theme of anxiety resulting from the specters of communism and war in Korea. Crookes's comments in 1950 about the worrying effects of the Cold War on children and the home were instructive, particularly as the Committee for the Study of War Tensions in Children was concerned about the effects of media on personality growth. Chapter 3 discussed the committee's view that nuclear defense films such as *Duck and Cover* provoked anxieties and insecurities in children, potentially leading the young toward the kind of anomie or nihilism that was exemplified by the teenage gang leader Artie West in the youth film *The Blackboard Jungle*. In the film, West claims he has been led to a life of crime because the alternatives are conscription or obliteration.

Although the twin themes of healthy personality and social anxiety at the 1950 conference blurred at times, the call to provide for child welfare was both welcome and worrisome, given the slow pace of advance in the previous twenty years. The Children's Charter, created after the 1930 White House Conference, emphasized the need to safeguard the child's "personality as his most precious right"; the Child Welfare League, established in 1921, focused on care inside and outside of the home. League members remained concerned, however, about facilities for African American children: significant differences in black and white child welfare were prevalent in northern cities; institutions for African Americans in Louisiana were overcrowded and poorly staffed; there were three times as many hospital beds in Florida for white children than for black; and black children in Maryland who were diagnosed with mental illness were put "in institutions for delinquents or for the adult mentally ill" because there was no dedicated institution for them.[46] The social psychologist Kenneth Clark also spoke at the conference about the damaging effects of segregated classrooms on the aspirations and self-esteem of African American children, a view that directly informed the challenge to school segregation of the National Association for the Advancement of Colored People. There were modest improvements in welfare provision for African Americans during the 1950s. But in 1960, when another White House conference focused on the social opportunities available to children and teenagers, it appeared as if the 1950 conference had brushed over many of the most difficult social problems.

The two White House conferences tacitly reinforced the norms of the nuclear family and heterosexual citizenship, but the second conference realized that poverty and broken homes can have deleterious effects on the well-being of young children.[47] Divorce rates were fairly low, actually decreasing during the 1950s (marriages also dropped slightly, after the postwar boom) and then not rising significantly until the second half of the 1960s. A 1948 report suggested that the chances of divorce in childless marriages were dramatically higher than in marriages with children, while advice columns in the *Ladies' Home Journal* emphasized that the wife should accommodate herself to the sexual needs of her husband to sustain a happy marriage.[48] But the fact that births to unmarried women rose steadily during the 1950s suggests that the model two-parent family was not viable for many Americans, with almost 200,000 babies born to single mothers in 1957 alone. Rickie Solinger points out that single, pregnant young women in the 1950s were "treated as deviants threatening to the social order," even if the typical story for white and black mothers, and for middle-class and working-class single mothers, diverged quite considerably.[49] Solinger bases her reading on such comments as this one, from Sara Edlin, author of *The Unmarried Mother in Our Society* (1954): "[Society] regards illegitimacy as an inroad on the family's stability and permanency, and repels it by ostracizing the unwed mother."[50] If things were difficult for single and divorced mothers, they were even trickier for children who inherited the stigma of illegitimacy or who were caught up in an emotional and financial battle between warring parents. Partly in response to these patterns, the Child Welfare League issued a public statement in 1957 as a reminder that the child's needs were primary, pointing out that foster care and adoption are socially responsible courses of action for children who lack proper parental support (even though there was a dispute at the time about whether information on the child's biological parents should be released to adopting parents, for fear that the new parents might project anxiety and envy onto the child).[51]

Although the home could be a haven for a sickening child, many parents looked to supportive facilities in the community for help with children who reacted badly to their domestic situation or who were prone to extreme behavior. Child welfare centers have a long history, going back to the mid-nineteenth century and the Children's Hospital in Boston, with its Christian message of care and strict routine. From the 1920s onward, many centers carried forward progressive initiatives of personal hygiene and the fight against infant mortality.[52] For those lucky enough to live close to a welfare center or have the means to pay for private care, there was growing demand in the mid-1950s for treatment and supervision of maladjusted children, despite concerns that more harm than good could come of intervention by a psychiatrist or welfare officer.

One of the most interesting specialist schools was the Southard School, established in 1926 by the Menninger family in Topeka, Kansas, as an attempt to fill a care gap for children who had personality disorders or were suffering from emotional imbalance. Realizing that they would probably operate at a loss in terms of fees they could charge for young inpatients, the Menningers initially accepted children with many different conditions, many of them loosely diagnosed as schizophrenic. The Menningers became more selective in their admissions policies during the 1940s, shifting to children of "average and superior intelligence," and later focusing their "recruitment efforts on the unusually bright," with the option of using foster families to offer an alternative support network.[53] The Menningers did not have much experience with child psychiatry, though, and another center became the most public face of child care after the war: the Sonia Shankman Orthogenic School. The school was affiliated with the University of Chicago, which appointed Bruno Bettelheim, an Austrian émigré, as its director in 1944. Bettelheim's reputation for treating autistic children was to suffer following the publication of his 1967 *The Empty Fortress*, but his earlier publications *Love Is Not Enough* (1950) and *Truants from Life* (1955), sponsored by the National Institute of Mental Health, offered a progressive view of how the Orthogenic School could provide an alternative support structure for children with behavioral and emotional difficulties. The school neatly illustrates the tensions between authority and collaboration in postwar therapy. Like the Southard School, the residential Orthogenic School took in children of normal or higher-than-normal intelligence between the ages of six and fourteen, "free of physical disorder" but suffering "from severe emotional disturbances that have proved (or are expected to prove) beyond the reach of the common therapeutic techniques."[54]

In the opening pages of *Love Is Not Enough*, Bettelheim argues that routine or mundane behavior can actually turn out to be a child's most significant activities, but he was concerned that such activities can become skewed or distorted when "short-comings in [a child's] upbringing" or home environment conspire against him or her.[55] Clearly stating that he did not believe in any such thing as "a typical child," Bettelheim sought to help "severely damaged" children "solve those problems which prevented them from succeeding in life," with the aim of helping them return home within two years.[56] Practicing a mixture of preventive psychology, psychoanalysis, and the acting out of everyday activities (based on John Dewey's conception of progressive education), Bettelheim was eager to ensure that Orthogenic School personnel were "free of conflict" so as not to project unresolved neuroses onto already troubled children. The therapeutic goal was to help children better integrate themselves into their environment and to become more aware of their developing ego; an overprotective and cloying parent can be harmful to a child in setting up false expectations, but so too can unpredictable or absent parents, or an overcrowded environment.

Bettelheim viewed the opposing psychic forces within a young child from a perspective similar to Erikson's, but he also outlined different modes of behavior—ranging from withdrawal to acting out. Whereas René Spitz emphasized "mother-love" in his work at the University of Colorado (see chapter 5), Bettelheim stressed that love, however important, was often not enough for a troubled child. The Orthogenic School was not designed as a surrogate home, nor were the staff members there to take the place of parents, avoiding extreme forms of maternal approval or paternal censure in their interactions with the children. Although Erikson stressed developmental change, the key word for Bettelheim was "integration." This was a common-sense goal, but it was quite conservative as well.

A cynical reading of Bettelheim's practices might suggest that the children needed to accommodate to the Orthogenic School's regulations. It had an open-door policy and placed an emphasis on the children as active learners. But according to his biographer, Nina Sutton, Bettelheim idealized the therapeutic environment, was often at odds with the staff, sometimes skirted the truth (such as when he put bars on the windows to prevent his charges jumping out), and was drawn to stories with neatly packaged endings to help reduce the children's anxieties.[57] Readers experience *Love Is Not Enough* as a progressive view of educational psychology with a therapeutic aim of "living well with oneself and with others," accompanied by a series of realistic pictures (taken by the *Life* photographer Myron H. Davis) in which the group environment is given precedence over images of isolation, such as one photograph of a class where two children are slumped over their desks after "giving up in despair."[58] Readers at the time would have little evidence to doubt Bettelheim's account, but the description of the school in *Love Is Not Enough* and the four "successful" case studies presented in *Truants from Life* conflict against the realities of the school.[59]

Nevertheless, Bettelheim's account offered a riposte to Albert Deutsch's *The Shame of the States* two years earlier and, at least on the surface, chimed with those voices at the Midcentury White House Conference that wished to put child welfare center stage. And it was not just in the domain of literature that such reports could be encountered. In 1955, for example, an episode of the TV show *Confidential File* focused on a residential facility for emotionally disturbed children who "say no to life." Written by the journalist Paul Coates, *Confidential File* (1955–1959) was particularly interested in medical practice, looking to expose quackery and malpractice. But the 1955 episode "Childhood Mental Illness" had a largely positive tone, focusing on the Camino Real Hospital in Mountain View, California, and its therapeutic effects on a number of pre-psychotic children. The first half focuses on Judy, a young girl whose father is dead and whose mother has been committed to a mental hospital. Judy is not interviewed, so we rely on Coates and the Camino Real doctors to interpret her condition. She is described as being "alone with the rage that has so often been her companion, alone with her terror" as she destructively pushes toys and objects off a table. She is enveloped in a world of things rather than significant people: "Judy's world of play is one of rage and destruction and the doctor has no intention of pushing into that world, not yet." Coates feels that her condition results from a loss of "emotional sustenance," leading to a "warped" personality that cannot appreciate the care of her nurses. Following Erikson's and Bettelheim's emphasis on play, the program sees in Judy's play world a "special language" that gives a hint of her condition. Coates does not refer to Erikson's opposing modalities, but the music lightens as he announces that the "therapy has already begun" and outlines the beneficial effects of attentive care. Even though Camino Real operates "under the terrible handicap of inadequate facilities and insufficient trained personnel," the program upholds the belief that institutional care can provide an alternative to a broken home, especially as Judy starts to trust the nurses and expand her play world beyond objects.

Love Is Not Enough and the *Confidential File* episode provide optimistic pictures of pre-psychotic children, but there was an accompanying fear that some conditions could not be easily treated, particularly if left to progress for too long. Those difficult years between childhood and adolescence were a particular concern to both liberal psychologists like Erikson and Spock and Cold War conservatives. The Senate Subcommittee on Juvenile Delinquency, for example, was established in 1953 to investigate the role of mass media in the development of a criminal mind-set among the young. The anti-Freudian psychiatrist Fredric Wertham contributed to the subcommittee's investigation and capitalized on the "recurrent moral panic about youth behavior and mass culture" in his 1954 book *Seduction of the Innocent*, particularly expressing his view about the deleterious effects of comics and other forms of mass media.[60] Wertham's book did much to challenge the assumption that childhood was an innocent period not troubled by adult concerns. Rather, *Seduction of the Innocent* suggested that the child's mind could be manipulated and distorted by stories of crime, horror, and sexuality, especially when accompanied by suggestive pictures. Wertham was particularly concerned about horror comics, but he was even critical of superhero comics in which moral polarities are stable and starkly drawn: "This superman ideology is psychologically most unhygienic. . . . I have had cases where children would have had a good chance to overcome feelings of inferiority in constructive ways . . . if they had not been sidetracked by the fancied shortcuts of superman prowess."[61] Instead of offering instruction or life skills, Wertham believed that popular culture could invade the child's play world, erasing personal interaction with parents and siblings and provoking sadistic and aggressive fantasies.

Wertham reserved most of his criticism for comics, but he held television responsible for poor literacy rates, and he was concerned that some TV programs blended with the "worst aspects" of comic books.[62] Senator Estes Kefauver was also concerned that many children were watching programs intended for adults as well as those aimed at children; he felt that links might be found between viewing habits and delinquency. The congressional hearings of the mid-1950s were fueled by increasing concern about the causes of organized crime and led to "the mass media being placed on a list of twelve 'special areas' that were 'worthy of concentrated investigation because of their effects upon juvenile delinquency.'"[63] Kefauver received considerable media attention on this topic, especially in the lead up to his failed bid for the Democratic presidential nomination (he later became Adlai Stevenson's running mate). *Seduction of the Innocent* and the hearings jointly created a widespread suspicion of the harmful messages and effects of mass media. Wertham was sensitive to the "paradox" of the child—in the sense that life history in childhood is mutable and more inwardly experienced than in adulthood—but he contributed to a reactive culture in which the child's voice remained mute, overlain by medical and sociological discourses.[64]

Adolescence and Delinquency

The myth of childhood innocence did not vanish in the 1950s but was complicated by the medical, social-scientific, and journalistic studies discussed above. Plenty of examples of innocent children and teenagers can be found in the mass media; for every mischievous Beaver in the sitcom *Leave It to Beaver* (1957–1963) there was a David and Ricky Nelson in *The Adventures of Ozzie and Harriet* (1952–1966) who suffered very few growing pains and experienced a straightforward trajectory to marriage (their real-life fiancées and wives were written into the series). But despite these innocuous representations of childhood and adolescence, child psychologists and educators increasingly worried about the mental health of teenagers, with "behavior deviations" and "adjustment problems" usually stemming from home or school (one account estimated that such problems affected a quarter of schoolchildren in the late 1950s).[65]

These concerns had also worried reformers early in the twentieth century and gave rise to tensions between custodial and therapeutic forces in the development of juvenile institutions, which grew in number during the 1900s and 1910s.[66] Concern about the consequences of poor parenting increased in the subsequent decades: lack of authority could easily lead to delinquency and crime, whereas overprotective parents might stimulate new anxieties in their children or push them to rebel through "nagging and monotonous encouragement," according to a 1955 report from the Joint Committee on Health Problems in Education of the National Education Association and the American Medical Association.[67] This report codified children—using the categories of "the Nervous Child," "the Timid Child," "the Meddlesome Pupil," "the Unhappy Child," "the Poor Student," "the Antagonistic Child"—and coached parents in responding to different behavioral patterns. The concept of the "troublesome child" ran from the Illinois Juvenile Court Act of 1899 and turn-of-the-century debates about welfare and crime through to educational programs such as the Cambridge-Somerville Youth Study community program, established in Massachusetts in 1935 to prevent delinquency among boys five and thirteen years of age. Nevertheless, the widespread worry that a troublesome child would develop into a delinquent adolescent was a distinctly postwar phenomenon.[68]

In his sociological book *One Million Delinquents* (1955), the *New York Times* education reporter Benjamin Fine claimed that delinquency was on a tragic upswing in urban centers, and he anticipated that there would be two million delinquents in the United States by 1960. Fine adopted the rhetoric of disease from anticommunist discourse, asserting that delinquency would become a "national epidemic . . . unless this cancer is checked early enough, it can go on spreading and contaminate many good cells in our society."[69] Many youth movies released between 1955 and 1958 reflect this concern for the teenager. Even as early as 1944, *Youth Runs Wild*—a quasi-documentary film based on a *Look* article, "Are These Our Children?"—documented teenage crime in a small town during World War II and promoted "juvenile citizenship" as a key component of nation building. Most often youth movies took an adult view of the perils of delinquency, following a trajectory toward punishment and resolution through implied or actual conformity. However, the most interesting examples offered a more balanced view and contributed to a debate about what lay behind the inflammatory criminological term "delinquency." For example, Nicholas Ray's *Rebel without a Cause* starkly dramatizes generational conflict by portraying Jim Stark's search for an alternative network of support when communication with his parents breaks down at home. Much has been written about the homoerotic charge between Jim (James Dean) and Plato (Sal Mineo), his male friend, partly deriving from one of Ray's early stories; but a more useful medical context for the film is Robert Lindner's 1944 book of the same name, for which Warner Brothers had bought the rights in 1946.

Lindner—a psychologist at the US Penitentiary in Lewisburg, Pennsylvania; a criminologist at Bucknell University; and a practicing psychoanalyst—was particularly interested in the fact that psychopathology could be detected in up to 20 percent of prison inmates. Echoing Hervey Cleckley's *The Mask of Sanity*, published three years earlier (see chapter 2), Lindner claimed that psychopaths are the "truly dangerous, 'hard-boiled,' 'wise guy' and least reformable offenders," differing from psychotics only in the absence of psychic disorientation.[70] He was also interested in the psychological masks that teenagers adopt, which he claimed often lead to extreme forms of regressive psychopathology, not dissimilar to criminal behavior. Lindner thought that psychopathology is likely to arise if personal freedoms are jeopardized or denied: "The psychopath . . . is a rebel, a religious dis-obeyer of prevailing codes and standards . . . a rebel without a cause, an agitator without a slogan, a revolutionary without a program."[71]

Whereas Erikson saw growing up as a developmental pathway toward maturity, Lindner thought that the rebellious teenager is unable to look outside himself: "All his efforts, hidden under no matter what guise, represent investments designed to satisfy his immediate wishes and desires."[72] Ray's *Rebel without a Cause* is not an adaptation of Lindner's book. Rather, it pushes the book's introspective mood further: instead of advocating a return to strong parenting, it points out that Jim's parents are no more able to look outside themselves than Jim is. Chapter 2 discussed how film noir created dark, fractured spaces for exploring extreme psychological responses to deceit, betrayal, and violence. Elements of film noir fed into Hitchcock's and Ray's films of the mid-1950s (they both produced noirs at the beginning of the decade), but in the empty swimming pool of an abandoned mansion toward the end of *Rebel without a Cause*, we see a potentially liberating space. In the swimming pool Jim, Plato, and Judy (Natalie Wood) discover, on both imaginative and visual levels, the possibility of an alternative family structure and a refuge from the stifling pressures of growing up in a myopic and intolerant society. On one level, then, *Rebel without a Cause* is a sociological film about delinquency; on another level, it explores the ambiguous social, psychic, and sexual spaces of the 1950s teenager at arm's length from parents and psychiatrists.

Lindner's dramatic prose was at odds with the more subtle depiction of youthful relationships in Ray's film. Indeed, when Lindner came to address widespread teenage rebellions in his 1954 Hacker Foundation Lectures, published as *Must You Conform?*, he resorted to rhetorical excess. Following his 1953 *Prescription for Rebellion*,

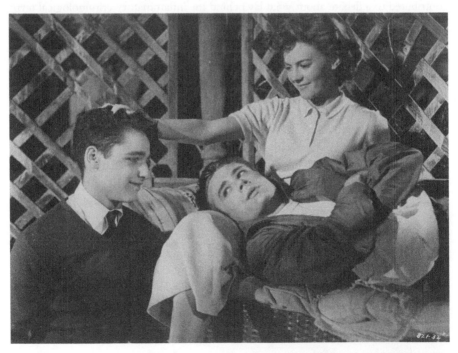

FIGURE 6.2   Jim (James Dean), Judy (Natalie Wood), and Plato (Sal Mineo) find their own space in an abandoned mansion. *Rebel without a Cause* (Nicholas Ray, Warner Brothers, 1955).

Lindner portrays young Americans as mutineers who "act out" their "inner turmoil"; they experience "a weakening or decay of psychic inhibitors, of mechanisms of control and restraint, so that their experience of teenage turbulence is immediately translated into overt behavior."[73] In his earlier book, Lindner used distinctly pathological language ("a sickness that destabilizes our civilization and immobilizes the hands that should cure it"), and he attacked the tendency to help individuals "adjust" to the present climate.[74] This destructive response to the Cold War climate is also a central theme in his Hacker Foundation Lectures, through which Lindner weaves medical, existential, and moral threads.

Paralleling the insight of J. D. Salinger's teenage character Franny Glass in her claim that going "bohemian" can be just be as fake as conforming, Lindner did not see rebellion as the antithesis to an accommodating other-directed personality, but as another version of conformity.[75] In their "abandonment of privacy," postwar teenagers adopt "a mass mind . . . a mind without subtlety, a mind without compassion, a mind, finally, uncivilized."[76] Lindner again conjures the figure of the psychopath driven by primitive desires, leading him to conclude that "the youth of the world today is touched with madness, literally sick with an aberrant condition of mind formerly confined to a few distressed souls but now epidemic over the earth."[77] Rather than contrasting the conformist with the deviant, Lindner argues that psychopathology often lies in mass behavior, "the slow and ominous advance of a psychic contagion."[78]

Lindner was not always so brash, though, and he was at his best in the case-study form. His interest in the disturbances of growing up found expression in a series of case studies he published in 1955 as *The Fifty-Minute Hour*. Abandoning the register of psychopathology, *The Fifty-Minute Hour* is sensitive to the therapeutic encounter in dealing with the "fragile web" of relationships that can often ensnare the individual into responding negatively or in self-destructive ways.[79] Instead of stressing the science of understanding the mind or the benefits of technology for extending human reach, psychoanalysis can offer "sympathetic comprehension" and "intimate, knowing communication between one being and the next."[80] For Lindner, in its emphasis on face-to-face communication and the tracing of life stories, psychoanalysis was a corrective both to the impersonality of mass society and to extreme forms of behavior that can spill over into psychosis.

The case study "Songs My Mother Taught Me" exemplifies Lindner's twin interests in criminality and adolescence. All five case studies in *The Fifty-Minute Hour* (including the most well-known, "The Jet-Propelled Couch," which was made into a *Playhouse 90* television drama for CBS in 1957) contain direct dialogue and close interaction between patient and analyst, but the narratives rely on Lindner's reconstruction of hidden stories. As with Bettelheim's idealistic account of the Orthogenic School, one might ask how real Lindner's cases are, but he was committed to getting close to the patient. In "Songs My Mother Taught Me" a late-teenage murderer, Charles, is initially described as possessing a "nonchalance and emotional flatness," combined with immature and inappropriate behavior.[81] He is held under psychiatric observation and diagnosed with "psychosis in remission, schizophrenia, with auditory hallucinations and homicidal trends," but this medical categorization does not offer an explanation for his criminal behavior.[82] A series of conversations reveals Charles's broken home, limited contact with his mother, and upbringing since the age of three in a sequence of religious orphanages, where he experienced sadistic beatings that pushed him to identify with his "tormentors" and to become what Lindner calls "an afflictor, delighting in giving pain."[83] Charles's antagonistic spirit is heightened when, at age eleven, he is plied with alcohol and beaten up by a gang. At thirteen he goes to live with foster parents on a farm, where he does odd jobs and is treated as little more than a farm animal before running away to find his mother. Charles is then sent to another home ("a way-station for youths who were expected to become criminals") and joins a vicious gang, soon becoming its leader.[84] He delights in victimization and bullying, often with a knife. When no more homes will take him, he rejoins his mother, but he drifts aimlessly before committing an opportunist murder of a young woman: he hits her sixty-nine times from behind with an ice-pick and then rapes her.

Intrigued by this case, Lindner started a course of analysis, surmising that his patient was living a "two-dimensional" existence, sealed off from the past. Avoiding hypnosis or narcotherapy for fear of precipitating another psychotic episode, Lindner realized that play techniques could have the most lasting effect on a young man who had not matured beyond his early stages. The bare outline of Charles's past helped to explain his murderous actions, but Lindner quickly learned that there is a lot more to the case. Through close interaction, the analyst stumbled on a clue to the patient's love-hate relationship with his mother. His interest in this medical box full of "tubes, vials, boxes, syringes, needles, capsules, clamps, pills, bottles" did not expose Charles as a secret drug addict; rather, it led Lindner to connect this to an earlier box belonging to his mother, which Charles had found when he was thirteen.[85] This box contained personal items, photographs, and letters (revealing Charles's father to be alive), together with his mother's wedding ring, on which he began to fixate. When living with his mother, Charles returned frequently to the box to finger the ring; one day, just before he is sent off to the farm, he plays with the ring, places it in his mouth, and uses it to masturbate. Afterward Charles is able to have sex with a prostitute only when he is in possession of the ring, which leads Lindner to conclude dramatically that he had undergone "layer after layer of further distortion—until he had become an adolescent, a veritable monster who could obtain satisfaction for his instincts and needs only through violence, perversion, and destruction."[86]

Although such moralizing language does not inflect his interactions with Charles, the closer Lindner comes to his patient's "secret," the more he feels his life is in danger, leading to the day when Charles grabs him by the throat. Charles is quickly removed to a mental hospital, but not before Lindner infers that the murder is a displaced act of aggression and an attempt by Charles to possess his mother. Rather than seeing this extreme behavior as aberrant, Lindner concludes that it stems from a lack of ego: "[Charles] became, for all intents, ego-less, an individual without a separate identity, hence a creature—not a person."[87] As Charles can express himself only through regression to childhood or extreme violence, Lindner realizes that the only effective therapy would be to help him to discover his ego—what Erikson would call path finding. However, this case implies that Charles is too deeply immersed in his psychosexual conflicts ever to be therapeutically released from them. In this way, "Songs My Mother Taught Me" is an instructive case study that reveals some of the deep-seated concerns about criminal behavior among adolescents, its complex causes, and the perils of a broken home. Lindner displays sympathetic understanding, but he nevertheless treats Charles as a puzzle to solve and seems unaware that he is digging up secrets that are likely to lead to a repeat of the murder, without techniques to protect against it.

On a broader level, this extreme story suggests a widening gulf between adults and teenagers, with the prewar youth of the adults seeming rosily innocent compared to the complexities that postwar teenagers were facing, and with cultural consumption (including television, comics, and rock 'n' roll) beginning to affect the psychology of the family. Many psychologists, including Bettelheim and Lindner, saw social integration as the therapeutic goal for emotionally scarred children and teenagers. But the psychologist Frank Riessman and others worried about the growing effects of child deprivation within urban communities (the proportion of "culturally deprived" children rose from one in ten in 1950 to one in three in 1960 in cities, partly due to migration, low socioeconomic status, and high percentages of orphans).[88] And still others, including Erikson, saw teenage rebellion as a necessary part of growing up, regardless of the stability of the family structure.

Writing in the mid-1960s, Bettelheim was concerned that adolescents could not test their "strength and vitality" because the silent generation of the 1950s gave them only a "vacuum" to push against, whereas David Riesman worried that adolescents who adjust to adulthood too readily are at higher risk of mental illness than those who rebel for a few years.[89] In a 1959 introduction to *The Vanishing Adolescent*, by the educator Edgar Z. Friedenberg, Riesman noted that "the American teen-ager, able to anticipate adulthood, so to speak, on the instalment plan, gives up too readily his search for significance, settling . . . for a pliable and adjusted blandness."[90] Friedenberg realized that there is no neutral word to describe late childhood and young adulthood: the term "teen-ager" (spelled with a hyphen at the time) is often patronizing, while "adolescence" is bound up with bourgeois discomfort toward amorphous sexuality, intensely personal behavior, and the morally corrosive effects of delinquency. Friedenberg was broadly in favor of adolescent self-expression and critical of the adult world, which he describes as being medically tranquilized:

> A society which has *no purpose* of its own, other than to ensure domestic tranquillity by suitable medication, will have no use for adolescents, and will fear them; for they will be among the first to complain, as they crunch away at their Benzedrine, that tranquilizers make you square. It will set up sedative programs of guidance, which are likely to be described as therapeutic, but whose apparent function will be to keep young minds and hearts in custody till they are without passion.[91]

For Friedenberg, this kind of overmedication leads to a soft, plastic culture that encourages the rise of the other-directed character type outlined in *The Lonely Crowd*. The problem of growing up among a tranquilized generation is that a young person who speaks out is often seen as dissident, whereas secrecy is linked to disaffection and conspiracy. Nevertheless, writing at the end of the 1950s, Friedenberg believed that the "adult empire" was "tottering" and would soon make way for "increasingly democratic relationships," in which differences between adults and teenagers were already starting to blur through new modes of interaction. Indeed, conflict could actually be seen as a positive rather than a merely destructive force; according to Erikson's model, conflict might lead to a "higher synthesis" away from the containment and cooperation of the Eisenhower years.[92]

Friedenberg's study importantly locates within adolescence two qualities that were commonly denied to the young: "the capacity of tenderness toward other persons" and "the respect for competence."[93] Rather than downgrading tenderness to a facet of immature and transitional relationships, Friedenberg saw evidence of empathy, mutuality, and heightened perception that are often lost in the working lives of adults; the villain, according to him, is not wayward youth but "hostile social processes" that either goad the adolescent "into hostile action" or overwhelm teenagers and lead to weak or restricted egos.[94] Simply put, Friedenberg worried that discipline, intolerance, and misunderstanding can force the young into accepting a predetermined course. Recalling Erikson's epigenetic model of crises and path finding, only an autonomous agent—one who is able to feel for others, develop competencies, and think for him- or herself—can develop an ego robust enough to carve a course between conformity on the one hand and self-destructive rebellion on the other.

Friedenberg's book offered a positive, at times romanticized, version of the American adolescent with the rare capacity to be "spontaneous, emotionally responsive, and genuinely interested."[95] He cherished self-expression and the capacity of the young to represent themselves in new and challenging ways, but he realized that the child needs to develop a strong ego to help facilitate what Erikson called an "ego identity."[96] Friedenberg was critical of the myopia of schools and other institutions that erode such capacities, but that does not mean that he underestimated the importance of schools for providing important educational building blocks. However, *The Vanishing Adolescent* steers a course between outlining, on the one hand, a therapeutic culture that could help nurture authentic teenagers and identifying, on the other hand, those social ills—crime, alcoholism, and drug addiction—to which teenagers can often fall prey without supportive structures. Friedenberg pays some attention to class differences, but overall he presents a generalized picture of (largely male) late 1950s adolescents, who are in danger of vanishing because there is nothing tangible against which they can define themselves. This stark picture of wasted youth tallied with Paul Goodman's strident claim in *Growing Up Absurd*, published a year later, that "our abundant society is at present simply deficient in many ways of the most elementary objective opportunities and worth-while goals that could make growing up possible."[97]

As the next chapter explores, issues of class and race came increasingly to the fore in reports and studies in the late 1950s and early 1960s, even if most sociological and psychological studies continued to focus on the "typical teenager"—as did a March 1958 *Ladies' Home Journal* article on "Our Teen-Age Drug Addicts." The article's authors pointed out that delinquency most commonly appears in "crowded neighborhoods" in big cities around the age of sixteen: "The typical teen-ager user lives in a poor neighborhood, where family life is disrupted, where the population is deprived and disorganized."[98] The use of the word "disorganized" here is interesting, given the emphasis that the Eisenhower administration placed on social and family organization as the foundation of a healthy environment. The article notes that no long-range study had been written about teenage addiction; most previous work focused on alcoholism and addiction in later life. The authors argue that there are no clear links between delinquency and addiction, but they also note that when addiction arises, it is often due to lack of recreational facilities, inadequate schooling, and meager job prospects. They point to the example of the Riverside Center in New York as a unit offering a halfway house for up to 140 young addicts, but requiring additional psychiatrists and social workers to bring about a "lasting cure." The article called for infrastructural improvements, but it also acknowledged that young addicts must "resist the invitation to oblivion" offered by drugs.[99]

Such interest in drug and alcohol use among teenagers indicated a shift in focus on adolescents at the end of the decade. The overriding theme of juvenile delinquency at the 1960 White House Conference on Children and Youth marked the move away from a psychological interest in the damaged child and his or her parental relationships toward an appraisal of "the inability or unwillingness of the existing social, economic, and political system to offer impoverished youth a legitimate chance for a decent standard of living" (this viewpoint contributed to the passing of the Juvenile Delinquency and Youth Offenses Control Act in September 1961).[100] This trend also refocused attention on class and race, but the shift toward a sociological and educational perspective overlooked the elisions that still existed in some clinical circles, such as the assumed link between alcoholism and homosexuality and the psychological dynamics of "growing up absurd," as Goodman called it in 1960, in which adolescent sexuality was often at odds with stable gender roles.[101]

Sex and Sexuality

Delinquency among 1950s teenagers was often linked to gangs and crime, but it was also often—either explicitly or implicitly—related to sex. When rock 'n' roll emerged in the early 1950s, many adults feared that the new, heavily rhythmic musical style would unleash latent sexual energy among the young that would be impossible to control, as portrayed in the genre of teenpic movies that began around 1955. Thomas Doherty argues that, despite their common subject matter, teenpics are hard to classify; within a single film, positive expressions of youthful exuberance and the need to retain parental discipline were often at odds with each other. The liberal message in *The Blackboard Jungle* (released a year after *Brown v. Board of Education* made classroom segregation unconstitutional) is that the teacher, Mr. Dadier, must find a way of bridging traditional methods of education and the interests of his racially mixed class. This message was flanked, on the one hand, by a scrolled warning at the beginning of the film stressing that this dysfunctional school was not typical of the US educational system and, on the other hand, by the violent reaction of young movie audiences in the United States and United Kingdom (ripping up cinema seats in some venues) that closely identified with the rebellious characters.[102] Although teenpics often emphasized normative heterosexuality as a precondition for a stable marriage and family (Dadier's safe marriage and his wife's pregnancy are threatened by hate messages sent by Artie West, the worst of the delinquents), within the transition from childhood to adulthood were conflicting sexual energies, frustrations, and desires to which discourses of normality could not do justice.

Cold War suspicions did much to regulate sexual identities, particularly when rumors at the end of the 1940s suggested that a large number of employees in the State Department were homosexual. Within a culture of "homosexual panic" (a term introduced to psychiatry by Edward Kempf in 1920 and then codified in *DSM-I* in 1952), Republicans claimed that "sex perverts" and "sex deviants," as they called them, were a threat to national security—a trend to which McCarthy was to add his voice, claiming that both communists and homosexuals were "twisted mentally or physically."[103] The fear that homosexuals and other dissidents were lurking unsuspected in Truman's government led many Americans to express their unease about what two *Saturday Evening Post* writers called "creeping neurosis" in the July 1950 article "Why Has Washington Gone Crazy."[104] Political and moral malaise was often linked to psychopathology, particularly by right-wing critics who feared a "homosexual-Communist conspiracy" that would lead to sexual anarchy and possibly the complete breakdown of social order.[105] Despite the political intentions of such claims, Kyle Cuordileone observes that these concerns unintentionally helped to bring homosexuality to public attention, combining with Alfred Kinsey's reports of 1948 and 1953 to reveal a much more variegated sexual landscape than many Americans, both conservatives and liberals, could tolerate.

Although normative sexuality was reinforced throughout the 1950s in the form of the nuclear family and strictly demarcated gender roles in the white-collar workplace, a range of sexual orientations became more visible due to the waning of censorship in the film industry, newly sexualized fiction, and media chatter. Representations were frequently conflicted, though, and explorations often tentative. One good example of this mode is Robert Anderson's quasi-autobiographical 1953 play *Tea and Sympathy*, directed on Broadway by Elia Kazan and made into a film by Vincente Minnelli in 1956. The film version of *Tea and Sympathy* tells the coming-of-age story of the seventeen-year-old schoolboy Tom Lee (John Kerr). We are told early on that Tom's parents divorced when he was five (in the tricky age range that Erikson and Spock warned about), and that he had been brought up by a maid—that is, until his father fired the maid after finding out that she has taught Tom how to sew and cook. Sent to a New England boys' school, Tom finds that his love of poetry, music, and the theater sets him apart from the other boys, who are interested in sports and male bonding. Overseen by the housemaster Bill Reynolds (Leif Erickson), the school has little room for alternative modes of behavior. Tom finds an outlet by befriending Laura Reynolds (Deborah Kerr), the housemaster's lonely wife (in the play, in contrast to the film, Tom's friend is a young male teacher who is dismissed for purportedly bathing naked with the schoolboys). Tom and Laura have both suffered loss: Tom's mother is dead, Laura's eighteen-year-old husband was killed during the war. When the other school-boys discover Tom sewing with the faculty wives on the beach, they name him "sister boy" (he is called "Grace" in the play) and seek to humiliate and bully him because he is not a member of the "Subcommittee on Masculinity," which Reynolds jokes about with the other "regular fellas." Tom's misery is compounded by the sadistic house-master and Tom's weak and disapproving father (who also wants him to be a "regular guy"), and his position in the school becomes less and less tenable—particularly when Laura is forced to withdraw her affections when she realizes that Tom is danger of falling in love with her.[106]

The film suggests that Tom confuses his need for maternal care with romantic love, which he tries to act out with Laura. When she points out the impossibility of an affair, Tom mistakes this as another rejection—or a "sending away," as he describes it—that directly echoes his childhood experience. In desperation, Tom attempts to prove his manhood with a local café girl, but he spirals into depression and tries to take his life, just as Laura's marriage falls apart under the weight of her husband's

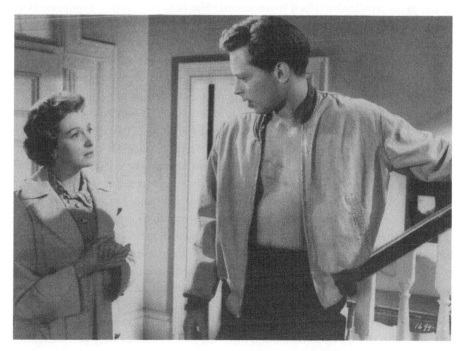

FIGURE 6.3 Laura Reynolds (Deborah Kerr) offers sympathetic words to the bullied Tom Lee (John Kerr). *Tea and Sympathy* (Vincente Minnelli, MGM, 1956).

constrained gender role. In a story marked by melancholy and loss, Tom's sexuality is less important than the long-term effects of an absent mother and an intolerant boys' school obsessed with masculinity. Laura's tenderness toward Tom is physically enacted one night in a nearby wood, paralleling the alternative imaginative space of the swimming pool scene in *Rebel without a Cause* (in Anderson's play, the scene occurs in the dormitory). This act offers Tom the self-worth that the educational system fails to provide, as well as an intimacy that looks beyond roles tightly defined in terms of gender and age (although, paradoxically, it confirms Tom's sexuality as "normal"). Interestingly, there are no figures of medical authority in the film; the counseling role falls to Laura, but she is expected in her position as a "faculty wife" to simply offer "tea and sympathy," and she is deterred by her husband from going too deeply into any of the schoolboys' teenage problems. The film's melodramatic mode also codifies Tom's potential homosexuality: it is framed in terms of an intolerant masculinist society embodied by the schoolboys, the macho practices of Bill Reynolds, and Tom's small-minded father, leaving Laura and the café girl as transitional relationships in Tom's heterosexual maturation. When we see Tom in the film's prologue and epilogue (not included in Anderson's play), he is presented as a well-adjusted adult and a published author who reflects on his youthful feelings for Laura, seemingly without many lasting psychological scars from his sadistic treatment.

This might suggest that cultural practitioners (especially film directors) were too nervous to deal with trends that pushed boundaries of acceptability, despite Elia Kazan's 1956 provocative (albeit heterosexual) film *Baby Doll* (with a Tennessee Williams script) and, six years later, Stanley Kubrick's adaptation of Vladimir Nabokov's 1955 novel *Lolita* (Kubrick was constrained by censorship laws to tone down the sexual obsession of a middle-aged academic for the fourteen-year-old Lolita). This conservative leaning is reinforced by Robert Corber's and Jackie Byars's readings of film noir and social problem films. Although both genres tackled challenging subject matter, the authors argued that the films tended to stigmatize homosexuality (Corber) and banished deviancy in favor of the "celebration of the family" (Byars).[107]

However, to see 1950s culture as simply reinforcing a model of sexual and family normalcy would be to simplify a broad spectrum of scientific enquiry and cultural representation in the decade, responding to a much longer tradition of interest in sexual interactions and their social, moral, and medical meanings. In the early twentieth century, such interactions were often charged with moralistic language, linked to the spreading of venereal disease or social ills associated with prostitution. The New York physician Prince Morrow, in his 1904 book *Social Diseases and Marriage*, tried to focus attention on science rather than ethics, but moral disorder and disease were commonly combined, even in Morrow's own work as an influential figure in the social hygiene movement.[108] The American Social Hygiene Association (formed in 1913 and soon afterward renamed as the American Social Health Association) promoted reproductive health and sex education, but it often did so with a missionary zeal, including one campaign for blood testing before marriage and another for chastity in young women. Reacting against such moralism, in the 1920s the National Research Council began to sponsor scientific research on the biology and physiology of sex, with a particular emphasis on hormones and genetics. This field of research provided the historical context for Alfred Kinsey's biological interest in sex, although his institutional home at Indiana University meant that his research was conducted at a remove from the National Research Council program.[109]

Kinsey's specialism was in classification and taxonomy, most clearly demonstrated in his extensive study of gall wasps in the 1930s and his book on a thousand species of plants and ferns, *Edible Wild Plants of Eastern North America* (1943). Although Kinsey was fascinated by the varieties of genetic types and was deeply interested in anatomy, physiology, and human sexuality, he was not a theoretical figure in the strictest sense. Nevertheless, through his two most famous books, *Sexual Behavior in the Human Male* (1948) and *Sexual Behavior in the Human Female* (1953), he became one of the most influential scientists of the postwar period, with the 1948 volume selling 200,000 copies in the first two months. Kinsey's initial stimulus was the dearth of published studies on sexuality, and he and his coauthors claimed that hitherto "we have been as handicapped as one might be if he attempted to understand the process of digestion before he knew anything of the anatomy of the digestive organs, or attempted to understand respiratory functions without realizing that the lungs and the circulatory system were involved."[110] Rather than publish a detailed clinical study on extreme cases of sexuality, Kinsey wanted to document common practices across a wide population sample. He pursued his projects rigorously and without an explicit social agenda, but his findings were anathema to moral crusaders, religious leaders, and those who argued that close relationships should be based on love, rather than sex.

Expanding the questionnaire-based approach of the decade-long study *Factors in the Sex Lives of Twenty-two Hundred Women*, published by the social reformer Katherine Bement Davis in 1929, Kinsey based his taxonomic study of sexual variety on a detailed interview format and sampling surveys. In 1941 he received funding from the Rockefeller Foundation (the foundation had sponsored the social hygiene movement in the 1920s) that enabled him to assemble a team of researchers, consult with specialists, and travel widely across the country in the 1940s. Paul Robinson calls the recorded interview "Kinsey's most brilliant creation, an authentic tour de force in which every scrap of sexual information available to memory was wrenched from the subject in less than two hours."[111] Rather than pure biology or a fixed identity position constrained by birth, sex and sexuality became lived experiences that could be recorded. Kinsey looked for consistency of response and tried to iron out exaggerations and understatements across a range of over five thousand interviews for each book, but some detractors claimed that his data was skewed "to heighten the prominence of 'deviant' behavior."[112] Kinsey was eager to be comprehensive in his sampling (although most of his interviewees were white), but he was not as concerned about repressed experiences or transference between interviewee and interviewer as a Freudian researcher would have been.

A number of critics, including psychiatrists and psychoanalysts, complained that Kinsey's view of sex was too narrowly mechanistic; instead of addressing issues of fantasy and neurosis, he reduced dreams to simplistic versions of wish-fulfillment or aversion scenarios, and he favored a biological model of health based on sexual outlets.[113] Although he was interested in the interviewee's voice, Kinsey largely ignored the psychodynamics of the interview scenario and relied heavily on statistical data. But in the scale of his research, he looked beyond typical or mean responses and refused to buy into rigid definitions of sexuality in order to assess how environmental factors condition individuals to restrain from or partake in certain kinds of sexual activity. Rather than pathologizing homosexuality, Kinsey used variety and variance as his guiding lights, revealing a continuum of sexual practice that challenged respectable gender models and exposed activities deemed peripheral or dangerous to the sanctity of marriage. Kinsey's findings did not go unfiltered into the public domain, however: the *Journal of the American Medical Association* commissioned two reviews (one was positive, the other critical) of Kinsey's second volume, and the *Ladies' Home Journal* popularized his findings, but, as Jessica Weiss notes, the "message of similarity" between the sexes "remained muted, drowned out by experts who . . . classified women's sexual responses as more emotional than physical and slower to develop than men's."[114] The backlash, particularly to the volume on women, stemmed from the evidence that sexual practices were more plentiful and diverse than commonly represented, together with Kinsey's tendency to downplay the emotional dimension of sex.[115] Published three years before Grace Metalious's best-selling *Peyton Place* looked behind the façade of middle-class respectability in a small New Hampshire town, Kinsey's second report, on female sexuality, was so controversial that the threat of a congressional inquiry led the Rockefeller Foundation to withdraw its funding in 1954.

For many mainstream commentators, Kinsey was a dangerous libertarian, a view fueled by his public statements on the variety of sexual practices and his 1949 argument to the California Subcommittee on Sex Crimes that sex offender laws needed limiting.[116] However, for homosexual communities Kinsey was a sexual liberator, and his work offered an intellectual bulwark against aversion therapy—widely practiced in the 1950s, especially in response to homosexuality, transvestism, and alcoholism. Guided by tenets of behaviorism and Ivan Pavlov's laboratory work on conditioning, the aversion therapist used mechanical, chemical, or electrical stimuli to turn an individual's positive triggers into negative ones, focusing particularly on erectile stimulation. Problems with patients becoming acclimatized to mild electrical shocks led some therapists to use stronger shocks or a combination of techniques. Aversion therapy was practiced in both the United Kingdom and United States. Its results were mixed, but it was clear that this kind of therapy veered toward authoritarian punishment; such a reeducation of the senses put self-worth at risk, even for patients who volunteered for the therapy.[117]

Kinsey's first book provided evidence that 37 percent of men had some homosexual experience, evidence that led the Californian erotic writer and tattoo artist Samuel Morris Steward (an "unofficial collaborator" on the male sexuality book) to claim in 1983 that Kinsey "blasted the country wide open," raising consciousness about sexual practices and provoking discussion in the mass media.[118] According to

Steward, Kinsey became a savior figure for gay communities in Chicago and Los Angeles, and an antidote to the police control that Steward links closely to the intolerance during the McCarthy period. Such state-sponsored control can be traced back to a number of political moments: Undersecretary of State Sumner Welles's resignation in 1943 from Roosevelt's administration, following rumors of his homosexual activity in Cuba and with African American train porters; the strict control of Truman's National Security loyalty program of 1947; and Eisenhower's ban on "sex perverts" becoming federal employees in his Executive Order 10405 in 1953.[119] Given these Cold War concerns about loyalty and dissidence, and the fear that homosexuality might spread like an epidemic (Senator Kenneth Wherry claimed that "one homosexual can pollute a Government office"), it was not surprising that there was a congressional investigation into Kinsey after he published *Sexual Behavior in the Human Female*.[120]

After the publication of the book on the human male, Kinsey acquired a reputation for seeking out interviews with onanists and sadomasochists, as well as drug addicts, criminals, hustlers, and artists such as the art curator Monroe Wheeler, novelist Gore Vidal, poet Allen Ginsberg, playwright Tennessee Williams, filmmaker Kenneth Anger, composer Ned Rorem, and dancer Ted Shawn.[121] Many thought that interview subjects drawn from homosexual and artistic subcultures skewed Kinsey's sample away from middle-class norms and practices. But although commentators have questioned the validity of Kinsey's sample, the neutrality of his interview techniques, and his hobby of collecting erotica (some of it was shipped from Europe), his overriding interest was to develop an alternative classification system for sexual variation, particularly for homosexuality, which remained coded as a mental disorder by *DSM* until 1973.

Kinsey's links with the Beat writers offered a potent interface between science and the arts that resisted the centripetal cultural pull of the mid-1950s. His initial contact was with Herbert Huncke, a key figure in the criminal underworlds of Chicago and Manhattan in which drugs, petty crime, prostitution, and diverse forms of sexuality were intertwined. When Kinsey met him in New York City in 1945, Huncke gave him a number of interviews (the first cost Kinsey $10), which he described as a form of therapeutic unburdening "of many things that I'd long been keeping to myself," including homosexual encounters as a young boy.[122] Huncke introduced Kinsey to a number of interview subjects who lived around Times Square, including William Burroughs and the young Allen Ginsberg.[123] Ginsberg thought that Kinsey was a pioneer in the emerging "sexual revolution" and believed that he needed statistics to preserve his scientific "credibility" (Ginsberg agreed to be filmed with his lover, Peter Orlovsky, and went back to the Sex Institute in Indiana in the mid-1960s for that purpose).[124]

Ginsberg was an important contact for Kinsey and is an appropriate figure to bring the diverse currents in this chapter together for three main reasons: the emergence of his homosexuality at an early age; his relationship with his mother and her mental illness; and his attempts to develop a mode of self-expression that would bypass normative categories. Ginsberg realized that he was gay at nineteen (if not before), at which time he had his first homosexual experience and an erotic liaison with Jack Kerouac on the Manhattan waterfront.[125] He was more sexually active in his early twenties, but initially he felt uncomfortable with his sexuality and often sordid. He even wrote to the radical therapist Wilhelm Reich and consulted a Reichian therapist in Newark, New Jersey, for three months before they parted because of Ginsberg's insistence on smoking marijuana.[126] Increasingly unhappy (and after being charged for petty crime), in 1949 Ginsberg entered the Columbia Presbyterian Psychiatric Institute, where he felt "spiritually or practically impotent in my madness" over the course of several months, during which time a psychiatrist tried to convert him with heterosexual fantasies of marrying and having a family.[127]

His sexual orientation took its own course, but in Ginsberg's mind it was often linked to a form of "craziness": partly a sense of being uneasy with himself but also, as he was to express in his long poem "Howl," a way of looking beyond the surface of things. In a journal entry from September 1955, he wrote the fragment "My mind is crazed by homosexuality"; three years earlier, he had reflected on the ambiguity of the word "crazy" and its obscuring of physical, psychological, and sexual categories.[128] In a journal entry from April 1952 he describes a dream in which he was accompanied by a friend's dog and "a boy with no legs from the madhouse" who tried to drive a car but kept crashing it.[129] Here "crazy" refers variously to the physical disability (no legs), the psychiatric institute ("the crazy house"), and the sexual insult "fairy" that was used by the police in his dream, shuttling across a spectrum of assumed afflictions.

The second dimension is Ginsberg's intensely idiosyncratic relationship with his mother, Naomi; their family was a compelling example of one that did not fit into a normative pattern. A member of a Russian immigrant family that settled in Newark in 1905, Naomi joined the Communist Party in the late 1910s and later became a branch secretary. But she suffered from bouts of mental illness, including depression, suicidal delusions, hypersensitivity, and auditory hallucinations. This led her husband, Louis, to commit her to the private Bloomingdale Sanatorium when Allen was a young child in the late 1920s and, following a failed suicide attempt, again in the late 1930s, during which time she underwent electroshock treatment. Her illness continued through Allen's childhood and teenage years, eventually leading to the collapse of her marriage and her institutionalization at the large Pilgrim State Hospital, which had been established on Long Island in 1931. Because Naomi was violent and difficult to control, in 1947 the hospital recommended that she undergo a prefrontal lobotomy; the consent form was left for Allen to sign due to his parents' divorce, and when later he went to the hospital to visit Naomi, she was unrecognizable to him.[130] Following years of incarceration, on the day of Naomi's death in 1956, Ginsberg wrote in his journals: "My childhood is gone with my mother. My memory becomes less clear. My body will go. There is no me left."[131] On another occasion he retreated from his biological age of thirty to express an infantlike need for his dead mother: "I have no mother's belly left to crawl back to under the covers."[132]

Ginsberg's mother was immortalized in his long, five-part poem "Kaddish," completed in 1959 (the kaddish is a Jewish prayer, often recited by a son mourning for a lost parent). Tony Trigilio notes that Ginsberg begins the poem by fusing a description of an early morning walk around Manhattan with the memory of his mother walking around the immigrant parts of the city fifty years earlier.[133] Trigilio reads "Kaddish" as Ginsberg's "desire to multiply, rather than fix, meaning," to move beyond normative conceptions of the nuclear family and pathological views about momism and oedipal relationships.[134] In the second section of the poem, Naomi's mental illness, her incarceration, and the sexualized (possibly incestuous) union between the son and mother are combined in a vision of what lies beyond the normative. This does not diminish the small boy's fright ("I lay in bed nervous . . . shaking"), or the waywardness of the mother's delusions, or Allen's pain of seeing his mother years later in Pilgrim State Hospital (which treated about 25,000 patients at the time).[135] The poem blends mourning and social critique: Naomi's bohemian outlook is partly the inspiration for the poem (she used to walk around the house naked when Allen was a child), but so are her communist views, prophecies, and fears of persecution. Ginsberg's free verse and fragmentary sound patterns reflect this attempted escape from social strictures, leading to a spiritual vision in the final two parts that focus on his mother's eyes and the intersection of earth and sky.

Last, and most important, Ginsberg was a creative writer, blending sexuality and psychiatry in imaginative ways. Reacting against the half-expressed unease of many writers in the mid-1950s, Ginsberg's language is nearly always excessive; his use of extended lines, hyphenated clauses, and epiphanic apostrophes immerse the reader in words that move in many different directions. Just as Ginsberg was desperate to avoid being pinned down as a sexual or psychological type, so his language works to free the self, to see beyond the ordinary, and to look beyond the present moment into the past and future. In the first three lines of "Howl," this prophetic voice allows him to see at dawn "the best minds of my generation destroyed by madness, starving hysterical naked," but also a beatific vision of "angelheaded hipsters burning for the ancient heavenly connection."[136] Sexuality is both corporeal and transcendent, and psychosis is worsened by psychiatric apparatus ("concrete void of insulin metrasol electricity hydrotherapy psychotherapy occupational therapy pingpong & amnesia"), but the experience of madness can also facilitate a new way of seeing ("who thought they were only mad when Baltimore gleamed in supernatural ecstasy).[137] The poem's third part brings these themes together in its paean to Ginsberg's friend Carl Solomon, whom Ginsberg had met in the Columbia Psychiatric Institute in 1949 after Solomon, a follower of Antonin Artaud, had committed himself as a nihilistic avant-garde gesture. "Howl" was partly stimulated by Solomon's return to psychiatric care in 1956 at the same hospital as Naomi. In the poem, Pilgrim State Hospital is transformed into "Rockland," suggesting both an immovable object and a comforting cradle; the poet repeats "I'm with you in Rockland" nineteen times to offset "the void" brought on by aggressive psychiatric therapies that pushed Solomon into an ontological space in which he felt simultaneously everywhere and nowhere, as expressed in his 1950 essay "Afterthoughts of a Shock Patient."[138]

Ginsberg's poetry was written in part to assault the closed categories that he and other Beat writers detected as the pervasive structure of institutional thought and practice in the mid-1950s. The white-collar fictions discussed in the previous two chapters expressed unease at constraining organizational forces, whereas Ginsberg's poetic voice is both penetrating and prophetic. Such insights became increasingly frequent in the early 1960s, when writers like Sylvia Plath and Richard Yates looked back on the mid-1950s with a few years of hindsight and found the means to critique institutional practices through the characters of Esther Greenwood in *The Bell Jar* and John Givings in *Revolutionary Road*. However, Ginsberg was in the thick of things when he wrote "Howl" and "Kaddish," and—along with his friend William Burroughs, the poet Frank O'Hara, and the social thinkers Mills and Goodman—he was able to see beyond surfaces to the oppressive structures within.[139]

The experiential dimension was vital for Ginsberg, as a homosexual Jew with a communist mother growing up during the Cold War. Personal experience was also central to his poetry: his experiments with excessive language and elongated breath patterns force readers to immerse themselves in the text rather than contemplating it from a safe distance. Trigilio notes that Ginsberg was distrustful of all language that is ignorant of its own textuality; citing a line Ginsberg wrote with Carl Solomon in the Columbia Psychiatric Institute—"beyond a certain point there can be no spoken communication and all speech is useless"—Trigilio argues that when Ginsberg's speech stops (in the hymnlike "Footnote to Howl" and the closing section of "Kaddish"), it is usually an active and creative silence, rather than an unknowing one.[140] "Howl" is often upheld as Ginsberg's major contribution to postwar literature, but "Kaddish" is more important for understanding the close relationship between the triumvirate of issues explored in this chapter: growing up, sexuality, and mental illness.

PART THREE

Reorganization

1961–1970

7 Institutions of Care and Oppression

John F. Kennedy's inauguration on 20 January 1961 promised a brighter future than many liberals thought possible during Dwight Eisenhower's eight years in the White House. Medical progress in the 1950s had been patchy, and the historical record does not credit Eisenhower with forthright medical reform, even though he established the Department of Health, Education, and Welfare (HEW) in his first term as president and tried to push a health reinsurance bill through Congress in 1954–1955, without success.[1] Presidents Kennedy and Lyndon B. Johnson fare better in the history of health reform because important legislation was signed on their watch, but it should be noted that Eisenhower followed through on President Harry Truman's pledge of additional federal funds to conduct more medical research, increase the number of hospital beds, improve rehabilitation facilities (particularly for veterans), and extend training for nurses. Some of Eisenhower's plans were stymied by members of his own administration. For example, his belief that the polio vaccine should be made available to all Americans who needed it was opposed by HEW Secretary Oveta Culp Hobby, who feared that the result would be the arrival of socialized medicine through the back door (instead, she wanted the states or the public to pay for the vaccine).[2] Although Eisenhower's record is less impressive on race, gender, and poverty, by signing the Health Amendments Act in 1956 he stressed the "critically important" care of the mentally ill, and on 7 April 1959 he publicly observed World Health Day, with its focus on mental health.

It is tempting to overplay the shift from Eisenhower to Kennedy as the key moment in the therapeutic revolutions that this book is tracing, but the different tone and impetus given to healthcare in the early 1960s should not be underestimated. If the 1950s was marked by a deference to political and medical authority, regulated forms of social organization, and a centripetal pull toward the cultural center, then thinkers from the late 1950s onward found ways to kick against institutional oppression and to reformulate health and illness as points on a psychosocial continuum where the sick could retain their agency and an active place within the community. We can think about this shift as one from rigid "organization" under Eisenhower to a more flexible "reorganization" during Kennedy's and Johnson's administrations, with healthcare at the fore. The centrifugal push of new social and cultural movements meant that the health narrative of the 1960s is more pluralistic and diffuse, as much about grass-roots activities, participatory communities, and the philosophy of holism as it is about federal initiatives. Nevertheless, it is with national politics that this chapter begins—specifically, speeches made by Eisenhower and Kennedy in 1961–1962.

Transitions in the White House

Eisenhower's farewell address, given three days before Kennedy's inaugural address, is remembered for its powerful image of a military-industrial complex, which had been emerging through the Cold War years despite Eisenhower's plans in the mid-1950s to scale back defense spending. He did not explicitly locate healthcare within this nexus, but his comments on science could be read to include medicine, which was fast becoming the nation's third largest industry in terms of personnel and which was tightly controlled by the American Medical Association (AMA), in its role as the official body of scientific medicine.[3] The tone of Eisenhower's address was somber, fueled by the fear that large-scale investment in the military and the scientific establishment was starting to shift the priorities of the government. This was a particular concern within the field of scientific research. Eisenhower believed that "the solitary inventor . . . has been overshadowed by task forces of scientists in laboratories and testing fields," and he feared that the rise of a "scientific-technological elite" could hijack public policy.[4] The outgoing president warned that balance should be maintained "between our essential requirements as a nation and the duties imposed by the nation upon the individual; balance between the actions of the moment and the national welfare of the future." Within this context of balance, his criticism of elites and systems and his emphasis on "national welfare" struck a caring note. The farewell speech can be read as the continuation of Eisenhower's campaign to increase hospital care and improve maternal and child health, but these were also the words of a retiring president facing old age with a frail physical constitution.

Perhaps in response to Eisenhower's address, Kennedy's inauguration speech on 20 January focused on protecting national freedom against external threats. He mentioned health issues only in passing—"Let both sides seek to invoke the wonders of science instead of its terrors. Together let us explore the stars, conquer the deserts, eradicate disease, tap the ocean depths, and encourage the arts and commerce"—as a long-term project that he believed would extend far beyond his term in office.[5] However, in his "New Frontier" speech at the Democratic national convention in July 1960, Kennedy had called for improved healthcare for the elderly (hospitalization rates for those over age sixty-five were three times higher than for the population as a whole), as well as the development of schools and the need to redress unemployment. His progressive message was an attempt to tackle the "dank atmosphere of 'normalcy'" that he associated with Eisenhower and Nixon, but he was also, implicitly, challenging the normative medical model that had been dominant in the 1950s. We might be skeptical of Kennedy's rhetorical flourishes at the Democratic convention, when he needed to appeal to a broad electorate, but his commitment to the needy, sick, and dispossessed was genuine—a commitment that was reinforced when he formed the Peace Corps two months into his presidency to help poor and undeveloped nations with infrastructural problems, including those related to healthcare.

Kennedy himself had long suffered from a range of physical ailments. He had contracted scarlet fever at age three. He had had appendicitis, tonsillitis, jaundice, and pneumonia as a teenager in the early 1930s, followed by bladder and prostate difficulties in the early 1940s and then malaria and sciatica caused by his war experiences. His malaria led to adrenal insufficiency, which in turn caused him to develop Addison's disease in the mid-1940s, resulting in immune deficiencies, bronzing of the skin, and an intensification of chronic back pain.[6] While campaigning for Adlai Stevenson in the mid-1950s, Kennedy spent six weeks in the hospital. Although he suffered from only minor illnesses during his 1960 presidential campaign and appeared healthier than Richard Nixon (who had an injured knee and looked slightly unkempt in the first of the live television debates), Kennedy's health was actually quite fragile.[7]

During his truncated term in the White House, Kennedy had two physicians (one was a female doctor, Janet Travell), as well as access to a number of medical specialists. His medication included codeine sulphate, procaine, Ritalin, steroids, and cortisone—the drug critiqued in the *New Yorker* article "Ten Feet Tall" and Nicholas Ray's film *Bigger Than Life* in the mid-1950s (see chapter 5), but now supported by a better case history. It is purely speculative that Kennedy's political vision was influenced by the "well-being, energy, cheerfulness, optimism, concentrating power, and hyperactivity" related to continued cortisone use, but it is clear that he was not a well man and might not have lived into his fifties.[8] Robert Dallek comments that "when he ran for and won the presidency, Kennedy was gambling that his health problems would not prevent him from handling the job," and others have speculated about whether he would have been capable of a second term.[9] He regularly wore a back brace and relied on crutches in private, and his physicians argued about whether or not immobilization with injections or regular exercise would be the most therapeutic treatment.[10] Nevertheless, in 1960, dubbed Mental Health Year by the World Health Organizations, many Americans (although only just enough to get Kennedy elected) were confident that they would receive better healthcare than in the past decade.

The Kennedy family had other reasons for focusing their energies on medical care: John's younger sister Rosemary was born with a cognitive impairment, probably after she suffered oxygen deprivation during birth. There is some debate about the actual circumstances. According to one account, the nurse (who was perfectly capable of delivering the baby) held back the birth, waiting for a male doctor who had been delayed—which led Laurence Leamer to place the blame squarely on "patriarchal modern medicine" with its "white-coated omnipotence."[11] Although physically active as a child, Rosemary experienced some dexterity problems, forgetfulness, and reading difficulties (probably dyslexia), and her frustrations at times erupted "in an inexplicable fury" (possibly epilepsy).[12] Largely educated at home, Rosemary's condition became more pronounced as she matured sexually, leading her father, Joseph Kennedy, to agree to a prefrontal lobotomy at St. Elizabeth's Hospital in Washington, D.C. Lobotomies were still in their infancy in the early 1940s, and Rosemary's parents had been warned of the risks, despite Dr. Walter Freeman's promotion of the benefits and successes of his new surgical practice. The results of the lobotomy were disastrous, leaving Rosemary "permanently incapacitated."[13] Two facts added to the psychological and neurological damage of the procedure: Rosemary was not clear about the nature of the surgery, and before 1941 lobotomies had been performed only on schizophrenics and the chronically depressed (such as the lobotomy performed on Tennessee Williams's older sister, Rose, in 1943), not on individuals with developmental disabilities.[14] After the operation, Rosemary was moved to a psychiatric hospital in New York State called Craig House, and then to St. Coletta's Catholic School in Jefferson, Wisconsin. Leaked stories claiming that Rosemary was teaching mentally retarded children at St. Coletta's ironically masked the truth of her institutionalization and lobotomy. The full picture did not emerge until 1962, two years into the Kennedy administration, and even then Joe Kennedy claimed that her developmental difficulties stemmed from childhood meningitis.[15]

Rosemary's treatment and parental guilt are probably two reasons why her father chose to concentrate his investment in research on mental illness through the Joseph P. Kennedy Jr. Foundation and to establish a Catholic memorial hospital in Hanover, Massachusetts. But, as Edward Shorter makes clear, the real shift toward a focus on cognitive disability took place in the late 1950s, when John's younger sister Eunice started to collaborate with her husband, Robert Sargent Shriver Jr. (the first director of the Peace Corps), and Robert E. Cooke (a pediatrics professor at Johns Hopkins University and later a significant figure in John Kennedy's healthcare team), and she pushed to establish the first President's Committee on Mental Retardation in 1961. Eunice was the family member most involved in caring for Rosemary; she was particularly interested in helping disabled individuals lead active lives (resulting in the first Special Olympics, held in Chicago in 1968); and she helped her presidential brother to form the National Institute for Child Health and Development in 1962.

When Kennedy spoke to the press in October 1961, he noted that mental health "strikes those least able to protect themselves," and he pointed out its prevalence compared to diabetes, tuberculosis, and infantile paralysis.[16] Perhaps reflecting on Rosemary's permanent separation from the family, he emphasized the isolation that many sufferers of both mental illness and cognitive disability experience, "forgotten except by the members of their family." Kennedy's language was both sympathetic (stressing the lack of "public understanding") and aggressive ("I believe that we, as a country, in association with scientists all over the world, should make a comprehensive attack"), as he sought to align the national agenda with the priorities of the World Health Organization.[17]

The most important speech Kennedy made on mental health was his "Special Address to Congress on Mental Illness and Mental Retardation" on 5 February 1963, which *Time* called "the first presidential message in history that dealt solely with the twin blights of mental illness and mental retardation."[18] The president called for "a wholly new emphasis and approach to care for the mentally ill," prompted by the 1961 report of the Joint Commission on Mental Illness and Health, *Action for Mental Health*, which focused on the "untreated and inadequately cared for."[19] Elements of the speech stem directly from this report, particularly the need to redress inadequate conditions in large overcrowded state hospitals and for major investment in treatment services at the federal, state, and local levels.[20] Kennedy hoped for new research on medical and genetic causes of mental illness; better training of medical and auxiliary personnel; and improved facilities, to reduce the huge number of inpatients (45 percent) who were incarcerated in hospitals for more than ten years. He wanted to reduce the number of cases by 50 percent within two decades; many of them would be treated as outpatients, so they could remain in their homes with support from their community. The speech was largely focused on outlining the role of community health centers for the mentally ill and promising specialist training and personnel to care for those with cognitive disabilities. In so doing, the president stressed the importance of a well-informed and supportive community to safeguard the health of the nation. This emphasis on community remained strong up to the signing of the Community Mental Health Act that autumn, which focused on establishing outpatient services for small to medium-size communities across the nation.[21]

This evidence supports the image of Kennedy as a crusader, fighting for the nation's health with a specific program—in contrast to the more piecemeal programs under Eisenhower. Early signs of the trend toward deinstitutionalization were visible in the late 1950s in care of those with chronic conditions, such as Anne Emerman—a young quadriplegic who used a wheelchair and was released from Goldwater Memorial Hospital, in New York City, as an "experiment in independent living" (she went on to complete a master's degree at Columbia University).[22] And in the second half of the 1950s, the National Institute of Mental Health stepped up its pamphlet campaign with the aim of reducing the stigma of mental illness by targeting readers among the general public.[23] However, despite Kennedy's making the right noises on public health and his engaging with broader cultural views of medicine—for example, he attended a preview screening for the Senate of the 1963 United Artists film *The Caretakers*, which promoted drug treatment over aggressive surgery—many Americans were skeptical that his plans were any more progressive than Eisenhower's.[24] Some conservatives believed that "legislative inaction" would block health reform, but many were still worried about the specter of socialized medicine.[25] For example, Ronald Reagan, then a Hollywood actor, released a record in 1961 under the sponsorship of the AMA. In the record, called "Ronald Reagan Speaks Out against Socialized Medicine," he attacked Truman's national health program and argued that "subsidized medicine would curtail Americans' freedom." Although Reagan looked back to the Truman years, many state hospitals had changed little during the 1950s, which added to Kennedy's sense of urgency in developing community-based services. This was the right time for reform, but its slow pace was sobering—prompting Milton Roemer, a professor at the University of California at Los Angeles, to proclaim in 1967 that institutional problems were "a consequence of the crazy quilt of a fragmented nonsystem of health service delivery in our country."[26]

Perhaps Kennedy was right, however, when he said that the path to change would be a long one. Kennedy's campaign was just part of the therapeutic revolution of the 1960s, which saw a slow transition from large, state-run hospitals toward a more diffuse system of patient care. Improvements in outpatient facilities and the redeployment of medical and psychiatric social workers did not happen overnight, but between the mid-1950s and the mid-1970s, the proportion of mental patients who were institutionalized fell sharply, from 77 percent in 1955 to 8 percent by 1975, as outpatient and community-based care grew rapidly in the mid-1960s.[27]

The third section of this book marks this broad trend away from large, state-run hospitals and normative models of health to a more pluralistic model of healthcare and organic interpersonal language to describe health and illness. It is certainly tempting to tell a progressive story of health policy in the 1960s, starting with Kennedy's mental-health campaign and continuing through Johnson's signing of the Social Security Act of 1965, with its two amendments to President Franklin D. Roosevelt's 1935 Social Security Act that established Medicare and Medicaid to provide health insurance for the elderly and the poor. The culmination of a decade of healthcare reform and federal legislation was the Developmental Disabilities Services and Facilities Construction Act of 1970, and when that act was passed, 75 percent of public facilities for what were then called "mentally retarded" inpatients had been built within the previous twenty years.[28] But we need to be wary about imbuing this narrative with too much optimism. Despite these advances, problems of social stigma, inequalities in health provision relating to region and race, bureaucratic red tape, overly aggressive surgery, and the psychology of damage marked the 1960s as much as they had the previous decade. Therefore, part 3 of this book will strive to give a balanced account of public health in the 1960s, where realist and progressive accounts of the postwar therapeutic revolutions are mutually informing.

In particular, this chapter will focus on the provision of institutions, especially those focusing on mental health. The movement toward the development of outpatient facilities and the influence of thinkers who saw psychiatry as an oppressive practice and mental hospitals as "total institutions" akin to prisons mark a break from the previous decade. However, new studies of healthcare in the early 1960s, personal accounts of therapeutic treatments, theories of damage, and diverse social factors complicate this notion of a single rupture, revealing that institutional care and oppression were entangled in the early part of the 1960s. In order to trace these complex relationships, I start by examining new health research in the early 1960s—particularly urban conditions and healthcare for African Americans—before looking closely at critiques of medical institutions. Erving Goffman's *Asylums* (1961) was one of the decade's most influential texts on the incarceration of patients, and it offers an intellectual framework for the discussion of two cultural texts that critique institutional power relations from the inside: Ken Kesey's novel *One Flew over the Cuckoo's Nest* (1962) and Samuel Fuller's film *Shock Corridor* (1963). These studies, in turn, raise broader issues about regionalism, poverty, and race, which I deal with from a more sociological perspective in the final section of the chapter. Karl Menninger predicted that the most pressing postwar problem would be treatment of minorities; responding to Lillian Smith's 1944 interracial novel *Strange Fruit*, he commented that "to be complacent about the greatest social problem in America is surely a form of passive suicide."[29] But it would take another fifteen years before clinical attention focused centrally on "the other America," as Michael Harrington called the broad sector that had been forgotten or denied a voice in the years following World War II.[30] As this chapter makes clear, the relationship between ethnicity and class began to play an increasingly important role in the redefinition of health and illness in the 1960s—a focus that helps to illuminate problems of medical philosophy and provision that persisted well beyond the decade.

New Health Research

Albert Deutsch concluded his historical survey of American mental health from colonial times to the end of World War II with the ideal of "well adjusted citizens, where the personality is permitted to develop naturally and freely, where the individual is given a sense of personal worth and dignity, and where his activities and ambitions are integrated with the development of group life."[31] First published in 1937 and updated in 1945, Deutsch's *The Mentally Ill in America* narrates an upward curve "from the ideal of repression to the ideal of prevention . . . from manacles to mental hygiene," but Deutsch admits that "a mantle of mystery still hangs over a large area of mental disorder." Two phrases here are worth further attention: "group life" and "from manacles to mental hygiene." Rather than stressing the personal autonomy that David Riesman had advocated in the 1950s, Deutsch makes his goal integrated behavior within a group. He does not define the group dynamic, but the seeds of a community model of health are present in the final pages of the book. The second phrase is central to Deutsch's heroic narrative, but in a study that largely ignores questions of race, the rhetorical link to slavery is particularly poignant given that mental health provision for African Americans was in a crude state in the 1940s and 1950s.

Deutsch's next book, *The Shame of the States* (1948), gave mental hospitals the label of "snake pits": understaffed, badly organized, and unsanitary. Truman's and Eisenhower's investments in improving the standards of public hospitals were partly attempts to undo the negative public perception of the institutions as snake pits. But, although there were marked improvements in the care provided in state hospitals during the 1950s, the quality range was huge at the beginning of the 1960s, and the experiences of inpatients varied widely. Mortality rates in state-run institutions decreased considerably; although people with Down syndrome often died before the age of thirty, patients with epilepsy, tuberculosis, heart defects, and related secondary infections could all be treated more easily than they could before World War II. Life expectancy in the institutions also rose considerably for children with mild to moderate cognitive and developmental disorders, who were less likely to be institutionalized for the long term, while the increase was much smaller for severely retarded patients, who were more likely to reside in institutions, many of which had unsanitary conditions and bad nutrition. Countering Deutsch's image of snake pits, Gerald Grob notes some positive reports, though, such as a 1955 survey of Warren State Hospital in Pennsylvania, which recorded that the number of patients released from institutional care within the first year rose rapidly across the first half of the century.[32]

One account—first published in May 1950 in the *Ladies' Home Journal* and published on its own later that year—did a great deal to help change perceptions of the therapeutic benefits of specialist institutions for caring for congenital or developmental disabilities. This account was the novelist Pearl S. Buck's *The Child Who Never Grew*. In it, Buck describes the helpful treatment of her daughter, Caroline, at the Vineland Training School in southern New Jersey. Established in 1887 as the New Jersey Home for the Education and Care of Feebleminded Children (the institution underwent numerous name changes), Vineland was a private research and training school that helped patients with cognitive and developmental disabilities to live on their own. Vineland pioneered intelligence testing in the 1910s, and in the interwar period it developed a Social Maturity Scale to calibrate self-help skills, communication capability, and social competence to better assess which modes of therapy best suited a particular child or young adult. This helped the staff to focus, where possible, on each patient's individual needs.

Buck's autobiographical essay was stimulated by her work on the board of the National Mental Health Foundation and proved helpful to parents and caregivers of children with what was then commonly referred to as mental retardation. She wrote candidly about stigma, inferiority, and feelings of imprisonment: "The silence of the parents infects all the children and sorrow spreads its blight. The child himself, poor little one, feels, though he cannot comprehend, his own inferiority. He lives in surrounding gloom. . . . His shadow falls before him, wherever he goes."[33] Written in a sentimental style, with only the occasional lapse into stigmatizing language (a child with Down syndrome is described as "unfinished"), the story is written from the perspective of a loving mother and a budding philanthropist (royalties for the book were donated to Vineland).[34]

When Buck committed her daughter to Vineland in 1929, at the age of nine, she found an attentive and well-staffed institution that provided Carol (as she was commonly called) with the developmental care that Buck felt ill equipped to give at the time. Carol's condition had gone undiagnosed in China, where she was born; it manifested itself as arrested development around her third year, accompanied by a short attention span and constant screaming, leading to years of frustration for her mother. Buck contrasts the progressive routine of Vineland with conditions in a state institution, which she described as "an abode of horror. The children, some young in body, some old, were apparently without any minds whatever. . . . They were herded together like dogs. They wore baglike garments of rough calico or burlap. Their food was given to them on the floor and they snatched it up."[35] A few years later, that particular hospital had improved, but it was another institution to which Buck took Carol: Vineland, with its "warm and free and friendly" atmosphere and "pleasant" buildings.[36] The homelike conditions of Vineland did not prevent Buck from feeling like she was abandoning her child, nor did it ease her sense of suffering for the children: "They were here for life, prisoners of their fate."[37] The narrative recounts Buck's coming to terms with her decision, discovering more about Vineland's therapies, and finding comfort in the experience that Carol's "life, with others, has been of use in enlarging the whole body of our knowledge."[38]

Although Buck's account is of great historical importance, equally significant is the fact that she hid her daughter from public attention for twenty years. In his biography of Buck, Peter Conn notes that "she systematically avoided any mention of her daughter in the autobiographical sketches she provided to publishers and journalists"; she defended herself by claiming that she was protecting Carol's privacy, but she might also have been protecting her own reputation as a popular author.[39] Nevertheless, *The Child Who Never Grew* is arguably the most important postwar text to chart a mother's coming to terms with her daughter's retarded condition (later confirmed as the genetic disease phenylketonuria) and for raising public awareness.[40] Although Vineland was a private institution and Buck championed philanthropic investment, she noted the importance of well-run state hospitals, as long as they were not merely "custodial" institutions "apt to degenerate into something routine and dead."[41] She was very eager to act on her experiences: she did volunteer work for Vineland, raised funds to build a new dormitory, and later became chair of the institution's board. She was also chair of the Pennsylvania Commission on the Handicapped, and in 1964 she established the Pearl S. Buck Foundation to support children born to American servicemen and Asian mothers in China.

The account of Vineland in *The Child Who Never Grew* supports the generally positive account of private institutions in the postwar period—even though Diane Arbus's 1970 controversial photographic portraits of inpatients in nearby Vineland Developmental Center (established in 1888) suggest that, twenty years later, many of the patients were still unable to communicate or interact meaningfully. However, a number of progressive institutional practices began in the mid-1950s, allowing patients to take an active role in their therapy. This trend was led by the British psychologist Maxwell Jones during World War II to better care for veterans suffering from war neurosis. It was most fully realized in 1947 in the Industrial Neurosis Unit (renamed the Social Rehabilitation Unit in 1954) at Belmont Hospital in Southwest London, run by the Ministry of Health and focusing on "the chronic unemployed neurotic."[42] Practices at Belmont included active discussion groups, social and vocational roles for patients, and ongoing links with the outside community. Patients were usually released between two to four months after they were admitted, results that Jones insists could not "have been achieved in individual psychotherapy and hospitalization alone."[43] Jones's model of a therapeutic community was transferred directly to the West Coast of the United States when he took up a professorship at Stanford University and started publishing in America in the early 1960s. Such a community had been established in Oakland, California, by Harry Wilmer in 1955–1956 as a center for naval and marine corps personnel serving in the Pacific, and at the beginning of the 1960s, Jones and Wilmer collaborated on a "comprehensive mental health service" in San Mateo, later described as "the prototype for which a great deal of Kennedy's Community Mental Health Act of 1963 was based."[44]

Jones could cite a positive example of a state-run institution in the United Kingdom, but the story was very different in the United States, particularly for families that could not afford the kind of annual fee that Vineland charged Pearl Buck. For many patients who had no relatives to care for them after treatment, there was little choice of institution or chance of release; those who were released were likely to be readmitted after a short time. The experience of poor, nonwhite Americans, particularly those living in small towns or rural communities in the South or West, tended to be worse: poor roads and transportation, together with meager medical services, meant the chances of being restored to a regular life were much slimmer. Those whose conditions were moderate to severe were likely to face a lifetime in a hospital or psychiatric ward, with no therapeutic trajectory that could help them to develop productive social relationships. Viewing National Health Survey statistics from the late 1950s, Harrington concluded that, in terms of health service, "the poor are physically victimized in America."[45]

In the early 1960s medical researchers became more interested in the specific environments that shape the illness experience of individuals and groups, defined in terms of class and race.[46] A precedent was set by a pioneering 1939 report titled *Mental Disorders in Urban Areas*, which considered how cases of schizophrenia in inner-city Chicago were shaped by environmental factors, focusing particularly on the relationship between "social disorganization" in specific communities and the "mental disorganization" of individuals with certain psychogenetic tendencies.[47] Issues of housing density, zoning, migration, and race feature in this 1939 report, but the shift to consider sociogenic factors did not become pronounced until the early 1960s, as Daniel Matlin explores in *On the Corner: Black Intellectuals and the Urban Crisis* (2013). Even though many studies published in the early 1960s relied on the 1950 census data or on research conducted in the early 1950s, this move toward particularism is one of the key shifts across the decades—although, as we will see below in the third part of this book, tensions between the general and the particular ran through the 1960s.

Following the Regionville study of 1954 (discussed in chapter 5) and the institutional studies *Social Class and Mental Illness* (1958) and *Family and Class Dynamics in Mental Illness* (1959), the major longitudinal study of mental health of the early 1960s was the Midtown Manhattan Study.[48] This sociological survey of psychiatric provision in a bounded area of New York City marked the shift toward examining specific topographies, with close attention to postwar urban conditions. Published in 1962, the Midtown Manhattan Study adopts a medical and psychiatric framework to provide a "broader understanding of social forces operating on the generality of people, nonpatients and patients alike."[49] The investigators supplemented official data by conducting over fifteen hundred home interviews in 1954 with a broad sector of midtown residents. Their findings were threefold: "emotional disability" was far higher within an urban setting than previously thought; the need for psychiatric help was greater than the services available; and "those most in need of such services had by far the least access to them," particularly the poor and elderly. Linking these findings, the study concludes that the gap in access to care was "highly discriminatory."[50]

This report, *Mental Health in the Metropolis,* was published the same year as *The Other America*. Whereas Harrington focuses on the "economic underworld of American life" in overlooked regions, the Midtown Manhattan Study adopts a more specific topographical perspective on a cross section of New York City, looking closely at demographics, housing, and population density.[51] There are some parallels between the two texts. For example, Harrington comments that the suburban boom of the late 1940s and 1950s meant that it was easy to overlook life in the inner city: "The failures, the unskilled, the disabled, the aged, and the minorities are right there, across the tracks, where they have always been. But hardly anyone else is."[52] The Midtown Manhattan Study focuses primarily on population density but also notes the ethnicity of European immigrants, who made up a third of the midtown inhabitants. Although the study reveals homogeneous traits within these national groups in terms of religion, socioeconomic status, and age-related conditions, it concludes that there are too many heterogeneous factors (such as language, family composition, and ethnic mix) to assert much more than that it is not easy to generalize about immigrant mental health.

This emphasis on heterogeneity also starts to emerge in housing and health studies of African Americans. Postwar explanations of the state of African American families often drew on psychiatric language to diagnose a generalized black experience, represented either in terms of pervasive stereotypes (as in Otto Klineberg's 1944 *Characteristics of the American Negro*) or the dynamics of the African American family. Most famously, in *The Negro Family in the United States* (1939), the sociologist E. Franklin Frazier proposed that the major social problem facing black families was one of disorganization, which could be traced back to the experience of slavery and pathological racist attitudes. Frazier pointed out the dangers of delinquency and broken homes as well as the damaging effects on black communities, writing in a follow-up study in the late 1940s that "life among a large proportion of the urban Negro population is casual, precarious, and fragmentary. It lacks continuity and its roots do not go deeper than the contingencies of daily living," especially in urban localities.[53] He noted that in the mid-1920s, poverty and the lack of health services were fundamental socioeconomic problems for both urban and rural blacks—a point emphasized in the psychiatric text *The Mark of Oppression* (1951), even though its authors, Abram Kardiner and Lionel Ovesey, acknowledged that postwar facilities in New York City were better than the national average.[54]

Manhattan was not the only site of urban deprivation for African Americans, despite a 1961 report in the *New York Times* that claimed Harlem "tops the city in mental hospital admissions, psychiatric cases, active tuberculosis, infant mortality, illegitimate births . . . and runs high in substandard housing."[55] Bonnie Bullough encountered a graphic example of such urban health problems while working as a public health nurse in Chicago's South Side in the early 1950s:

> In 1953, rats mutilated and killed an infant in an area next to the district in which I was working. In my own district, they chewed the hand of a small black newborn infant [living with his mother and three siblings] in a dug-out basement under a dilapidated row house . . . his hand was a bleeding mass of mangled flesh. [The mother] took her baby to Cook County Hospital for emergency care [but it] was more than an hour away by bus.[56]

When Bullough tried to intervene, public officials said they could do nothing about the rats nor offer alternative accommodation for such a poor black family. Many families doubled up in order to escape bulldozers during urban renewal projects, but that just added to the overcrowding in slums and the potential for disease and infection. This led Vern Bullough and Bonnie Bullough to conclude that poverty and race made a disastrous combination for such families: "They faced poverty, discrimination, and an inadequate health care delivery system. It was an impossible combination."[57] Reflecting back thirty years later, the authors noted that "discrimination related to poverty and ethnicity [was] lessening and becoming more subtle," but there was no heroic story to tell about progress in health provision for poor ethnic groups in the 1950s and 1960s.[58] For instance, in the mid-1960s, visits by physicians were significantly more common for whites than for members of other ethnic groups (4.5 versus 3.1 visits a year), while tuberculosis continued to be more prevalent in poor ethnic families, leading some "white reactionaries" to view "black tuberculosis as a harbinger of racial degeneration."[59]

Kardiner and Ovesey's *The Mark of Oppression*—based on twenty-five psychodynamic case studies—was republished in 1962, with a preface reflecting on readers' responses to the 1951 edition. The authors point out that many readers rejected their findings about the links between race, poverty, and stigma "on largely emotional grounds because they found them too painful to accept."[60] They saw oppression as being much greater than the experience of one race and, taking their cue from Frazier's study of urban pathology, they contributed significantly to the discussion of personality damage and how institutional racism can promulgate racial inferiority, self-hatred, and aggression. Nevertheless, the 1961 edition begins with a more upbeat message: in the ten years since the first edition, the civil rights movement had demonstrated that social transformations and new communities could help to unseat deeply ingrained inferiority complexes.

Part of the problem of assessing the provision of health care for African Americans before the 1970s is that statistical studies tended to use only the classifications of white and nonwhite. For example, the 1963 report titled *Health Progress in the United States* charted trends in mortality, birthrates, and healthcare from 1900 to 1960. Other reports published in the early 1960s, including the New York statistician Benjamin Malzberg's *The Mental Health of the Negro* (1963), tended to rely on data that were ten years old. Malzberg's work followed earlier statistical studies such as the 1940 survey of nearly 90,000 cases by the Massachusetts physician Neil Dayton, in *New Facts on Mental Disorders*.[61] Malzberg's study focused on admissions to New York State mental hospitals during 1949–1951. Using census data going back to the mid-nineteenth century, he had noted in 1930 that "the foreign-born apparently always had a rate of mental disease higher than that among natives."[62] But instead of generalizing, Malzberg was very interested in the specificity of ethnic experience, which led him to publish subsequent reports on Jews (1960), African Americans (1963), and Puerto Ricans (1965), and to consider variations in other ethnic experiences of mental facilities (1966). Malzberg was aware that his studies gave only a partial snapshot of mental illness based on first admissions. But they did show that admissions among African Americans actually declined during the 1940s, which he attributes to improved living standards in New York, although he recognized that migration to New York from the South was a complicating factor. For this reason, he realized that his figures did not apply to other US states, where healthcare facilities were scarcer.[63]

Other reports paint a bleak picture of mental health care for African Americans. For example, one from 1950 pointed to an increase in mental illness among migrating blacks that mostly went untreated and that was related to higher rates of alcoholism and suicide in northern cities.[64] A 1979 HEW report estimated that the rate of decline of inpatients after 1950 was much slower among blacks than whites, while the rate of psychotic conditions among black male inpatients rose from 17 percent to 19 percent in the 1960s and rose much more significantly among black female inpatients, from 25 percent to 40 percent.[65] In addition, only 2 percent of physicians were African American in the early 1960s—a subject dramatized in the Twentieth Century–Fox film *No Way Out* (1950), featuring Sidney Poitier as a young doctor working in a prison ward and having to contend with violent racism.[66] And as there were even fewer black psychiatrists, the therapeutic situation could easily be complicated by racial factors. This was particularly true of psychoanalysis, where the majority of recorded case studies are of Protestant or Jewish patients and where the transference dynamic could easily be destabilized by racial expectations.[67] An additional problem was that with an implicitly racialized (that is, white) norm of health, any marked deviation could be seen as psychotic behavior.[68] Although Kardiner and Ovesey noted that retaliation could actually be seen as an adaptive response to white norms, not until later in the 1960s were aggression and rage among ethnic groups seen as potentially therapeutic responses.

Frazier's reading of the disorganized black family persisted into the mid-1960s, but President Kennedy's stress on community health was to shift the emphasis away from the pathology of the individual to a more diffuse notion of health within a group setting. The problem with this view was that institutions were slow to respond, and statistical reports always a few years behind. There were only a few reports in the mainstream press dealing explicitly with race and illness in the early 1960s. Compulsory sterilization practices in Virginia for the "mentally unfit" in order to regulate sexual behavior (practices often targeted at African Americans) came to public attention in the early 1960s.[69] And the shooting of the black civil rights activist Medgar Evers by Byron de la Beckwith, a forty-two-year-old white fertilizer salesman, in June 1963 was one high-profile case (Beckwith was quickly moved from mental hospital to prison). Unknown to the public until significant media coverage in July 1972 was the forty-year research project carried out by the US Public Health Service in Tuskegee, Alabama, in which four hundred poor male black sharecroppers with syphilis were, from 1947 onward (fifteen years into the study), denied penicillin in the name of medical science. There had actually been articles about the Tuskegee project published in medical journals, but the fact that the men did not know that they were part of an experiment, or that they could be treated, showed clearly that medical ethics had been violated—in this instance, within a racialized framework.[70]

Following earlier exposés such as the reporter John Bartlow Martin's feature "Inside the Asylum" for the *Saturday Evening Post*, which labeled mental illness "America's No. 1 health problem," Michael Harrington released his widely read *The Other America* and Erving Goffman published *Asylums*, his bleak picture of mental hospitals as "total institutions" from which, like the urban ghetto, there was no way out.[71] Although both Harrington and Goffman desired reform, these accounts were diametrically opposed to Kennedy's progressive vision. If Kennedy wanted to get the nation moving again, as he stated in his fourth presidential debate with Nixon in 1960, institutional stasis and aggressive therapeutic practices would need to be radically changed. The fact that Goffman did his research for *Asylums* at St. Elizabeth's Hospital (assisted by a grant from the National Institute of Mental Health), where he was a physical therapist's assistant in the mid-1950s—the very hospital where Kennedy's sister Rosemary had undergone a prefrontal lobotomy in 1941—adds historical poignancy to Goffman's study. I discuss that work in the next two sections of this chapter, alongside Ken Kesey's novel *One Flew over the Cuckoo's Nest* and Samuel Fuller's journalistic film *Shock Corridor*.

On the Inside: Fieldwork as Critique

Asylums portrays the mental hospital as a form of institutionalized incarceration, in which patients "together lead an enclosed, formally administered round of life" akin to that in a prison.[72] Goffman identified five types of "total institution": (1) those for the "incapable and harmless" (homes for the blind and orphaned); (2) those for people with diseases that are a threat to the community (mental hospitals, leprosy colonies); (3) those established to protect the community against danger (prisons, POW camps); (4) those geared toward "worklike tasks" (army barracks, boarding schools); and (5) "retreats from the world" (monasteries, convents).[73] This range of institutions is admittedly broad and has been criticized because it blurs voluntary and enforced membership, but Goffman was interested in the intensity of the patient experience in the face of bureaucracy, routines, and daily practices.[74] The topography of the institution was particularly important for Goffman—as it was for Maxwell Jones, who sought flexible architectural spaces as an alternative to the oppressively rigid structures of large state hospitals.[75] Drawing an analogy with prisons, Goffman argued that in these tightly controlled spaces, individuals are treated as "blocks" to be managed through surveillance and a strict hierarchy of command; "social mobility" is "grossly restricted"; and communication is regulated by wardens and curfews.[76] A patient's feelings of demoralization might be triggered by the lack of meaningful exchange between staff and patients, and a machine-like hospital system can often intensify these feelings of alienation and contribute to the erasure of the patient's identity.

The first pair of four essays that comprise *Asylums*—"On the Characteristics of Total Institutions" and "The Moral Career of the Mental Patient"—had been published before, the first in a collection on *The Prison* in 1961 and the second in the journal *Psychiatry* in 1959; these essays were repackaged with two others, "The Underlife of a Public Institution" and "The Medical Model and Mental Hospitalization." In

Asylums, Goffman's criticism was leveled at both the inhumanity of these authoritarian systems and their duplicity: on the surface they "present themselves to the public as rational organizations," but they are structured along caste lines and geared to bend the inmate or patient to the system, molding a modified or diminished self that the individual accepts in order to survive.[77] The response is usually passivity and compliance; any sign of dissidence is likely to be met with a reprimand or, in the case of mental illness, packaged as part of the medical condition rather than as a genuine response to an enclosed environment. Critics have objected to this totalizing picture because it lacks specific case studies and pays little attention to race and gender.[78] The fact that Goffman did not offer any examples of patients or inmates successfully negotiating the institutional machinery was partly due to the absence of a depth model of the mind in his work, which contributed to Goffman's pessimistic view of a hostile system in which the incarcerated self is reformed with little reference to prior or future identities. However, offsetting this bleak vision, in the third essay of *Asylums*, he acknowledges an "underlife" through which patients can maintain (or regain) agency despite the strict rules, noting that "our sense of personal identity often resides in the cracks."[79]

Goffman's insights were most clearly dramatized in Ken Kesey's early countercultural novel, *One Flew over the Cuckoo's Nest*—which was influenced by the stories of brainwashing coming out of the Korean War that were illustrated in Richard Condon's 1959 novel, *The Manchurian Candidate*. But Kesey's novel is largely based on patients whom he had met at a Veterans Hospital in Menlo Park, California, near Stanford University where he had voluntarily tested LSD and had worked as a psychiatric aide in 1960–1961. Kesey was deeply affected by the patients on the ward at Menlo Park. He wrote to his friend Ken Babbs that many of the patients were "all twisted out of shape by so many years" in the hospital; some he only knew "by the empty eyes, like the eyes are holes spiked in the shell and all you can see inside are the dilapidated organs."[80] Kesey's book is often placed alongside Thomas Szasz's *The Myth of Mental Illness* (1961), with its suspicion of the therapeutic apparatus and its critique of institutionalized psychiatry, but the description of the "Combine" and institutional "machinery" in *One Flew over the Cuckoo's Nest* more clearly resembles *Asylums*.[81] Roger Loeb has taken issue with Kesey's depiction of the mental hospital as a machine, particularly his exaggeration of the "mechanistic coldness" and the tyrannical rule of Nurse Ratched, commonly referred to as "Big Nurse."[82] Heavily influenced by discourses of momism and dominant and submissive roles, Kesey's story is about the subjugation of a ward of chronic and acutely ill patients by the sadistic Big Nurse.

Importantly, the story is told in the first person from the perspective of an inmate who is half Native American, Chief Broom Bromden, whom the other patients and the staff assume is mute. Kesey was drawn to Native American culture, reflecting his backwoods Oregon roots and interest in primitive cultures, but he also was keenly aware of the dispossession and maltreatment of Indians, especially over land rights. Echoing the insight of Holden Caulfield at the end of J. D. Salinger's *The Catcher in the*

Rye about the benefits of keeping silent (an institutionalized Holden seems to oppose analysis when he says "don't ever tell anybody anything"), Bromden's strategy for survival is to keep his thoughts on the inside by pretending to be deaf and dumb.[83] Bromden has been in the hospital for over fifteen years, but it is unclear why he is there. His admission might be linked to the disappearance of his tribe (the Columbia Gorge Indians), but we find out that the tribe's land had been purchased by government agents and that his father had also been a patient and had been ground down by the system.

The tyrannical rule of the Big Nurse over Bromden and the other male patients is disturbed one day when Randle P. McMurphy enters the ward. There is no clear health reason why McMurphy should be there; it seems simply to have been a better choice for him than being imprisoned for petty crime. Kesey admitted that McMurphy is a fictional character "inspired by the tragic longing of [the] real men" he had worked with at Menlo Park.[84] McMurphy had been a war hero: he had fought in Korea, where he escaped from a communist prison camp (for which he was awarded a Distinguished Service Cross), revealing a resourcefulness and tenacity that helps him to subvert the rules of the Combine. He has seen hard labor, as shown by the scars on his strong hands, but he is also a reckless gambler, at times "frantic," and not a good judge of limits.[85] McMurphy's rebellion is overt: he flaunts rules and challenges Big Nurse's regime. This is in direct contrast to Goffman's account of an "underlife" in which patients retain their own identity through covert means. Bromden fits better into this underlife role; by avoiding the surveillance of Big Nurse, he tries "to foul her equipment up as much as possible by not letting her see my eyes—they can't tell as much about you if you got your eyes closed."[86] But the danger is that the "fog" of the hospital, which prevents patients from thinking clearly, might affect Bromden's ability to survive on his own terms. In the course of the novel, McMurphy returns vitality to Bromden, helping him to recover his thoughts, to see "some good in the life around" him, and, eventually, to escape.[87] But this sharing of a life force is at the expense of McMurphy's own well-being; his final punishment is a lobotomy, a drastic treatment that he had earlier acted out.

As Kesey was eager to stress, the book is clearly a work of fiction, but the system that the patients endure closely resembles Goffman's model in *Asylums*. The Combine works via fear, dressing up disciplinary procedures as therapeutic ones. Whereas Hall Bartlett's 1963 film *The Caretakers* favorably contrasts group therapy to the sadistic methods of the head nurse, Lucretia Terry (Joan Crawford), in *One Flew over the Cuckoo's Nest*, Big Nurse humiliates the patients during group therapy and is quick to resort to aggressive procedures such as electroshock treatment and, in McMurphy's case, lobotomy.[88] Although Big Nurse's hold over the patients might seem total, Kesey employs certain literary techniques to undermine her regime, and his style is diametrically opposed to the subdued white-collar fictions of the 1950s in its heightened emotions, dark comedy, and the hallucinogenic quality of the prose (related to Kesey's LSD experiences at Menlo Park and his prominent role in the West Coast drugs scene in the mid-1960s). The novel belongs within the genre of the modern Western, with McMurphy's wanderlust (Bromden is intrigued by the map-like markings of the new patient's palms), the critique of rigid systems of organization in which patients become "mechanical puppets," the revitalizing role of nature (symbolized by McMurphy's smell of "open fields" and the recreational therapy of the patients' fishing trip), and, at the end of the novel, Bromden's dramatic escape from the hospital.[89]

Through these means, Kesey goes beyond Goffman's identification of institutional structures and the coping devices of survival to offer an alternative mode of therapy.[90] McMurphy is constantly laughing, described by Bromden as "tromping up and down the halls and laughing out loud in meetings and singing in the latrines."[91] Although he is no philosopher, McMurphy associates laughter with an authentic sense of self, commenting that he has not "heard a real laugh since I came through that door."[92] Laughter is both an act of defiance and therapeutically empowering, making the patients feel better about themselves and helping to restore their sense of masculinity. As a Western, the novel tries to restore rugged masculinity from its diminished status due to the domestic softening of mid-1950s suburbia (see chapter 4) and in contrast to the sadistic but sterile tyranny of Big Nurse. It does not do this by promoting single-minded individualism, but through a communal spirit that wells up from below rather than being artificially induced from above. This emphasis on masculinity reconnects the patients to a life force that the machinery of the Combine is eager to neuter, particularly through the mortifying practice of lobotomy—described in the novel as a form of frontal lobe castration.[93]

Such an emphasis on distinct "roles" echoes Goffman's work on the structure of social encounters. In *The Presentation of Self in Everyday Life* (1956), Goffman describes how individuals "perform" a self by manipulating masks appropriate to various social situations. Reality is maintained through the appropriate choice of mask, and "well oiled" impressions of self-mastery enable "the firm self . . . to emanate intrinsically from its performer."[94] This dramaturgical method of presenting the self is at the heart of Goffman's theory of social performance. It does not mean that the "true" or "authentic" self is presented; indeed, it might lead to the contrived or cynical manipulation of socially respected masks.[95] Maxwell Jones was eager to keep these social roles open within new therapeutic communities, but Goffman examines scenarios where such masterful performances are prohibited or when the machinery of performance breaks down. In *Asylums*, he writes of the ways in which patients or inmates are "stripped of the support" offered by stable social arrangements and are forced to accept the loss of their "identity kits."[96] In *One Flew over the Cuckoo's Nest*, Kesey dramatizes this process of mortification at the hands of Big Nurse, brought about by what Goffman describes as "a series of abasements, degradations, humiliations, and profanations of self," but Kesey holds onto the notion of an authentic self based on autonomy, mobility, and imagination.[97]

Although Kesey can be accused of misogyny in the caricature of Big Nurse, the novel attempts to break through the restrained tone of much 1950s fiction, pointing out the necessity but also the potentially tragic consequences of nonconformity. But this is not the whole story. Laughter and camaraderie are proposed as humane thera-pies, enabling the patients to coexist as a community and find new ways of being.[98] For a novel published in 1962, this balance between individualism and community is a potent mix. It echoes Goffman's insight that "our sense of being a person can come from being drawn into a wider social unit; our sense of selfhood can arise through the little ways in which we resist the pull."[99] It also aligns Kesey more closely with the therapeutic communities of Jones than with Szasz's "myth of mental illness" model. And Kesey's search for alternatives and meaningful communal actions can be linked to President Kennedy's dual emphases on getting the country moving and community care.

Literary critics applauded the imaginative reach of Kesey's novel, and the work sold more than a million copies during the 1960s. But there were two major criticisms of Kesey, based on what was seen as an exaggerated view of a mental hospital and on the caricature of a ward nurse who seems to gain pleasure out of subjugating her patients. The first criticism stems from these exaggerated techniques, but it is also closely related to responses to the first theatrical adaptation. When the novel was adapted for stage by Dale Wasserman and performed on Broadway in 1963–1964, with Kirk Douglas as McMurphy, its dark humor was mistaken as a parading of the patients in a stigmatizing freak show. A *New York Times* reviewer thought that the comedy was in bad taste and that the dramatic pattern was undermined by "a crazy-quilt of wise-cracks, cavorting, violence and histrionic villainy" (similar criticisms were made of the 1971 stage version).[100] These criticisms do not neutralize Kesey's and Goffman's critiques, but they raise questions about whether any such totally enclosed institution actually exists. However, Kesey's exaggeration can be read as a literary and ideologi-cal strategy to urge readers to respond to an oppressive system that masquerades as a caring one. Moreover, although there is a barrier between outside and inside in *One Flew over the Cuckoo's Nest*, the novel uses the microcosm of the mental hospital as an analogy for social relationships at large. In this way, it foreshadowed another account of medical relationships, published two years later.

In contrast to Goffman's bleak picture of total institutions, this 1964 publica-tion, *The Psychiatric Hospital as a Social System*, offers a more benign "cultural sub-system" of "patterned relationships."[101] Sponsored by the Veterans Administration, the fieldwork for this study was carried out in a neuropsychiatric hospital in Virginia in 1951–1952, so the findings were not very current. The team of researchers studied a chronic ward and an admissions ward, focusing on particular roles ("social," "aso-cial," and "isolate"), group dynamics, and the social structure of the wards. Although the patients passed through the admissions ward fairly quickly, the study reveals marked similarities in behavior on the two wards, with "acceptance-rejection" and "dominant-submissive" relationships the two most prominent dynamics.[102]

These relationships mirror those dramatized in *One Flew over the Cuckoo's Nest*, but whereas Kesey tends to elide conditions (he has just two categories, "chronics" and "acutes"), *The Psychiatric Hospital as a Social System* finds that the community dynamics differ markedly depending on personality type, clinical condition, and prior social roles.

Adopting new roles might prove therapeutic for some patients, but finding a consistent role in which the patient feels comfortable might be the best technique for others. Albert Wessen's study differentiates the "restrictiveness" of hospitals from the punitive practices of prisons, but the ultimate goal, according to Goffman, would be to develop a therapeutic community within hospitals that could increase the patient's motivation rather than creating what the research team called a "completely conditioned patient" with habituated behavior.[103] The book also mentions another technique that would have met with Jones's and Kesey's approval—"permissiveness" (a technique also recommended by David, an intellectual patient, as a way of dealing with the chronic schizophrenia of a withdrawn patient, Lisa, in Frank Perry's 1963 film *David and Lisa*)—but Goffman spares only a few lines for the therapeutic benefits of that technique.[104]

A more balanced view of this 1964 study on the variety of institutional roles is that the border between the inside and outside of institutions was more permeable than *Asylums* suggests—particularly during the early 1960s, when outpatient facilities and community support were being taken more seriously. This change in approach was demonstrated by a community health project initiated in 1953 by the Harvard School of Public Health and sponsored by the National Institute of Mental Health, whose goal was to examine rehabilitation of outpatients after hospitalization. The projects' leaders sensitively acknowledged that:

> Psychiatric rehabilitation should be concerned especially with optimal restoration of social roles and social functioning. . . . The doors of the hospital are not one-way exits into the community used solely by persons restored to health and able to take up active instrumental roles and assume the full responsibilities of communal life. Instead, they are doors used by both the sick and the well—and revolving doors at that.[105]

Nevertheless, the bleak picture of state institutions as places of incarceration continued into late 1960s, as evidenced by the welfare investigator Frank Leonard's brutal exposé of an overcrowded metropolitan institution in his novel *City Psychiatric* (1965) and Frederick Wiseman's film *The Titicut Follies*, which aroused considerable controversy when it was in 1967. Wiseman focused this (his first) documentary, filmed over twenty-nine days, on incarcerated individuals who were both inmates and patients at Bridgewater State Hospital in Massachusetts. One review in *Life* noted that Wiseman "relentlessly pursues the horrible truth of a horrible situation" and that he offered "no easy outs" for viewers. Nevertheless, the reviewer suggested that Wiseman deliberately creates moments when we realize that the inmates "are uncomfortably like us, their behavior only an exaggeration of that state we are pleased to call normal."[106] Perhaps for this reason, the film was banned a year later for purportedly violating Massachusetts privacy laws, a ban that was upheld by the Supreme Court even though filming had been cleared with staff and patients at Bridgewater. *The Titicut Follies* depicts patients living in crude conditions—many of them in solitary confinement and force-fed by staff members who treat them with utter disdain—and it offers an uncomfortable illustration of an institution where flexible roles cannot flourish.

On the Inside: A Journalist's View

Goffman's influential account of pernicious institutional structures and Kesey's literary exploration of muted voices within them suggested to readers that psychiatric hospitals were sealed units, with no way in except through committal. Although Walter Freeman, the champion of transorbital lobotomy, published *Psychosurgery and the Self* in 1954, outlining the effects on the patient's sense of "self-continuity" and promoting the therapeutic effects of psychosurgery (which he argued could release the patient from morbid symptoms and the grip of the past), the details of electroshock treatments and psychosurgery in the 1940s and 1950s remained mysterious to the general public.[107] There were rumors that the psychological problems of the film actress Frances Farmer had worsened after she had been diagnosed as a paranoid schizophrenic and given electroshock treatment in Western State Hospital, Washington, in the mid-1940s. Concerns about the procedure were substantiated by Sylvia Plath's account of it in her quasi-autobiographical novel *The Bell Jar*, when Esther Greenwood experiences being "burned alive all along [her] nerves."[108] Plath portrays Esther as a victim of an authoritarian system and likens her electroshock treatment to the Rosenbergs' electrocution for Cold War espionage in 1953. Esther is an apolitical character, but this analogy is not dissimilar to the way in which Allen Ginsberg—in his autobiographical poem "Kaddish"—sees his mother's psychiatric treatment ("with your eyes of shock / with your eyes of lobotomy") as an assault on her communist beliefs (see chapter 6).[109] Accounts of psychiatric treatment became increasingly politicized in the 1960s, but the literature of psychological damage goes back to the early 1950s, with Ralph Ellison's exploration of the social effects of electroshock treatment on African Americans in the period between the two world wars, based on Ellison's work with Harry Stack Sullivan in the mid-1930s and at Lafargue Psychiatric Clinic in the mid-1940s. Although the Lafargue Clinic could be seen as an enabling space in the heart of Harlem, psychiatric treatment in Ellison's Invisible Man is much more threatening: the surgeon promises that the patient will remain "physically and neutrally whole" after the treatment, but the unnamed protagonist feels the "pulse of current smashing through [his] body," leaving him "disconnected" and "remote" from himself, as if all his limbs had been "amputated" and his thoughts lost in a "vast stretch of clinical whiteness."[110]

In addition to these literary accounts and psychological and sociological studies by Goffman, Bruno Bettelheim, and Robert Jay Lifton that explored the debilitating effects of institutional regimes on patients' well-being, regional journalists were becoming increasingly interested in mental illness and the enclosed environment of psychiatric hospitals. A thirteen-part television series on community services for the mentally ill, *The Changing Mind*, was broadcast in St Louis in 1959; a program called *The Face of Despair* was aired in Sacramento in 1960; and a series on mental retardation, *The Twilight World*, was produced in Oklahoma City in 1964. In print, *Harper's* ran a special supplement in October 1960 titled "The Crisis in American Medicine," which included a piece on "Tomorrow's Hospitals" that began "American hospitals are in deep trouble" and called for "sound economic and social planning."[111] In 1961 the journalist Michael Mok wrote a piece titled "I Was a Mental Patient" for the *New York World-Telegram*, in an effort to improve conditions in New York hospitals; and in the summer of 1959 Jack Nelson, a journalist for the *Atlanta Constitution*, published a series of reports on the long-term maltreatment of patients at the State Hospital in Milledgeville, Georgia.[112] The hospital had opened in 1842 in response to the passage of a Georgia state bill to create a "State Lunatic, Idiot, and Epileptic Asylum." A century later, Milledgeville was the nation's largest psychiatric hospital with over 120,000 patients, but it had only forty-eight doctors in the late 1950s and no trained psychiatrists at all. A disregard for patients, the use of unqualified staff members to administer anesthesia and insulin treatment, experimental drug practices, alcohol abuse, unsanitary conditions, and burying dead patients in the grounds were among the practices that Nelson exposed at Milledgeville—reporting for which he was awarded the Pulitzer Prize in 1960 and that was featured in a 1963 issue of *Time* with the title "Psychiatry: Out of the Snake Pits." A few years later, Rosalynn Carter noted that conditions at the hospital remained far from perfect. But, due to an official inquiry and new funds pledged by Governor Ernest Vandiver, by the mid-1960s the hospital was employing fifty psychiatrists, nurses, and occupational therapists, and release rates of patients had increased.[113]

Within this context of investigative journalism, Samuel Fuller's film *Shock Corridor*, released in 1963, takes a journalistic—some would say a tabloid-style or sensationalist—approach to psychiatric treatment. Fuller had worked as a newspaper reporter in the 1920s for the *San Diego Sun*, specializing in crime reports; in the 1930s and 1940s, he turned his hand to writing pulp fiction. After he became a filmmaker in the 1940s, he saw his films as "front page material" designed to provoke the reader—in the same mode as Ken Kesey, but cranked up a notch.[114] The film historian Lee Server calls *Shock Corridor* "hyped-up, unpredictable, grotesque, tasteless, embarrassing and scary . . . alternatively electrifying and unbearable."[115] It pushes viewers into thinking about the fine line between sanity and psychosis, and it suggests that vain ambition and an oppressive system could combine to shock a sane man into permanent psychosis. The film is deliberately rough around the edges; produced in black and white, with three grainy color dream sequences on 16mm film, *Shock Corridor* took two weeks to shoot on a limited budget.

The film is not based on a contemporary journalistic exposé. Rather, it was inspired by Nellie Bly, a late-nineteenth-century journalist who posed as a patient in order to enter the mental hospital on Blackwell's Island (now Roosevelt Island), located in the East River between Manhattan and Queens.[116] The film tells the story of Johnny Barrett (Peter Breck), an undercover reporter who thinks he can win the Pulitzer Prize if he solves a murder that has been committed in a southern mental institution. To gain admittance to the hospital, Johnny pretends that he has schizophrenia and has attempted to sleep with his sister—a role he asks his reluctant girlfriend, Cathy (Constance Towers), to play. He has assistance from his newspaper editor and his psychiatrist, Dr. Fong, but portents of doom are present from the beginning, with an epigraph from Euripides about madness, shadows reminiscent of film noir, Johnny's strained relationship with Dr. Fong, and sexual tension between Johnny and Cathy.

Just as it does in 1940s film noir (see chapter 2), space plays a major role in *Shock Corridor*: many scenes hem Johnny in, before and especially after he has been admitted to the hospital. Fuller presents a classic example of Goffman's total institution, although it appears more disorganized than the strict regimes described in Goffman's and Kesey's texts. The film takes its title from the hospital's central thoroughfare, where patients are "free" to walk, converse, and display themselves in "public." But they are not in control of the masks they wear, except for Johnny in the early stages of his hospitalized life. In an attempt to track down the murderer of a former patient named Sloan, Johnny interviews three resident patients, but this is less the central focus of the film than the hospital community as a microcosm of the nation: the "shock corridor" masquerades as a relatively free space, but it is where psychoses manifest themselves most clearly.

The three patients Johnny interviews are Stuart, a former farm boy and Korean War veteran; Boden, an atomic scientist; and Trent, an African American patient who has turned into a hater of his own race and an admirer of the Ku Klux Klan. Each one has a psychotic condition that is linked closely to his social status, and Johnny has to play particular roles to get close to them. Stuart's experience in Korea has pushed him to retreat into the past, where he imagines he is a Confederate Civil War general. Boden's work on the atomic bomb has triggered his regression into an autistic, childlike state where he scribbles diagrams that could reveal scientific secrets and communist plots, or might merely represent the confused expressions of a lost man. Trent's condition is the most disturbing of the film; he alternates between suspicion that Johnny is an infiltrator and a sense that they are co-conspirators in a plot. When we first meet Trent, he is hidden by a sign reading "Integration and Democracy Don't Mix, Go Home Nigger!," and we don't see the color of his skin. His story makes it clear that he has been the victim of racial discrimination at a southern university, and his extreme response has been to adopt the vindictive attitude of his tormentors. In line with contemporary clinical accounts of self-hatred that can often lead to "pugnacious and destructive" or "norm-violating" behavior, Trent believes he is a Klansman and wants Johnny to join him in starting a race riot.[117] Instead of identifying with an older African American patient in the corridor, Trent incites the other patients to join him in a brawl.

Trent's behavior is disturbing because it is so extreme, particularly for 1963. Boden and Stuart regress into private worlds related to their experiences as veteran and physicist, but Trent's fantasy of being a white supremacist has direct social consequences in the context of the white southern backlash to racial integration. Not only is Trent's psychological damage clear to see, but his disturbing language suggests that he has undergone a psychotic splitting of the self. Writing about the broader condition of split-self syndrome in black patients, the educational psychologist Jocelyn Landrum-Brown notes that such "splitting appears to be the result of having

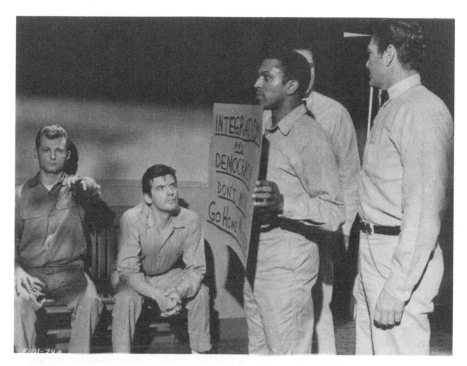

FIGURE 7.1   Johnny Barrett (Peter Breck) contemplates Trent (Hari Rhodes), who incites racial hatred. *Shock Corridor* (Samuel Fuller, Allied Artists, 1963).

internalized negative messages about their racial differences and the result of a desire to disown those differences in order to feel accepted and valued."[118] This stems from Trent's experience of discrimination, but in a hospital full of blurred identities, he stands out as an extreme reminder that the syndromes on display relate directly to the outside world. His incitement of race hatred and attempt to lynch another black patient reveal that this hospital is not equipped to deal therapeutically with such a deep-rooted psychosis or to address its root causes.

Johnny's behavior in the hospital does not go unpunished: he receives electro-shock treatments and at one point is confined in a straitjacket. This is also the punishment for Dale Nelson (Stuart Whitman) in the Twentieth Century–Fox film *Shock Treatment* (1964), in which Nelson, a skilled actor, masquerades as a patient in order to investigate a homicide in a mental hospital. The hospital is a scene of Cold War secrecy (a sleeping pill is called "Number 4"), psychiatric interrogation, and control of patients by drugs: the ward psychiatrist, Dr. Edwina Beighley (Lauren Bacall), experiments with a catatonia-inducing drug that is described as being "far beyond LSD or anything else they use today." When Nelson is caught spying on Beighley, he is punished with high-voltage shock therapy; a sustained aerial shot shows Nelson's convulsions as he is pinned to the bed by orderlies and leather straps. The sadistic Beighley follows up the shock treatment by injecting Nelson with the psychotropic drug (previously tested only on animals) to convince the court that he is "a catatonic

schizophrenic with only periodic phases of mobility." Although Nelson retains
moments of lucidity and he eventually manages to escape from the hospital with
a female patient with whom he has fallen in love, he struggles to control his actor's
mask in a climate of hallucinations, paranoia, and pernicious authorities.

Johnny Barrett's treatment in *Shock Corridor* also makes him increasingly paranoid: he hears voices in his head, and he starts to believe that Cathy really is his
sister. As in *Shock Treatment*, Lisa Dombrowski identifies role-playing as the central
motif of *Shock Corridor*. Cathy is well-read and immaculately dressed, but she earns
her living as a stripper at night and reluctantly sustains the pretense that she is Johnny's sister; Johnny tries to cling to his powers of reason and retain his journalist's
objectivity, while appearing "unbalanced enough to be believable and trustworthy in
the hospital."[119] The more time Johnny spends as a patient, the more his inner voice
becomes strained and fragmented; he becomes forgetful and has to try hard to keep
his thoughts clear and purposeful. The fog that pervades the hospital in *One Flew over
the Cuckoo's Nest* becomes a cacophony of noise, screams, and voices in *Shock Corridor*, which makes the film overwhelming to watch—as if Fuller wants the viewer to
experience a version of Johnny's psychosis. Johnny's cracked voice and split-self seem
central to Fuller's aesthetic, which borrows from the literary tradition of Southern
Gothic, reflecting the tropes of illness and disability in the fiction of Carson McCull-
ers and Flannery O'Connor. However, Fuller's film has little meaningful to say about

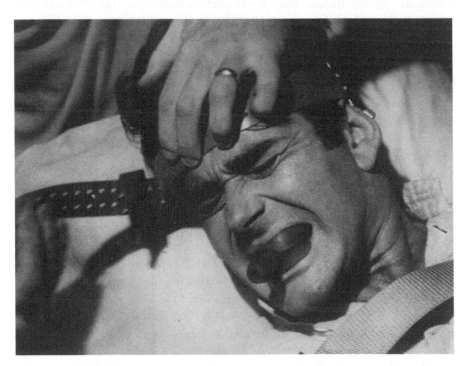

FIGURE 7.2   An institutionalized Dale Nelson (Stuart Whitman) receives aggressive
therapy. *Shock Treatment* (Denis Sanders, Twentieth Century–Fox, 1964).

schizophrenia and confuses it with multiple personality syndrome (now referred to as dissociative identity disorder), a mistake also made in the 1956 film *The Three Faces of Eve*, in which Joanne Woodward plays a mental patient with three distinct personalities that she is unable to control.

The detection plot of *Shock Corridor* is less important than the psychological strains placed on Johnny. He learns the name of the killer fairly soon, but he keeps forgetting it as the overload of noise drowns his thoughts. Following each of the patient interviews, the film cuts to a grainy dream sequence in which the tempo slows and the natural world is glimpsed, suggesting that the only contact with the outside is through dreams and fantasy. Dombrowski notes that the film conflates "what is real and what is imagined," as the dreamlike color imagery is closely linked to "moments of lucidity" that "startle viewers . . . into an awareness of the patients' subjective experiences," in an environment where words prove inadequate.[120] As Johnny's psychosis intensifies, so the camerawork "abandons any pretense to maintaining a unified presentation of time, space and action": rain pours down on Johnny in the hospital, and "sound effects of thunder and lightning heighten the subjectivity, while an optical lightening strike cues a series of low-angle color shots of overflowing waterfalls."[121] Johnny recovers his senses enough to remember the identity of Sloan's murderer, but during his investigation—and precipitated by supposedly therapeutic disciplinary practices—his formerly stable ego completely collapses.

When we see Johnny back in Dr. Fong's office at the end of the film, he is completely catatonic, speechless, and impervious to Cathy's desperate embrace. When he raises his arm stiffly to a horizontal position, it signals that he has a deep-rooted psychosis that will require intensive medical care. Johnny may have won the Pulitzer Prize for exposing a murderer in the hospital, but it is at the expense of his mental health. Ironically, his outstretched arm may never be able to grasp the prize he desires, and the implication is that he will have to return to the hospital, this time with a permanent psychosis. Thus, the journalist has lost his two most important gifts: his ability to coolly observe and to find words to describe his story. The film blames the regime of the mental hospital, but it also implicates the psychiatrist, newspaper editor, journalist, and girlfriend—all of whom collude in a plot that blurs a much-needed inquiry into institutional practices with cinematic sensationalism.

On the Outside: Region, Race, and Poverty

The previous two sections of this chapter have shown the ways in which sociologists, writers, and filmmakers began to expose institutionalized psychiatry in the early 1960s by representing the inside operations of mental hospitals. The hospital communities in *One Flew over the Cuckoo's Nest* and *Shock Corridor* are quite different, but both sets of patients are beleaguered and belittled by systems that regulate their behavior. These are very different communities from the ones President Kennedy envisaged, particularly as patients and hospital workers often colluded in the systems for fear of punishment or out of lack of opportunity to do otherwise. Kesey wrote that the black orderlies in his fictional hospital are "sulky and hating everything, the time of day, the place they're at here, the people they got to work around," as he tried to capture the mood of nonprofessional black hospital workers, often employed because their labor was cheap.[122] Similarly, orderlies in a later novel by Richard Yates, *Disturbing the Peace* (published in 1975 but set in 1960), are employed to sedate the patients and distribute cigarettes to keep them from revolting. Although Randle McMurphy and Johnny Barrett's heroic (or possibly vainglorious) attempt to exert pressure from within the institutions, external social forces contributed most to institutional changes, particularly for African Americans and the poor. Extending earlier discussions in this chapter, it is to these two topics—race and class—that this chapter now turns, in order to assess the patchy provision of healthcare that Kennedy, Johnson, and reformers were faced with in the first half of the 1960s.

As discussed above in this chapter, the major conceptual problem for African American mental health after World War II is that it was often defined against a (usually unacknowledged) white ideal of health. Therefore, trying to pass as white or being resentful and aggressive toward a white patriarchal doctor or the largely white establishment could be seen as forms of psychosis.[123] The "social pathology" model of black mental health suggested that the white ideal was always out of reach, but it remained the tacit norm against which ethnic deviance was measured. In 1952 the Martinique psychiatrist Frantz Fanon called this type of pathology a "corporeal malediction," which he linked to feelings of inferiority and racial damage that tend to be intensified within a medical institution where black "unreason" was countered with white "reason."[124] Goffman also portrayed the worst forms of psychiatric hospitals as institutions of slavery, where the relationship between staff and patient was often one of master and slave, or colonizer and colonized. The patient's response to this might be withdrawal from the situation ("prison psychosis"), rebellion (often punished by electroshock treatment or lobotomy), colonization (accepting life on the inside), or adaptation (acting out the role of the "perfect inmate").[125] All four responses might be seen as maladaptive for a black patient, but the ontological significance of the response differs depending on patients' social and economic background, their age, the racial dynamics of their community, the severity of their illness, and circumstances within the hospital. Goffman leaves open the possibility that patients could retain a secret life, hidden from hospital surveillance. Fanon describes this as a slipping into corners—"I remain silent, I strive for anonymity, for invisibility"—but he did not see it as a therapeutic existence.[126] Indeed, the racial realities of hospitals, particularly in the South, were likely to compound rather than ease any preexisting mental illness.

Class and region proved almost as important as race for defining the medical experience of African Americans. Malzberg's statistics on admissions to mental hospitals in New York State, for example, reveal a firm relationship between strong income and good health: illness was least frequent for those in "professional and technical occupations" who had high levels of education, and it rose "to a maximum among laborers" and other jobs associated with low esteem.[127] According to statistics from 1949–1951, fewer than 5 percent of admitted African Americans were in the financially "comfortable" category (with "resources sufficient to maintain self and family for at least four months"), compared to 66 percent in the "marginal" category, and nearly 30 percent who were considered "dependent" ("those lacking in the necessities of life, or receiving aid from public funds, or from persons outside the immediate family").[128] Malzberg notes that afflictions and class were closely related: 64 percent of patients with senile psychoses were dependent, whereas only 11 percent of manic depressives and 21 percent of people with dementia were in this category.[129] The one illness that bucks the trend was manic depression, which was more common among those with high levels of education, both white and black.[130]

Karen Kruse Thomas has done a great deal to map African American health in the South up to the Supreme Court's ruling in *Brown v. Board of Education*, but early detailed health data on African Americans in southern states is hard to come by, partly because research into hypertension, stress, nutrition, allergies, industrial injuries, and social discrimination among poor black southerners was thin until the mid-1960s.[131] These restrictions were partly because low-income southern states were regularly ranked in the bottom ten states for healthcare (about twenty-five years behind facilities in the Northeast), but they were also due to the effects of segregation, which meant that only severe cases of disease among African Americans were likely to receive hospital treatment.[132] However, the gap in mortality rates between high-income and low-income states narrowed in the 1950s, and the health standards of African Americans generally improved after World War II, leading a 1963 report to note that the "health gap" between whites and blacks was "due primarily, if not entirely, to environmental rather than hereditary factors."[133]

Twenty years earlier, the Swedish economist Gunnar Myrdal—in his influential account of African American culture, *An American Dilemma* (1944)—thought that economic development among black Americans was key to improving their health, but Myrdal said little substantive about healthcare, despite resorting to the language of pathology in places.[134] The postwar picture for African Americans was actually quite mixed. The decline in deaths from tuberculosis and other communicable diseases meant that the chief causes of death among nonwhites were heart and cardiovascular disease, cancer, influenza, syphilis, and homicide.[135] Although deaths from syphilis declined with the availability of penicillin, cancer rates went up, particularly among people without easy access to medical facilities for early diagnosis. In terms of mental health, studies of state hospitals in Virginia and Ohio revealed that there were more admissions of black patients than whites over the forty years leading up to 1955, particularly among people with low socioeconomic status.[136] And ten years later, a pioneering study of poor black neighborhoods in Nashville conducted by Meharry Medical College revealed that four in every ten residents "presented themselves as being in unstable or neurotic categories."[137]

The AMA recognized racial problems within the medical profession as early as 1950, just at the National Medical Association (founded in 1895 to represent African American physicians) entered a more politically active phase, including challenges to the inadequate provision of hospital care to African Americans after 1957. However, the AMA and HEW were slow to act. The lack of opportunities for black physicians and discriminatory practices against black staff members and patients continued into the 1950s and 1960s, leading to a "negro medical ghetto," as the *Journal of the National Medical Association* put it in 1957.[138] There were 3,800 black doctors in the United States in 1951, and 5,000 in 1960 (blacks made up about 1 in 5,000 American doctors at that time), and the number of all-black hospitals had fallen by nearly 50 percent between the mid-1920s and mid-1940s.[139] After World War II, fewer than eighty all-black hospitals served 9.6 million southerners, and the ratio of black physicians to patients was just over 1 for every 7,500 in North Carolina, but only 1 for every 18,000 in Mississippi.[140] Even northern cities like Philadelphia ran a "racially dualistic medical community"; discriminatory practices were common throughout the country; there were fewer black physicians working in largely white hospitals in the 1950s than in the 1930s; and only a small fraction of the 1,300 nursing schools trained black nurses.[141] Some progress was made in northern cities like Detroit and Chicago in the early 1950s, but institutional problems were more endemic in the South, where change came slowly even after the Supreme Court's 1954 *Brown* decision. The *Brown* ruling specifically affected racially segregated education, but it was widely viewed as bringing to an end the premise of separate but equal public provision of services, including healthcare facilities and training.[142]

President Truman's Commission on Higher Education set out the vision of abolishing separate education for white and black students, but it was two years after *Brown* before any black students were admitted to Vanderbilt University, for example, and not until 1966 did two male black students enter the University of Alabama School of Medicine (no female blacks studied there until 1971).[143] Before *Brown*, African American students could study medicine at only two universities: Howard University College of Medicine in Washington, D.C., and Meharry Medical College in Nashville, Tennessee. After *Brown*, the number of internships from these two universities allowing black graduates to work in white hospitals rose from eight graduates in 1947 to forty-six in 1956.[144] Fifty medical schools nationwide were accepting black students by 1956, but sixteen southern schools did not admit blacks in 1956 (ten fewer than in 1948), and barriers to black students at southern medical schools persisted into the 1960s. Although Vanderbilt University had cooperated with Meharry on Operation Heartbeat to encourage high-school students (both white and black) to take up medicine, Vanderbilt did not agree to open its doors to black applicants until May 1962; even then, it did not admit suitably qualified black undergraduates until 1964 and did not actively recruit them until 1965, after the Civil Rights Act became law.[145]

Hardly any African Americans studied psychiatry in mid-century, and there were only a small number of practicing black psychiatrists until the 1960s.[146] Howard University established a Department of Psychiatry in 1952, appointing Ernest Y. Williams as the department's head, but Meharry did not have such a department until 1961; its new curriculum then combined "sociology, anthropology, psychology, and the role of religion while giving adequate coverage of nutrition, sexuality, and lifestyle." The department quickly became one of the most progressive academic units in Tennessee: it opened a twenty-four-hour outpatient clinic in 1964, emphasized the importance of "the patient in the community," and pioneered holistic patient care.[147] The story for psychology was similar. The eight southern states housed 16 percent of the nation's population in the mid-1950s but had only 6 percent of its psychologists, and only 1.5 percent of all psychology PhDs were awarded in the South.[148] Attempts to increase the number of qualified psychologists included a proposal that the Southern Regional Education Board provide a five-year grant to Fisk University in Nashville "to channel more Negro students into doctoral work in psychology."[149] Fisk had pioneered a sociological approach to health issues in the 1930s by using health habit questionnaires among children in local black schools, and, like Meharry, it was eager to extend health education into the community. Through this five-year grant, Fisk planned to become a hub for postgraduate research for all black students taking their first degree in Kentucky, Virginia, or Tennessee.[150]

These developments occurred against the backdrop of the Hospital Survey and Construction Act of 1946 (also known as the Hill-Burton Act), which required that all hospitals receiving federal aid provide beds and services for nonwhites, but which often led to racially separate facilities (or "deluxe Jim Crow," as segregated wards were called).[151] The act permitted separate facilities for the different races as long as they were equal, but in practice black patients were often kept in poor facilities, housed in distant wings or basements.[152] Even after *Brown*, desegregated hospitals proved to be a major obstacle in extending fair healthcare to all southerners, and it took a full decade—following court cases in Greensboro and Wilmington, North Carolina, and the passing of the Civil Rights Act—before southern hospitals were fully desegregated. Eisenhower was criticized by liberals for the sluggish speed at which *Brown* was implemented, and similar criticisms were made of the Hill-Burton Act, which permitted separate but equal hospital provision in practice if not in spirit. This inaction was not helped by the 1953 opposition of HEW Secretary Oveta Culp Hobby to the desegregation of military schools, and Hobby was also fairly passive about enforcing the Hill-Burton Act.

Indeed, the tensions between segregation and desegregation in schools caused immeasurable psychological damage to children, partly because of the white backlash to segregation but also because school principals and teachers underestimated the effects of desegregated classrooms. It was clear that both segregation and desegregation each brought their own psychological stresses. In a series of court cases in the early 1950s, the National Association for the Advancement of Colored People highlighted the psychological damage caused by classroom segregation, supported by evidence gathered by Kenneth and Mamie Clark in a series of doll tests that they conducted in the late 1930s in both segregated and integrated schools. This evidence was also presented at the White House Midcentury Conference on Children and Youth in 1950—and the subject of psychological damage was later imaginatively explored in Toni Morrison's debut novel, *The Bluest Eye* (1970), in which an eleven-year-old black girl, Pecola Breedlove, growing up in Lorain, Ohio, in 1941, desires Caucasian eyes like those of her white doll.

In contrast, an article in *Psychiatry* in 1953 estimated that the consequences of both legal and tacit desegregation include social devaluation, severe emotional stress, and weak ego development among African American children (often complicated in cases of poor or low-status families).[153] Eight years later, the child psychologist Robert Coles moved from New England to the South to conduct interviews with black schoolchildren in Atlanta and New Orleans (and in schools in North Carolina, Tennessee, and Arkansas) to assess the psychological effects of legal desegregation after *Brown*. In a short report in 1963—preceding by four years the first volume of his Children of Crisis series, the account of his fieldwork in the South—Coles describes a talented black girl who had been transferred to a desegregated school in Atlanta but had to return to her own black school because "she was suffering from insomnia, depression and cumulative fatigue."[154] It is unclear whether this was the direct result of desegregation or family problems, but Coles saw that anxiety, gastric disorders, migraines, loss of appetite, and low self-esteem were all consequences of her classroom experience.

Michael Byrd and Linda Clayton have argued that although federal health initiatives improved access to healthcare across the black community, "these measures, with their serendipitous, sometimes positive, effects on long-standing maldistribution and public health problems exacerbated by race and class segregation and discrimination, proved to be too little and too late."[155] Even after the Civil Rights Act, discrimination continued: only eleven of the thirty-nine southern hospitals visited by the Civil Rights Commission in 1965 had "achieved any substantial degree of desegregation," and HEW was held accountable in 1966 for not vigorously enforcing the spirit of the Civil Rights Act.[156]

This rather bleak summary is a counterweight to Kennedy's optimism in the early 1960s, but it also skips over progressive training programs at Meharry and Fisk and local initiatives in the mid-1950s that led to more positive accounts of southern medical facilities. For example, a Governor's Conference on Mental Health met in Detroit in February 1954 to reflect on the condition of medical treatment and after care, and the delegates realized that more support was needed in southern states. However, later that year, following conferences in Atlanta (in July) and Boca Raton, Florida (in November), the executive director of the National Mental Health Committee, Mike Gorman, claimed that "the South is the first region to mount a cooperative attack upon mental illness, but the idea is catching on rapidly in other parts of the country."[157] The National Association for the Advancement of Colored People was also very active in ensuring that the Hill-Burton Act did not lead to a two-tier health system: the association attempted to block proposals in the early 1950s for segregated hospitals in Atlanta and Memphis, and it held annual meetings for healthcare practitioners between 1957 and 1963 to discuss racial integration, to which members of the press were invited.[158] In August 1963 (the year that Emory and Johns Hopkins Medical Schools changed their admissions policies to accept black students), John Kenney Jr., the retiring president of the National Medical Association, gave a rousing speech on medical civil rights at the association's Los Angeles convention, outlining how the group had attempted to close the racial loophole in the Hill-Burton Act, detailing discussions with the AMA and Vice President Johnson on employment opportunities for black physicians, and calling for solidarity to ensure that race would not continue to divide the medical profession.[159]

Of course, the major economic and medical divide that was hardest to breach in the South was between urban and rural. Half of rural Americans lived in southern states, and many of them had worse healthcare facilities in the 1940s and 1950s than their parents had had before the Great Depression. Although the growing African American middle class in Nashville and Memphis experienced marked improvements in medical support after the war, the division between urban and rural southerners—who, according to Edward Beardsley, lived almost entirely outside existing health systems—meant that change in the South occurred at varying rates (there were only twelve physicians in rural North Carolina in 1945, compared to nearly a hundred and twenty urban physicians).[160] This account tallies with the 1948 report titled *America's Heath*, which focuses on rural health and is less positive about the South than other regions in terms of current provision and future directions of healthcare. Fifteen years later, there were marked improvements, particularly in maternal and infant care, but the focus on urban facilities and medical schools meant that Atlanta was more similar to Chicago than it was to small-town Alabama or backwoods Arkansas. Michael Harrington's *The Other America* and the photojournalist Robert Frank's *The Americans* (1959)—his dramatic account of his trip through the South and West—explored outlying and neglected regions of the nation, and President Kennedy had aligned the public misunderstanding of poverty with misconceptions about mental illness.[161] But it was not until three years after President Johnson had called "for a national war on poverty. Our objective: total victory" that the progressive story about healthcare in the South was given a reality check.[162] It took two poverty tours of the South in 1967, the first including Robert Kennedy and the second Robert Coles, to reveal a large number of unfed and malnourished children and poor rural families who were suffering from tuberculosis and syphilis.[163] And not until the appearance of a report titled *Hunger USA* (1968), the 1968 CBS documentary *Hunger in America*, and popular journalistic accounts such as Nick Kotz's *Let Them Eat Promises* (1969) did poverty and the health effects of malnutrition in the South become a national concern.[164]

The state of medical provision for urban African Americans might have been better than for those in rural communities, but the Midtown Manhattan Survey made it clear that the difference was not great. Studies in New York City and Nashville in 1965–1966 linked ill health closely to hard-core poverty, unemployment, and unsanitary living conditions in urban slums—conditions not much different from Bonnie Bullough's description of a Chicago tenement in the early 1950s, quoted above in this chapter.[165] These conditions gave rise to a number of physical problems—cancer rates and heart disease were much higher in poor, inner-city areas than in rural localities—and psychological well-being was often at risk as well.[166] All this indicates that Kennedy's health reforms had a long way to go to make a substantive difference in the rural South or inner-city ghettos, and it emphasizes the significant lag between the reality of institutional care and Kennedy's vision of community medical support. This was partly because many health studies published in the early 1960s relied on research and data five to ten years old, but it was also because, as Kennedy realized, institutional practices were hard to change and federal reform needed time to trickle down to regional practice.[167] As chapter 9 elaborates, pioneers of localized therapeutic communities on the West Coast revealed progressive possibilities for outpatient care, but deep-rooted racial and economic issues meant that it would be difficult to fully roll out federal initiatives or to establish adequate outpatient facilities in all localities.

Although Allen Ginsberg tried to challenge silence and misperceptions on issues of sexuality and psychosis in his poetry and journals of the mid-1950s (as discussed in the previous chapter), it is clear that speaking out in the early 1960s was a pressing need—whether it is Chief Bromden who regains his voice toward the end of *One Flew over the Cuckoo's Nest*, Jack Nelson in his newspaper exposés on medical practices at the Central State Hospital at Milledgeville, Michael Harrington's work on the forgotten poor in *The Other America*, or civil rights initiatives geared to tackling discrimination in the hospital system. But, despite the deep-rooted infrastructural barriers to improving the nation's health, Paul Goodman's rallying cry of 1960 marked a moment of real possibility for postwar medical care: "One has the persistent thought that if ten thousand people in all walks of life will stand up on their two feet and talk out and insist, we shall get back our country."[168]

The Human Face of Therapy

HUMANISTIC AND EXISTENTIAL TRENDS

When President Lyndon B. Johnson addressed the nation for the first time on 27 November 1963, five days after President John F. Kennedy's assassination in Dallas, Johnson struck a reassuring tone. As vice president, he had often been of kilter with the Camelot culture of the Kennedys, and the two leaders had not always seen eye to eye. But in his televised speech, the new president claimed that his predecessor had been "the greatest leader of our time" and sought words "to express our sense of loss" at this "profound shock."[1] As well as promising to "continue the forward thrust of America," Johnson projected himself as a leader who aimed to put "ideas and ideals" into "effective" and "decisive" action, including Kennedy's "dream of care for our elderly—the dream of an all-out attack on mental illness—and, above all, the dream of equal rights for all Americans, whatever their race or color." This pledge to continue Kennedy's work with a "new spirit of action" was tempered by the mournful tone of a man who a week earlier had been very much in the shadows. Emerging from the speech are two attitudes: Kennedy's determination to act and Johnson's renewed commitment to "negotiate the common interest." The speech was not heavy with therapeutic language (it devoted more words to civil rights and the next tax bill than to healthcare), but Johnson's evocation of a spirit of "new fellowship" at a time of national trauma struck just the right balance between reflection, recognition, and progressive action.[2]

Johnson continued to emphasize community, perhaps even more than Kennedy had done. The new president's "War on Poverty" speech of March 1964 sketched out a Community Action Program that would "strike at poverty at its source" in both rural and urban localities aided by teams of volunteers; he announced a Work-Training Program for young adults between the ages of sixteen and twenty-one, following up on his work as vice president on equal employment opportunities; and he also announced a Work-Study Program to provide part-time jobs for those who could not otherwise afford a college education.[3] Johnson emphasized local plans motivated by grass-roots activism, but he also introduced the creation of an Office of Economic Opportunity, which would provide leadership for these initiatives. This has led some commentators to argue that Johnson's program was actually "a conservative application of structuralist observations," in his concerted attempt to get the poor back into the workforce.[4] But, despite reports coming out of the South in 1967 that poverty had not really been tackled, those living under the subsistence line decreased from 20 percent to 12 percent during Johnson's five years in the White House. Whether or not Johnson's determination to win victory over poverty could ever be realized (Nixon later accused him of using "inflated rhetoric that promises more than it can deliver"), it showed the humane face of politics in the years between the Cuban missile crisis and the escalation of the Vietnam War.[5]

The balance between central leadership and local cooperative ventures offered a different model of organization than the one endorsed by President Dwight Eisenhower's administration, epitomized by Johnson's conception of a "Great Society." This mode of social reorganization was an attempt to supersede a fixed hierarchical structure governed by a "power elite" (to recall the title of C. Wright Mills's 1956 book), replacing it with a series of interacting layers in which federal responsibility did not preclude local, grass-roots efforts, and governance was not at odds with civil liberty.[6] In this regard, in his speeches of 1964 and 1965, Johnson made use of therapeutic language, mixed with a brand of confident pragmatism, which took his presidential policies beyond mere extensions of those of his predecessor. Addressing a large audience at the University of Michigan in May 1964 (when Johnson was running for president in his own right), he stressed that the Great Society "is a challenge constantly renewed, beckoning us toward a destiny where the meaning of our lives matches the marvelous products of our labor."[7] The phrase "Great Society" might be dismissed as a slogan or a grand gesture (in 1966 Norman Mailer thought it was imbued with a "curious sense of happiness"), but Johnson's pledge was made equally to urban and rural Americans and was enacted through a rebuilding exercise designed to produce jobs and give communities a sense of local and national purpose.[8] Pollution and ecology appeared on the political radar for the first time in 1964 (stimulated by the publication of Rachel Carson's *Silent Spring* two years earlier and Lady Bird Johnson's interest in the beautification of the natural landscape); so did a concern that the nation's school systems needed reforming to ensure that nobody was too poor to receive an education and that school curricula could meet future national needs.

The amendment to the Social Security Act in 1965 was as important as the Civil Rights Act a year earlier, particularly the decision to add Medicare and Medicaid to the Social Security Act: Medicare focused on acute, noncatastrophic care for the elderly; Medicaid administered means-tested benefits for the poor.[9] Johnson thought that Medicare "foreshadowed a revolutionary change in our thinking about health care"; controversially, he called healthcare "a right, not just a privilege," and he pledged to invest $29 billion annually, up from $17.4 billion.[10] Federal spending on the poor doubled between 1960 and 1970, but the cost of Medicaid was to be shared between Washington and the individual states: Alabama, for example, received 75 percent of its Medicaid costs directly from federal funds, while California got 50 percent, and a later report on New York City estimated that combined federal and state investment was only 75 percent "of the costs of treating the newly entitled population."[11]

Johnson was proud of his work in combating physical and mental illness and in increasing the numbers of doctors, nurses, and hospitals, but the dramatic rise in public expenditure and the escalating costs of healthcare were the major reasons why Nixon wanted to scale back spending at the end of the decade. Nevertheless, welfare provision, civil rights, community action, and job opportunities were the cornerstones of Johnson's Great Society and, in combination, suggested that the nation was more caring than it had been ten years previously.[12] Johnson could be gruff, and he was at his best as a negotiator rather than an orator. Reviewing the president's 1964 book *My Hope for America*, Mailer considered Johnson a conservative leader with "double-barreled ideals" and a tendency to use "aggregate words" in the mode of a "communications engineer," while Herbert Marcuse was unconvinced about the domestic promises of the Great Society at a time when US defense policy militated "against progress toward higher forms of freedom and rationality."[13] But even Mailer and Marcuse begrudgingly credited Johnson for his sincere attempt to alleviate poverty, and Johnson was more enthusiastically described in the mid-1970s as "a very human president." In 1969, at a gathering to mark Johnson's departure from the White House, the historian James MacGregor Burns credited him with attacking domestic social ills "across the widest front, with every possible weapon."[14]

A New Fellowship

This human face of the presidency is very important for this chapter, in which I consider the ways in which Johnson's "new fellowship" can be seen to parallel developments in humanistic and existential psychology. These developments tended to privilege the patient's unique life world over rigid diagnostic frameworks, but they also looked beyond the individual to the ways in which new bonds could be forged within communities—what Philip Rieff called "commitment therapies," as distinct from "analytic therapies."[15] However, rather than seeing the tensions between the individual and community as irreconcilable, the thinkers addressed in this chapter—including Carl Rogers, Abraham Maslow, Harry Stack Sullivan, and Frieda Fromm-Reichmann—saw the two as mutually supporting, with existential aloneness closely related to the German philosopher Martin Heidegger's notion in *Being and Time* (1927) that "being-in-the-world-with-others" is an irreducible state of existence.

It would be tempting to see these interconnecting trends as a watershed in the postwar narrative, echoing Eli Ginzberg, who saw the Social Security Act as a discrete break in the story of postwar medicine. Ginzberg viewed 1961–1965 and 1965–1975 as distinct periods, with the latter marked by accelerating public expenditures and "heavy inflows of new dollars," before the fiscal crises of the mid-1970s.[16] However, I would argue that 1970 marks the most significant fulcrum, for reasons explored in the next chapter and the conclusion, but also because that is when Nixon started to scale back expenditures, in an "era of negotiation" as he outlined in his 1969 inaugural address.[17] The other major reasons why Ginzberg's periodization does not really work is that humanistic trends in the social sciences can be traced back to mid-century and that Johnson's health program was largely a continuation of Kennedy's plans. There were some new elements, such as Johnson's concern about the impact of pollution on health and the environment. These led to the Water Quality Act of 1965 and the Mental Health and Mental Retardation Act of 1966, which was designed to ensure adequate and equitable provision of mental health services at the state level for everyone, "regardless of religion, race, color, national origin, settlement, residence, or economic or social status."[18] However, the most visible way that Johnson helped to move Kennedy's community health care plans forward was through the neighborhood health project, which began in 1966 under the guidance of the Office of Economic Opportunity—a project to which I will now turn, to exemplify Johnson's "new fellowship."

A report on "The Bright Promise of Neighborhood Health Centers"—published in March 1968, the month when Johnson announced that he would not run for reelection following the Tet Offensive in Vietnam—suggested that out of all federal initiatives, the healthcare center scheme would be the most successful in tackling poverty. Thirteen family-focused neighborhood health centers had been established by the end of 1967, with more planned and $60 million of federal funding promised. The author of the report, Judith Randal, was very positive about the benefits of bridging the divide between "medicine's ability to deliver care to the whole community" and the "high quality service it can provide the relatively few": she wrote that the centers offered job opportunities for the poor and unemployed, training them to assist doctors and nurses or to become family health workers and laboratory aides.[19] Randal stressed the close link between illness and poverty as the central tenet of preventive healthcare, particularly in deprived localities such as Watts in Los Angeles, or the all-black town of Mound Bayou in Bolivar County, Mississippi, near the Arkansas border. With only three doctors for 40,000 African Americans in Bolivar County (there were nineteen doctors for the 19,000 white residents), the only previous healthcare facility for African Americans in Mound Bayou was a fraternally run Taborian Hospital, which had been established in 1942, with the proto–civil rights activist T.R.M. Howard as the hospital's chief surgeon for the first five years. Although the hospital also had directors of medicine and nursing, very few staff members had formal medical training and there were no ambulances.[20] The Taborian Hospital was successful in its own right as a grass-roots initiative, but a fully fledged medical center was not available until 1966, when the Delta Health Care Center was established. This health center offered emergency care in collaboration with local hospitals; it served an outpatient community, providing mental health and substance abuse facilities; and it provided financial assistance to those under the federal poverty line (42,000 people in Bolivar County were from families earning less than $3,000 per year).[21]

Although these new centers had to deal with regionally specific health problems (in Bolivar County, these included high infant mortality rates and malnutrition), Randal noted that the chosen urban and rural localities ("areas the doctors in private practice have found unrewarding") were not so distinct: sanitary problems in homes, overcrowding, and the transmission of disease were common to both. She saw that the centers helped to facilitate social change within communities—particularly those areas that had not traditionally had medical support (for example, the community-based Pilot City Health Center in Minneapolis began development in 1967, and Lowndes County, Alabama, received a health center planning grant in 1968)—and influenced university training. At places like Fisk University and Meharry Medical College, both in Nashville (see chapter 7), there was a growing realization that medical theory and practice in the community should be closely linked. And the University of Southern California, in Los Angeles, helped to establish a center in Watts in 1967, largely in response to the riots of 1965 in that neighborhood.[22] Randal cited warnings from the American Medical Association (AMA) and pharmacists that the neighborhood centers ran the risk of undermining free choice for those living within the centers' catchment areas, but she applauded Johnson's aim of having fifty centers by the end of 1968 and "the chain reaction this social experiment will set off" (there were eighty centers by 1973).[23]

The Neighborhood Health Center program was the most visible face of a caring government, and it was a success on its own terms, despite the cost. It stemmed from the Partnership for Health Act of 1966, which, as a report from the Department of Health, Education, and Welfare (HEW) put it, was born out of the realization that a "close cooperative effort would be required on the part of governmental, voluntary, and private organizations and agencies" to develop "statewide and areawide comprehensive" health facilities.[24] It was also part of a concerted attempt to return the human face to medicine as a caring profession, not only attempting to reconceptualize the patient's experience and the doctor-patient relationship, but also reconsidering conditions such as schizophrenia and depression that seemed to increase in frequency during the postwar years, as the later sections of this chapter will explore in relation to clinical and cultural accounts.

In addition to the realization that something needed to be done to improve care for patients, there was also a crisis in the image of the doctor in the early to mid-1960s, as ongoing developments in the Cold War threatened to replace the friendly family doctor with the more impersonal specialist or researcher. Kennedy's and Johnson's emphasis on community care attempted to check this trend, but it did not prevent "several dozen specialties" emerging in the related professions: one 1963 book found that "each specialty [was] budding with sub-specialties," many of which were reliant on "machines and techniques of dazzling variety and sophistication."[25] According to this view, the art of therapy had been replaced with a scientific model often bolstered by technology—which, as chapter 7 discussed, could be seen alternatively as the apparatus of care or that of oppression. The attempt to revive the art of the caring doctor was well expressed in 1963 by the editor of the *Lancet*, T. F. Fox:

> The teachers and the schools will have to decide whether they are content to produce a poker-faced technical expert who will attend to the faulty body as a garage technician attends to a faulty car, or whether, even in the modern world, they should still be producing doctors who will feel the same kind of personal obligation toward their patients as was felt by the old physicians. For my own part, I hold that our training lately has been far too much concerned with the body. . . . An education truly based on science as it has latterly advanced would pay far more attention to the emotions of the patient.[26]

In May of the same year, a *Time* cover story celebrated the American surgeon, with the message that "surgery now offers the first and the best hope of all."[27] And two years earlier, an article titled "The Doctor's Dilemma" conveyed the strong message that prescription drugs are subject to various safeguards before appearing on the market, but also that physicians should be knowledgeable and careful in their treatments.[28] Perhaps the most visible attempt to put a face on a caring doctor whom patients could trust was the character of Doctor Kildare in the television show of the same name. Nearly two hundred episodes of the show were broadcast on NBC between 1961 and 1966, with Richard Chamberlain playing the role of the handsome young James Kildare, a medical intern and later resident at a large urban hospital (Lew Ayres and Lionel Barrymore had made the same role famous on film screens in the 1930s and 1940s). Guided by an AMA advisory committee's desire to safeguard the reputation of the profession, the television version of Doctor Kildare balanced "hospital-based 'realism'" in terms of setting and equipment with melodramatic plotlines, while Chamberlain played Kildare as a responsible doctor and public servant who held patient care in high regard.[29]

In addition to concern about the male doctor's image, the early 1960s raised a different set of issues relating to female medical professionals and posed broader questions about the role of women (as doctors, analysts, and patients) in the history of medicine. For example, on the surface the CBS hospital-based series The Nurses (1962–1965) used a formula similar to that of Doctor Kildare, expanding on an earlier series, Janet Dean, Registered Nurse—which ran for thirty-nine episodes in 1954–1955 and was the first television show to have a female nurse as the main character. Not only was Ella Raines's character, Janet Dean, knowledgeable about medical matters, but she was smart, resourceful, and adept at solving cases. The series was endorsed by the American Nurses Association for promoting the profession—particularly in the last few minutes of each episode, when Raines spoke directly to the camera with a message that combined professional knowledge with common sense. One of the reasons why Janet Dean was an isolated example was because the medical profession remained a sector in which women were largely limited to supporting roles—as shown in 1964 when the two female characters in The Nurses series were joined by male doctors who offered assistance in applying medical ethics. If the series prompted questions about the autonomy of nurses, the case was worse for women doctors: only 6 percent of physicians were female in 1950, rising to only 7.6 percent (or 25,400) by 1970; and the American Medical Women's Association was marginalized until the early 1970s in terms of female representation in the AMA, even though women surgeons had been admitted to the Army and Navy Medical Corps in April 1943.[30]

After World War II, there was a marked increase in the numbers of female occupational therapists, social workers, nutritionists, psychologists, and nurses, but limited cultural representations of medical and scientific women reinforced the idea that professional women belonged in the supporting roles that they often took.[31] There were exceptions, such as Sara Murray Jordan, a well-published gastroenterologist at the Lahey Clinic in Burlington, Massachusetts, from 1923 to 1959; and Martha May Eliot, a pioneer in the field of children's health, the first female president of the American Public Health Association, and the only woman to sign the founding document of the World Health Organization. Theodora Abel is another important figure, particularly across the fields of experimental psychology, cultural psychology, and anthropology: in 1947 she became director of psychology at the Postgraduate Center for Mental Health in New York City, which pioneered community services and family therapy, and she was very interested in diverse cultural patterns displayed by Pueblo, Apache, and Navajo communities in New Mexico during the 1970s. In addition to the work of these figureheads, there were repeated reports about a major shortfall in personnel, and calls during the Cold War to increase the scientific and medical workforce.[32] But the historian Ellen More points to a 1957 report, *Womanpower*, which stressed "women's future role as teachers and nurses," reinforcing "old prejudices" and supporting the view that "women professionals had been used during the war only as a last resort."[33] It is not surprising that young female doctors, like Beneatha Younger in Lorraine Hansberry's 1959 play *A Raisin in the Sun*—about an African American family trying to escape the ghetto in Chicago's South Side—were such a rarity in postwar culture. Johnson's paternalistic presidency did little to help the cause of women, even though the banning of discrimination based on sex was included in his Civil Rights Act. In fact, this led the 1963 Presidential Report on American Women, which had been commissioned and researched during the Kennedy administration, to conclude weakly that "the advancement of women's legal rights would appropriately be pursued at the state rather than the federal level."[34]

Johnson's neglect of women's rights suggested that despite the caring face of his administration, something was missing. If medicine and psychiatry were to rediscover their therapeutic faces as healing arts, then something more than new health dollars was needed: a shift away from a Cold War mentality to a more caring interaction was one key element, together with a reassessment of the place of women and members of ethnic and racial minorities within the medical profession. The problematic relationship between women and healthcare reemerges later in this chapter, but the emphasis on face-to-face interaction in the mid-1960s can be seen to complement Johnson's stress on community and fellowship, fostering a shift from a normative account of health and pathology predicated on hierarchical structures of control to a more horizontal dynamic that focused on the patient's energies and capabilities. Erich Fromm detected that these "human proportions" were in danger of extinction with the emphasis on automation; for him, the "self-realization of humanity" could come about only if individuals took responsibility for their own and others' education (a positive form of self-love) and were willing to participate in small, face-to-face groups.[35]

This interest in humanistic psychology by theorists such as Fromm, Rogers, and Maslow is an important dimension of this chapter; so too are Erving Goffman's notion of "face work" (which he had outlined in the mid-1950s and which informed his sociology of the 1960s) and Kenneth Clark's psychological research with children and on the intimate relationship between identity and place. Complementing these strains of social psychiatry, the other major dimension discussed here is the influence of existential ideas on the medical humanities. Largely the domain of European and émigré intellectuals, existential thought emphasized the fundamental solitude of individuals and the need for people to accept the absurdity of the universe before they could lead authentic lives. These facts did not preclude a therapeutic community or the development of more flexible, open-door institutions, but existentialism suggested that illness could not be addressed simply as a public phenomenon to be solved through federal and state policy, with no acknowledgment of the very personal dimension to mental illness. As this chapter will discuss, the most important theorist of existential psychology was not a European émigré, but a neglected figure, who, I would argue, was central to American existential thought. The work of Ludwig Binswanger, a Swiss psychiatrist and one-time protégé of Freud, was translated from German in the late 1950s and early 1960s; Binswanger was promoted by Rollo May, and his thought linked laterally to Erik Erikson's research on the human life cycle and psychobiography.

Reflecting on the work of Binswanger, as well that of émigré and American practitioners, this chapter will explore humanistic and existential psychology as key inflections of the progressive therapeutic revolution of the 1960s, before returning to more specific issues—schizophrenia, depression, and suicide—that mark the mid-1960s as a particularly significant moment within the postwar cultural history of medicine. As well as reprising the discussion of African American healthcare in chapter 7, the later sections of this chapter develop earlier discussions of domesticity, gender roles, and growing up, particularly for people with medical diagnoses of schizophrenia and depression. Two of the most compelling fictionalized autobiographies of the decade, Sylvia Plath's *The Bell Jar* (1963) and Joanne Greenberg's *I Never Promised You a Rose Garden* (1964), offer interesting counterpoints to two other novels discussed in this chapter, Walker Percy's *The Last Gentleman* (1966) and James Baldwin's *Another Country* (1962), which deal with disorientation and depression on more diffuse levels. Johnson's community health program provides a historical framework for this discussion, and, as we will see, Johnson's own health problems and those of other high-profile public figures feature prominently in the medical story of the mid-1960s.

Humanistic Psychology

Humanistic psychology was formally named in Britain in 1958 and came to prominence in the United States in the early to mid-1960s, when practitioners sought to emphasize the primacy of experience.[36] William James had developed a pluralistic notion of experience at the beginning of the century, but James's brand of pragmatism was eclipsed by the rise of Freudian psychoanalysis between the world wars. However, there was a growing suspicion of psychoanalytic terminology in the late 1950s (Sidney Hook railed against "the monistic dogma of psychoanalysis" in a 1958 symposium at New York University[37]) and a renewed interest in James's phenomenological psychology in the early 1960s, as scientists realized that they need to become "sensitive observers" rather than systems builders, as James described in his 1896 essay "The Will to Believe."[38] I have argued elsewhere that the practitioners of a transatlantic mode of "romantic science"—including James, Otto Rank, Binswanger, and Erikson—did not flee from theory wholesale but looked to privilege personal experience rather than explaining the self on a deterministic level. Whether these thinkers were actually anti-Freudian is open to debate: Rank and Binswanger broke openly with key Freudian tenets, and the suspicion of Freud's emphasis on infantile sexuality ran through the medical humanities in twentieth-century America. Not only did these thinkers focus on the possibility of recreating the self in the present, but they discerned a therapeutic potential to positively reshape the environment by engaging in diverse therapeutic relationships and cultivating an ethical respect for others. Freud remained an important touchstone for these figures, but I would argue that he is not the influential presence among them that he is often assumed to be.

Two distinctly American thinkers, Rogers and Maslow, can also be positioned within this tradition. Rogers was influenced by Rank through his student Jessie Taft in the 1930s, and Maslow shared a similar critique of psychoanalysis, arguing as a student in 1932 that psychoanalysis "acts on the assumption that the individual is always wrong" and usually neglects the potential of individuals to transform their environment: he later called this "the sick half of psychology," to which he wanted to supply "the healthy half."[39] Both Rogers and Maslow were drawn to humanistic psychology, which focused on the possibilities of health rather than the limitations of sickness, but they arrived at this view from different intellectual paths. Maslow's influences in the early 1930s stemmed from anthropology and the cross-cultural studies of Margaret Mead and Ruth Benedict. In contrast, Rogers combined his early interest in theology (he considered becoming a Christian minister and studied at the Union Theological Seminary in New York in the mid-1920s) with practical studies on children (reflected in his 1939 book, *The Clinical Treatment of the Problem Child*), and he espoused a combination of Jamesian pragmatism and Rankian dissidence that broke from the scientific models Rogers encountered as a student at the University of Wisconsin.

The key for Rogers, as he outlined in *Client-Centered Therapy* (1951), was to build therapeutically productive relationships within a psychotherapeutic framework in order to "perceive as sensitively and accurately as possible all of the perceptual field as it is being experienced by the client."[40] There is a strong existential current in Rogers's work: he believed that the "suffering and the hope, the anxiety and the satisfaction" that fills "each therapist's counseling room" does not isolate the patient within a sealed inner life but offer paths of entry for the analyst.[41] "Client" for Rogers is a more therapeutically useful term than "patient," encompassing the kind of agency often negated by the implied passivity of sickness. Rather than the distant scientific figure represented by Dr. Brulov in *Spellbound* (see chapter 2), Rogers recommended that the therapist as counselor should actively develop a unique relationship with each client, "participating in [the individual's] struggle as deeply and sensitive as [the therapist] is able." In this vein, in the preface to *Client-Centered Therapy*, Rogers positions himself as a "midwife" in facilitating "a new personality," rather than piecing together the fragments of a past self by "thinking back" and "working through," on the Freudian model: "I stand by with awe at the emergence of a self, a person, as I see a birth process in which I have had an important and facilitating part."[42] Rogers took this emphasis on natality from Rank's work, while his interest in emerging patterns reflects the Gestalt writings of Paul Goodman and Frederick Perls.⁴³ There is also a sense that these new, emerging selves are pragmatically useful, enabling patients to overcome psychic hurdles or achieve new goals.

With his emphasis on self-development, Rogers was criticized by Rollo May and R. D. Laing for ignoring the demonic aspects of the self. Rogers did not entirely overlook psychic conflict or the "blind power" of life with its "tremendous capacity for destruction," but he nevertheless sought out "the opportunity for growth" in the face of social conformity.⁴⁴ He remained suspicious of medical diagnosis and behaviorism, as demonstrated by his 1956 exchange with the behaviorist B. F. Skinner, followed by a public debate between the pair at the University of Minnesota in June 1962.⁴⁵ However, Rogers argued that "cold and abstract" scientific models should not be abandoned outright because they "assist us in releasing forces that are warm, personal and complex"; although "science is slow and fumbling it represents the best road we know to the truth, even in so delicately intricate an area as that of human relationships."⁴⁶

Rogers had started to explore these ideas in his 1942 book, *Counseling and Psychotherapy*, which includes the first electronically recorded transcription of a course of therapy. In *Client-Centered Therapy*, Rogers further outlined his nondirective approach, ranging from play therapy among children and group therapy among adults, in which the analyst rarely intervenes or sets out a predetermined program. According to this model, the patient is not a puzzle to solve but a "co-worker on a common problem" and a hub of potentiality, which the therapist can help bring to realization by focusing on questions of the patient's significance and worth.⁴⁷ In order to reorganize the relationship between therapist and patient, Rogers would ask different questions than those posed by a Freudian analyst, emphasizing the growth, change, integration, congruence, and responsibility that are often bracketed off by analysts who are persuaded by a more strictly scientific approach. Whereas Goffman was drawn toward the roles people play in their private and public life that require a particular "face," Rogers was worried that role-playing (for both therapist and client) could be an inauthentic activity in which individuals "operate behind a front" and "tend to say things they do not feel."⁴⁸

Instances when public and private selves strain against each other (what Goffman called having the "wrong face or no face") would be examples of what Rogers called incongruence, as evidenced in the 1962 film *David and Lisa*, based on a 1961 case study and screenplay by the psychiatrist Theodore Isaac Rubin.⁴⁹ In both Rubin's case study and the film, the schizophrenic patient Lisa hides her face behind her hair and speaks only in rhyme; she can show her face only in the presence of David, a fastidious fellow patient with a phobia about germs, who breaks through Lisa's defenses by matching her rhyming speech patterns.⁵⁰ The camera work in *David and Lisa* is much more personal and intense than the objective style of many 1950s films; the camera lingers on the two patients' faces, opening up facial gestures and mannerisms in ways that are more expressive than actual words. This is a useful example for thinking about a Rogerian approach, particularly as Rogers believed that self-awareness and transparency are crucial if the individual is achieve a self-actualizing state, but he also believed that this sometimes requires an indirect route, as David finds in his encounters with Lisa. The individual might fear transparency because it can expose deep-seated neuroses or existential dread, but this fear would be more authentic than the cultivation of a composed face that conforms to a particular role in a "ritual game."[51]

Rogers realized that distortion, denial, and incongruence are common modalities in psychic illness, contrasting with a cohesive self that has the capacity to positively shape its environment, to meaningfully say "I am," and to balance autonomy with receptivity. This left Rogers open to the criticism that he was promoting an idealistic self in disguise and pandering to a brand of positive thinking—which led him to be adopted by the Christian pastoral counseling movement.[52] Rogers's defense was that he resisted idealized conceptions of the self in favor of an actual self that emerges from personal experience, but he nevertheless sidestepped common therapeutic problems. For example, he believed that strong transference leading to dependent relationships was rare in analysis; when such feelings arose, he was confident that an open, accepting environment would help the client to recognize "that these feelings are within her, they are not in the therapist."[53] Realizing that relationships should be at the heart of therapy, Rogers steered away from psychiatric treatment, so much so that when he established a counseling center in Chicago in 1945, he chose not to employ psychiatrists.

The reason why Rogers's work in the early 1950s is so important for the 1960s is that his humanist emphasis on self-actualization was strongly promoted by the

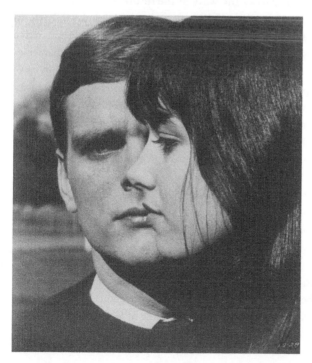

FIGURE 8.1   Lisa Brandt (Janet Margolin) allows David Clemens (Keir Dullea) to see her face. Publicity still for *David and Lisa* (Frank Perry, Continental Distributing, 1962).

American branch of the Association of Humanistic Psychology, which was launched at Brandeis University in 1961. Sometimes called a "third force" (following the "first force" of behaviorism and the "second force" of Freudian psychoanalysis, with its emphasis on the unconscious), humanistic psychology was heavily influenced by Maslow in the late 1950s and reflected Rogers's work in the 1940s and 1950s.[54] Although they were interested in actual experience, Rogers and Maslow had an idealistic bent, developing concepts of fullness to offset the rhetoric of deficiency in many clinical and psychological writings. But Maslow thought that Rogers fell into the trap of "overpsychologizing and under-sociologizing," and Maslow wanted to ensure that his "psychology of being" was creative on both individual and communal levels.[55]

In line with Maslow's plan to develop a social program for psychology, the Association of Humanistic Psychology launched its *Journal of Humanistic Psychology* in late 1963. The group held its first annual meeting in the following year in Los Angeles, at which Rogers was a keynote speaker, following the publication of his best-known book, *On Becoming a Person*, three years earlier. Rogers most often focused on the therapeutic encounter, but in the early 1960s he also became very interested in its social implications. For example, his consistent emphasis on openness was in direct opposition to covert Cold War political operations, and he thought that transparent foreign policy—in which vested interests, inconsistencies, and fears about the future could be acknowledged through open dialogue—was preferable to Cold War game playing.[56] In his keynote talk Rogers focused on the future, describing humanistic psychology as part of a developing trend in which "the subjective human being as an active agent . . . is to be a growing part of the wave of the future."[57] The talk followed Rogers's recent move from the University of Wisconsin to the Western Behavioral Sciences Institute, in La Jolla, California, where he started working with encounter groups—which explains why his talk focused on broader contexts rather than one-on-one therapy. Rogers thought that the core mission of the association was to challenge the "sterility of most present day psychological science" and to resist "the way in which man is treated as an object in present day behavioral science."[58] Rather than simply accepting the role of the association as a counter to the first and second forces of psychology, he explored the contribution that humanistic psychology could make to scientific knowledge and practice in addressing ontological questions that are often overlooked by medical practitioners. This form of connectedness—between art and science, practice and theory, knowledge and being—was a distinctive expression of the holistic practice that Rogers and others saw as a better model for the medical humanities than previous ones.

Existence and Being

European existentialism strongly influenced American social and psychological thought in the 1940s and became even stronger within the medical humanities in the 1950s and 1960s. This was partly because of the work of a number of émigré thinkers steeped in German existential ideas and often marked by the experience of war, such as Bruno Bettelheim and his fellow Austrian psychiatrist Viktor Frankl.

Bettelheim's *The Informed Heart* (1960) and Frankl's *Man's Search for Meaning* (1964) reflected their experiences in concentration camps during World War II. Existentialism inflected postwar thought in other ways as well: the Freudian dissident Otto Rank, for example—who spoke at the First International Congress on Mental Hygiene in Washington, D.C., in May 1930—wished to remodel psychoanalysis along philosophical lines and to rescue the "vital" human element from the scientific analysis of it.[59] Rank lectured widely at East Coast universities in the 1930s, promoting the "soular" (*seelisch*) dimension of human life and the "science of relationships," which he felt should motivate the individual to look beyond neurosis—an approach that Rogers called "relationship therapy" in 1942.[60] This philosophy of self-overcoming chimed with the cult of positive thinking, but Rank influenced broader humanistic currents in his attempt to go "beyond psychology" (the title of his posthumous 1941 book) and develop a "new vocabulary" that could do justice to the twin psychic drives of individuation and connection.[61]

As suggested above, another important figure for reshaping the research and practice of psychiatry and psychology in the late 1950s and early 1960s was the Swiss psychiatrist Ludwig Binswanger. His selected papers and case studies were first translated into English in a 1958 volume, *Existence: A New Dimension in Psychiatry and Psychology*, and additional work became available in North America in 1963 in *Being-in-the-World*, edited by the young American philosopher Jacob Needleman. May and Needleman did much to promote Binswanger's existential view of human life and mental health, particularly Binswanger's assault on what he called in a 1955 essay the "Magna Charta of Clinical Psychiatry." Established in the mid-nineteenth century, this "magna charta" explained Freud's early reliance on biology and natural science as the cornerstones of any legitimate scientific enquiry.[62] Binswanger was not the first Freudian dissident to influence American thought—Adler, Jung, and Rank all preceded him—but, despite his relative neglect now, he was arguably the most influential of these figures in 1960s America, offering a parallel to Rogers's and Maslow's humanistic psychology and more directly informing the psychiatric knowledge of schizophrenia.

Binswanger's disagreement with Freud was based on the idea of *Weltanschauung*. Freud thought that this term was a crude "philosophy of life" that provided a "unified solution of all the problems of existence," and he wanted to replace it with a biological model.[63] Binswanger disagreed, arguing that an existential branch of psychiatry would enable the analyst to overcome the natural-scientific bias of psychoanalysis and contribute to "the effort of psychiatry *to understand itself as science*."[64] This would represent the encroachment of philosophy on psychoanalysis in order to address the "total phenomena" of psychic life, enabling Binswanger to shift away from a biological study of "the 'sick' organism" toward a holistic understanding of the sick human being.[65] Thus, Binswanger prioritized the particularity of his patients' experience rather than fitting them into a fixed meta-psychological framework.

Binswanger took his intellectual cues here from Martin Heidegger, particularly his understanding that science addresses the "ontic" level of behavior, rather than the "ontological" level of being that can reveal the structures of existence. This switch from the ontic to ontological is expressed in Binswanger's 1946 essay "The Existential Analysis School of Thought" as a movement away from "discursive inductive knowledge" to a "phenomenological empirical knowledge," which demands that the analyst listen attentively to his patient.[66] Binswanger also wanted to dispense with the oppositions between subject and object and between mind and body, thereby overcoming the thorny philosophical problem of dualism that is likely to obstruct a person-centered approach. On this level, the Swiss gentile Binswanger shared with the Austrian Jew Martin Buber an interest in the plenum of existence: what Buber in *I and Thou* (1923) called the "I-Thou" relationship that differs from the instrumental "I-It" and narcissistic "I-I" relationships in emphasizing a quasi-mystical bond that connects human beings and that is marked by a respect for others.[67] Again using Heidegger as his guide, Binswanger also stressed interconnectedness in terms of *Dasein*, or "being-in-the-world." He argued that the scientific conception of a human "as a physical-psychological-spiritual unity" cannot address what it means to be in the world, whereas "existential analysis undertakes to work out being human in all its existential forms and their worlds."[68]

Binswanger was not unique in this regard: Harry Stack Sullivan and Frieda Fromm-Reichmann worked together in the 1940s (until Sullivan's death in 1949) at Chestnut Lodge Sanitarium in Rockville, Maryland, where they stressed communicative interconnections between analyst and analysand (and avoided medication) in an attempt to more fully behold their patients face to face, through methods of empathy that often arise outside regular channels of communication.[69] But Binswanger's importance rests on his case studies of female schizophrenic patients, published as *Schizophrenie* (1957). He approached each patient without theoretical preconceptions, in order to gain "insights into the *specific* ontological structure of our cases."[70] He saw schizophrenia as a disproportionate mode of being-in-the-world, characterized by delusions and grandiose ideas—not dissimilar to Ed Avery's cortisone-induced symptoms in *Bigger Than Life* (see chapter 5). Binswanger tried to dispense with normative taxonomies and focused on the life-world of his patients in an effort to reveal an underlying "world-design" that can be mapped despite disorderly behavior, but cannot be reduced to a scientific principle.[71] Two important case studies, "The Case of Ellen West" (1945) and "The Case of Lola Voss" (1949), exemplify such an approach, but they also address issues of social stigma, clothes phobia, bulimia, anorexia, and suicidal tendencies that had an impact on the fears and aspirations of these two patients.[72] Binswanger's analysis of his patients was not always successful, but he did succeed in focusing on the indivisibility of mind and body and on the possibility that individuals can transcend their ontic life, "climbing above it in care and swinging beyond it in love."[73] "Care" and "love" here are crucial elements: both involve a looking after the self and the capacity to transcend states of depletion or inertia. In this way, Binswanger developed a rather sketchy concept in Heidegger's work by seeing "being-in-the-world" as fundamentally a "being-in-the-world-with-others." Revealing his caring face, Binswanger cultivated an ethic of genuine sympathy that he hoped would lead to a creative analytic encounter, combining solidarity with a respect for the patient.

The reason why the Ellen West case study was important is twofold: first, it presented a detailed account of schizophrenia with tragic consequences (the patient's suicide); and second, the American Academy of Psychotherapists had a session focusing on the case at an autumn 1958 symposium. Organized by Rollo May and featuring Carl Rogers, this session debated Binswanger's method, the patient's condition, and her varied psychiatric treatment. Rogers was angry that Ellen West had been mistreated by her parents, physicians, and psychiatrists, arguing that the case is "an illustration" of isolation and loneliness taken to a "tragic point."[74] Ellen's sense that she exists behind a "glass wall" where people cannot hear her resonates with literary texts such as Ralph Ellison's *Invisible Man* and Sylvia Plath's *The Bell Jar* in their central metaphors of invisibility and entrapment. Rogers discerned in the case an exaggerated form of estranging loneliness, which results when an individual is unable to, or is prevented from, communicating "our real experiencing—and hence our real self—to another."[75] He believed that Ellen was experiencing an extreme form of loneliness, made worse because at "significant moments of [her] life, she was made to feel that her experiencing was invalid, erroneous, wrong, and unsound," and that her treatment foundered because "no one involved seems to have related to her as a person."[76] Rogers was in indignant mood, stressing that her doctors had projected a series of diagnoses onto Ellen (manic-depressive, obsessive-compulsive, melancholic, and, later, "suicidal, schizophrenic, and hopeless for treatment"), and he was evangelical in believing that she would have fared much better under his care. Rather than attempting to diagnose her condition, Rogers would have encouraged her to work out her depression, her body image, and her "love and resentment" toward her father (feelings inevitably projected onto the male therapist), and to openly experience her fears and self-doubt.[77]

Despite Rogers's emphasis on the fully-functioning person, Buber was critical of Rogers's treatment of the patient because he thought the emphasis on reciprocity could hide the institutional power base of therapy.[78] This criticism could be leveled at nearly all forms of practical therapy, but it does suggest that, in his emphasis on congruence and transparency, Rogers tended to overlook the structuring issues of transference and dependency. Alan Petigny takes a broader view, arguing that Rogers influenced the consciousness-raising of second-wave feminist activity in the early 1960s, particularly by his emphasis on personal growth and a nonjudgmental attitude toward others (a trend that Petigny also sees reflected in Maslow's work as far back as the late 1930s).[79] However, when we compare Rogers's view of the Ellen West case with his own treatment of female patients, some specific conclusions emerge. Two sessions—a transcribed session with a schizophrenic patient, Loretta (1958), and a filmed interview with a thirty-year-old divorcee, Gloria (1964)—illustrate his nondirect approach and his desire to avoid imposing a meta-psychological framework.[80]

In 1957 Rogers began a long-term research project on schizophrenia at the University of Wisconsin, involving chronic and acute schizophrenics and "normal" patients from the local Mendota State Hospital.[81] During that time, he came into contact with Loretta, a "paranoid schizophrenic" inpatient, who had been recently treated by two therapists (including the humanist psychologist Richard Felder, whose approach was close to that of Rogers). Loretta had "grown tired of talking to that doctor" (Felder) and felt that he was overlaying her thoughts with his own.[82] The institutional context is that Loretta is about to be moved to another ward, but she does not know if she is ready for this move. Screaming from an adjacent ward made it difficult for Rogers to sustain his empathic approach through his half-hour interview with Loretta, which largely revolved around her mistrust of the staff (especially a hospital worker named Anita, whom Loretta "didn't trust very far . . . because she's the one that put me on shock treatment") and her fear that she could end up like the patient scream-ing and banging in the background.[83] Not only does she feel let down and bewil-dered by the shock therapy, but the drug treatment (she mentions sodium amytal) has a somatic effect; she experiences a tickling sensation in her knees and restless feet, which (on Rogers's prompting) she interprets as a rerouted sensation that prevents her "from just batting my head against the wall." Rogers's empathic technique (with lots of nonjudgmental and reassuring "mm-hms") helps Loretta to regain her self-worth—"I think my head's too valuable to bat against the wall"—and to realize that some actions are futile or self-harming.[84] By the end of the interview, Loretta seems ready to change wards, but she remains confused about the possibility of returning home and suspicious of hospital rules, many which she believes are hidden from her.

Loretta's interview illustrates the value of nondirect therapy, as it helps her to regain her self-respect and to trust her own experience within an alienating insti-tutional environment. Rogers's technique assists Loretta in recognizing patterns of experience, structuring her thoughts and speech, and focusing her attention.[85] How-ever successful Rogers's interview with Loretta is deemed to be, the 1964 case of Glo-ria is commonly thought to be the best example of the Rogerian approach, described as "an astonishing demonstration of what in practical and experiential terms it means to be acceptant, empathic and congruent in a therapeutic relationship."[86] Gloria was seen by three consultants, including the Gestalt therapist Frederick Perls, but the half-hour she spent with Rogers was the most productive of the sessions. It opens with Gloria expressing her sexual frustrations as a divorced single woman and the gap between how she presents herself to her nine-year-old daughter and how she really is. Gloria is pushed to wrestle with feelings of guilt when she lies to her daughter, but all is not strife; later in the session she describes "utopian moments" (or what Maslow would call "peak-experiences") in which she feels whole and does not need to wear a particular face to match the occasion.[87] On a conceptual level, this would be a direct challenge to Goffman's idea of "face work," in which putting on a face is necessary to maintain ego identity, even in personal relationships. Rather than focusing on the gap between the public and the private self, Rogers reinforced the importance of self-acceptance, often repeating Gloria's words back to her in a slightly different form. Critics have identified a transference dynamic in the dialogue: Gloria refers to Rogers as a surrogate father after mentioning that she cannot communicate with her own father, and Rogers focuses on positive rather than negative aspects as if this would magically overcome Gloria's neuroses through positive thinking.[88] Nevertheless, the session demonstrates how the therapist can facilitate problem solving without pushing the patient in a fixed direction.[89]

One point on which Rogers and Binswanger would have agreed is that the patient's psychic landscape can be squeezed into a rigid medical and psychological framework only at the risk of harming the self. We saw an example of this in chapter 6, with Robert Lindner's case of Charles "In Songs My Mother Taught Me." In that instance, a potential breakthrough leads to a regression on the patient's behalf, resulting in his trying to strangle the therapist. The case of Gloria had a more positive outcome: she and Rogers became friends, and Gloria enrolled in one of Rogers's workshops two years after the initial session. One might argue that the cases of Gloria and Loretta were not as severe as those of Charles and Ellen West, where strong impulses—homicide and suicide—would have destabilized the empathic and communicative approach popularized by the clinical psychologist Haim Ginnott in *Between Parent and Child* (1965) and *Between Parent and Teenager* (1967). One of the problems of humanistic psychology is that it tended to focus on new possibilities rather than tackling neurological or medical issues that cannot be easily overcome through self-actualization and positive thinking. It also points to a more systemic problem of institutional therapy in the 1950s and 1960s, when most doctors and therapists were white males. The previous chapter considered the racial implications of this institutional dynamic, but it is clear in Gloria's case that the gender dimension was a complicating factor. With this in mind, I want to turn to an important literary statement on mental illness—Joanne Greenberg's *I Never Promised You a Rose Garden*—in which a female therapist treats an extreme case of schizophrenia.

Schizophrenia and Colliding Worlds

Schizophrenia was one of the most significant mid-century American illnesses, which had its roots at the end of the nineteenth century, when Central European interest in what was then referred to as dementia praecox traveled across the Atlantic.[90] One of the most influential early theorists was the Swiss psychiatrist Eugen Bleuler, who described schizophrenia in 1911 as a dynamic version of dementia praecox, which he believed was reversible with careful treatment. Bleuler's work was translated into English by A. A. Brill in the mid-1920s and resonated with the ideas of two other Swiss psychiatrists, Adolf Meyer (who emigrated to the United States in 1892 and became director of the Psychiatric Institute in New York, and whose methods influenced Harry Stack Sullivan) and Oscar Forel (who, together with Bleuler, had treated F. Scott Fitzgerald's wife, Zelda, in Switzerland in the early 1930s for a variety of physical and behavioral symptoms that amounted to a version of schizophrenia). Even though Zelda Fitzgerald suffered from eczema, asthma, fainting, nightmares, and erratic and sometimes violent behavior (including attempted suicide), schizophrenia was generally not considered dangerous until the 1940s, when it was increasingly linked to psychopathology and sometimes to homicidal criminality.[91] In popular culture it was often confused with multiple personality syndrome, so much so that in the Twentieth Century–Fox film *Three Faces of Eve* (1957), based on a clinical case study by Hervey Cleckley and Corbett Thigpen, it is hard to distinguish between the patient, Eve White, who involuntarily switches between three different personae, and the distortions of her inner world. One concern was that schizophrenic patients seem to be locked in, lacking a meaningful way to make or sustain relationships, either within a family or in a broader community.

Given the entrapment that many women experienced in the 1950s and early 1960s, it is not surprising that schizophrenia (especially when it was divorced from discourses of criminal psychopathology) was often linked to women's experiences. This gender specificity had a clinical grounding. In a 1963 article, the psychology professor Jules Holzberg noted a three-year-old investigation into schizophrenia published in the *Journal of Abnormal and Social Psychology*, in which 38 percent of 298 studies used exclusively male subjects, with only 5 percent exclusively female; many of the studies did not differentiate between the gender of their subjects.[92] This failure to attend to gender differences (with the exception of Freudian references to the oedipal complex) led Holzberg's team to deal with psychopathology from a gendered standpoint. Their conclusions were that female schizophrenics tended to elicit "more extreme moral judgments" than their male counterparts, and tended to "operate under the tyranny of a severe conscience."[93] Although the investigations did not address issues of body image, social desirability, and suicidal impulses, they suggest that the relationship between sexuality and schizophrenia had more profound consequences for women as regards parental relationships, self-regard, and stigma.

Often schizophrenia was a catchall clinical term for a distorted view of reality marked by delusions and paranoid hallucinations, but for women it was often closely bound up with developing sexuality. This is certainly the case for the alluring siren figure Lilith Arthur, played by Jean Seberg in the 1964 movie *Lilith* (based on J. R. Salamanca's 1961 novel), who has the capacity to seduce fellow patients and hospital workers—including a Korean War veteran, Vincent Bruce (Warren Beatty), who is trying to restart his career as a trainee occupational therapist in a clinic resembling Chestnut Lodge. Criminal behavior was also sometimes loosely linked to schizophrenic women who had been released (or escaped) from a hospital (as two 1965 reports documented), but it was more often linked to withdrawal, body image problems, and sometimes self-harm, as in the case of Ellen West.[94]

Schizophrenia was of particular interest for Sullivan and Fromm-Reichmann, who pioneered an existential and personal focus on their patients' life worlds. Sullivan published papers on schizophrenia and social psychiatry in the 1920s and 1930s, but his work became influential after his death, when the seminars he had given at Chestnut Lodge were published as *The Psychiatric Interview* (1954) and *Clinical Studies in Psychiatry* (1956). In contrast, Fromm-Reichmann arrived in the United States in 1935, following a period in the mid-1920s when she worked with her husband, Erich Fromm, to develop a therapeutic community for Jewish patients in Heidelberg. She later helped to form the Frankfurt Psychoanalytic Institute in 1929, and she practiced as a psychoanalyst in Berlin, before the rise of the Nazi party caused both her and Fromm to flee Germany (the pair effectively separated in 1931 but did not divorce until 1944).[95] Fromm-Reichmann worked for much of her American career at Chestnut Lodge. There, like Sullivan, she stressed the need for therapists to be adaptable and the importance of interpersonal communication (sometimes verbal, sometimes nonverbal) in drawing out the patient, on occasions augmented by "collateral information" garnered from relatives and friends.[96]

Prior to her relationship with Fromm, Fromm-Reichmann had worked in a German Army hospital during World War I and became used to dealing with severe cases of neurological and psychological damage, often linked to other medical complications. However, such experiences did not lead her to use drugs with her patients; instead, she worked hard to establish a close relationship with withdrawn and depressive patients. Wayne Fenton (who joined Chestnut Lodge in 1984) later described this as a practice in which "all interventions aim to minimize the effects of vulnerabilities, bolster adaptive capacities, and reduce the extent and impact of stress. . . . The strategic rosetta stone here is the therapist's capacity to shift gears, be flexible, and change roles with patients based on changing circumstances."[97] The Chestnut Lodge brand of psychodynamic therapy was not identical with Carl Rogers's client-centered therapy, but the two reflect the same humanistic philosophy. Through her attunement to the patient's unique life-world and her careful attention to detailed medical histories, Fromm-Reichmann detected schizophrenics' unique gifts, which were often misunderstood in conventional psychiatric diagnosis and treatment. This misunderstanding is starkly evident in the case of Zelda Fitzgerald: in the mid-1930s she had responded to psychodynamic treatment at the Sheppard and Enoch Pratt Hospital in Baltimore (where Sullivan had worked until 1930), but when she was admitted in the late 1940s to Highland Hospital in North Carolina, a course of insulin therapy led her to "hypoglycaemic shock and attendant convulsions and coma"—which was, ironically, the ultimate form of isolation leading to death.[98]

Fromm-Reichmann was based at Chestnut Lodge through the 1940s and 1950s, but her work came to public attention with the release of Greenberg's *I Never Promised You a Rose Garden*. Like Plath's quasi-autobiographical *The Bell Jar*, *I Never Promised You a Rose Garden* was published as a work of fiction in 1964 (it was first drafted in 1956) under a pseudonym. Greenberg used the name Hannah Green primarily to protect herself and her family, and she had to work hard to prevent her publisher, Henry Holt, from marketing the book as nonfiction.[99] In the book, Fromm-Reichmann is presented as Dr. Clara Fried, the analyst of sixteen-year-old Deborah Blau, a patient who is admitted to a Midwest hospital following an attempted suicide. The medical record shows that Deborah Blau (like Joanne Greenberg) was born into a Polish immigrant family in Chicago in the early 1930s. She possessed high intelligence as a child but was often compulsive and masochistic, tended to subjectivize, and was prone to random and inappropriate behavior. Her records mention a childhood operation to remove a tumor from her urethra (described as "the wrongness inside her, in the feminine, secret part"), as well as experiences of anti-Semitic cruelty by her baby sitter, neighbors, and schoolmates, and at summer camp.[100] In contrast to this brief medical case study and the initial diagnosis of schizophrenia, the novel relates Deborah's illness and treatment at length. In doing so, it shifts between narrative points of view—those of Dr. Fried (who is alternately baffled, intrigued, and impressed by Deborah), Deborah's parents (who display feelings of disbelief and rejection toward her), and Deborah herself, who is in her own distorted and isolated world.

The element that makes the book so engaging is Deborah's created world, Yr, with its own secret language, Yri (Greenberg's language was called Irian). Deborah views Yr as a much more attractive place than Earth; Yr is a place "where she is most alive" and where her imagination can roam free. This is the linguistic equivalent of the Mexican painter Martín Ramírez, who created a remarkable series of imaginative and vibrant drawings on a range of found and improvised papers over fifteen years (1948–1963), during which time he was institutionalized for schizophrenia in DeWitt State Hospital in Auburn, California.[101] But whereas Ramírez's images suggest a realm of inner freedom—his figures, creatures, patterns, journeys, and religious icons move creatively through time and space—Deborah's imaginary world is full of torments; its guardians are often cruel to her, and a censor controls her "speech and actions" to protect "the secret of Yr's existence."[102] However, despite its tyrannical hold, this alternative cosmology seems more real to her than the social reality with which her parents, teachers, and peers expect her to engage. The narrative relates Deborah's three-year institutionalization and her therapeutic encounters with Dr. Fried, but it also explores the midworld where these two worlds collide: Yr and the Earth, "where the ghosts and shadows lived."[103] Deborah even gives Dr. Fried an Yri name, "Furii, or Firetouch"; this is a mark of respect, but it also implicates Dr. Fried within Deborah's psychodrama, leading the doctor to engage with Yr even though she cannot fully understand its language.[104]

The story is based closely on Greenberg's own therapy with Fromm-Reichmann at Chestnut Lodge, starting in 1948. In the same year that Albert Deutsch published *The Shame of the States*, in which he bemoaned the condition of large state hospitals, Chestnut Lodge offered an alternative to them as a private institution tailored to the individual patient's needs. In Greenberg's book, published seven years after Fromm-Reichmann's death, Deborah Blau's schizophrenic symptoms were similar to the author's, and their treatments followed a similar course, taking both women from a pre-psychotic state to life as an outpatient and a college student within four years. Whereas Rogers's successes with Gloria and Loretta were based on short therapy sessions, Fromm-Reichmann's therapy took a lengthy course, with its avoidance of psychotropic drugs and the analyst's desire to understand the complex world of her patient, in which freedom from the real world and subjugation to inner demons were close companions. Gail Hornstein writes in her biography of Fromm-Reichmann:

> For Frieda, treatment of mental illness was like physical therapy after stroke: a painstaking exercise in hope. Improvement was unpredictable, and was often followed by relapse or deterioration. Recovery, to the extent it was present,

proceeded at an agonizingly slow pace . . . [but] a patient had to have at least one person who could imagine the possibility of his getting well. Frieda thought the reason most psychiatrists failed at their work wasn't because their methods were ineffective, but because they gave up too soon.[105]

The average length of stay in Chestnut Lodge was two years, and in Greenberg's case Fromm-Reichmann had to construct an extended course of intensive therapy over three years. Chestnut Lodge largely attracted local inpatients in the 1940s—the preponderance of them being women—who were cared for by a team of largely autonomous nurses, in addition to regular meetings (between four and seven per week) with a designated therapist.

The early exchanges between Fromm-Reichmann and Greenberg in the autumn of 1948 were attempts to understand the patient's secret universe, with its seven intersecting worlds and its own hermetic language that inflected Greenberg's poetry. Although she was relatively inexperienced in analyzing teenagers (and she consulted with the psychoanalyst Hilda Bruch on the topic of eating disorders), Fromm-Reichmann was careful not to push her patient further into her isolated world and struggled to find "a way into the terror without colluding in the sickness."[106] It helped that they were both Jewish (they shared jokes) and were of the same sex (they slowly built trust, without too many complications of transference), but the key element was that Fromm-Reichmann could value her patient's life-world as much as she recognized that the alternative cosmology was a response mechanism to medical and family problems. During the course of therapy, Greenberg claimed that as a five-year-old she had tried to kill her baby sister (Fromm-Reichmann saw this as fantasy or guilt displacement) and that she lost her mother for a time when she left home full of rage following a stillbirth in the family.[107] Hornstein takes these disclosures (and others, such as of self-harming) as a turning point in the therapy and a sign of Greenberg's realization that her punishment was unwarranted. But the bridge of trust that Fromm-Reichmann managed to build between the pair was the key to successful therapy, leading Greenberg to switch to outpatient status in 1951.

Another important aspect of the therapy was for Deborah to reorient herself toward others. The roots of her mistrust lay with her parents, who could not really move beyond incomprehension of what had happened to their daughter or why their "golden toy was flawed," first by the presence of a tumor and then by suicidal depression.[108] Deborah's response is withdrawal, often accompanied by silence (Greenberg's actual response was mistrust of the Chestnut Lodge staff and a reluctance to change her clothes). Relationships within the institution do not prevent Deborah from periodically "drawing away from the external world," and nor do they prevent her from trying to commit suicide (the first time with a metal lid, and later by burning herself), but she does form new personal bonds, primarily with Dr. Fried, but also within the psychiatric wards. After the first suicide attempt, Deborah is moved to the Disturbed Ward. This both terrifies her ("women were sitting bolt upright in bare chairs, and sitting and lying on the floor—moaning and mute and raging"), but it also comforts her because there was "no more lying gentility or need to live according to the incomprehensible rules of Earth."[109] In some respects, Ward D is more authentic than Wards A and B, where patients "whispered their little symptoms and took their sedatives and were terrified of loud noises or overt agony or towering despair."[110] Within this community Deborah senses freedom, but conversations there are often fractured and repetitive, and another patient repeatedly tries to break free in a "blind dash to the closing ward door as the dinner trays left."[111] Deborah insults one of her fellow Ward D patients, Carla, but is met with compassion rather than recrimination, a response that makes her feels abject but also teaches her a more important lesson than punishment or rancor would have done.

During therapy, Deborah develops other relationships—for example, with Miss Coral, a "tiny, white-haired lady" who returns to care after a period of remission. Getting beyond Miss Coral's "blank and expressionless face," Deborah admires her as a teacher of languages, and they develop a relationship in "loose moments between the closing of their separate worlds."[112] Although there are significant moments of regression (a brief transfer to Ward D after a move to Ward B and further suicide attempts), Deborah's newly formed relationships lead Dr. Fried to detect a movement away from the polarities of her earlier life: the domineering attitude of her father, the anxiety and guilt that accompanied her feelings toward her mother and sister, and the persecuting tyranny of Yr. Deborah starts to see "new colors" in the hitherto gray world around her and learns to "look into the face of people, to talk with them and hear them."[113]

Deborah's time in care was also part of her maturation, and it is less likely that an older patient would have had the same capacity to change. An interesting case to compare with Deborah is Mary Barnes, a British nurse who started therapy at age forty with suspected schizophrenia and entered the experimental community-based Kingsley Hall, in London, as an inpatient two years later; her developing talent for art helped her to make a full recovery. Deborah's institutional experience taught her that communication is an essential companion of creativity. This was also the case for Barnes, who—although she suffered from periodic regression—became well enough to write a book with her American ward psychiatrist, Joseph Berke, in 1971.[114] Therapy was not a matter of coaching Deborah to wear an appropriate public face, but of encouraging her to broaden her horizons. Rather than a "narrowing of her life-space," as Binswanger described it, it was a movement from the *idios kosmos* of the isolated dreamer to the *koinos cosmos* of a wider community.[115] All this does not mean that there is a neat therapeutic ending or that Fromm-Reichmann/Dr. Fried is a "magical doctor" who simply banishes Greenberg's/Deborah's demons, but the narrative indicates that humanistic therapy, with its emphasis on love and care, can succeed where invasive therapies fail.[116]

Beyond Depression and Suicide

The attempt to restore the human face at the heart of therapy is not as simple as this, though, particularly as the 1960s witnessed a spate of high-profile deaths, many of them following courses of treatment. Comparative statistics reveal that the rate of suicide in the United States in the mid-1960s was lower than those of Australia, Japan, and many Central European countries, and similar to the rate in the United Kingdom.[117] However, the suicides (or, in the first case, assumed suicide) of the actress Marilyn Monroe, the poets Sylvia Plath and Anne Sexton, the writer Ernest Hemingway, the actress and singer Judy Garland (in her case, an overdose rather than suicide), and the photographer Diane Arbus suggested intense pressures lurking behind the public face of creative artists. These figures experienced different pressures. Marilyn Monroe, for example, consulted a range of therapists, including the Los Angeles analyst, Ralph Greenson, who saw her as "a borderline personality: addictive, needy, impulsive, prone to bouts of rage and feelings of self-abasement compounded by sexual and emotional excess."[118] Linked to Monroe's unhappy childhood and the fragile mental health of her mother, Gladys Baker (she was committed to Norwalk State Hospital in 1933 when her daughter was seven), was her difficulty in sustaining a meaningful heterosexual relationship, compounded by problems she had experienced at an early developmental stage (she was raised periodically by foster parents). Common to all these cases was a deep-rooted depression, symptomatic of pre-psychotic schizophrenia in the cases of Monroe and Plath and a combination of anorexia and prescription drug addiction for Garland (lightly fictionalized in the character of Neely O'Hara, in Jacqueline Susann's *Valley of the Dolls*). Even though Diane Arbus believed, following Jean Paul Sartre, that suicide can be a rational affirmation of being, the fact that her suicide in 1971 came after a largely unbroken course of antidepressants (linked to bouts of hepatitis in 1966 and 1968) suggests that it was difficult to divorce suicide from full-blown depression, which was not then fully understood as a condition in its own right.[119]

Depression and anxiety were often associated with schizophrenia, but unlike the extreme disorientation of schizophrenia (what the art critic Hal Foster calls the "terror of collapsed boundaries and invasive spatiality")—depression was a common complaint that was connected to the growing interest in ordinary psychopathology during the 1960s.[120] Even Presidents Kennedy and Johnson suffered from depression. Kennedy's was linked to his physical afflictions, but it also was related to his family psychodynamics and the pressures of the presidency. His depression arose at the time of the assassination of South Vietnamese President Ngo Dinh Diem (three weeks before Kennedy's own assassination), and Arthur Schlesinger Jr. noted that Kennedy was "somber and shaken. I had not seen him so depressed since the Bay of Pigs."[121] Johnson's depression was more profound and long-lasting than Kennedy's and came to a head during the escalation of the Vietnam War. Johnson had experienced depression while he was a senator, following a heart attack from overworking in the summer of 1955, during which time his alcohol intake rose. A decade later, Johnson had another bout of depression after gallbladder surgery. But the most severe episode occurred during his final two years in the White House and was linked to insomnia, excessive displays of emotion, and an obsession with Vietnam that verged on the paranoid (perhaps not so distinct from what Hal Foster calls "a paranoid counter—a defensive projection [in] a world that is suddenly estranged and hostile").[122] According to Robert Gilbert, Johnson's decision not to run for a second term as president was bound up with what might be considered to be borderline psychotic moods that deeply concerned Lady Bird Johnson and Sam Houston Johnson, the president's brother, who also drank excessively.[123]

Given the escalation of the Vietnam War, Johnson's condition was linked to his fears of isolation and making wrong decisions at a time when no risk-free course of action was possible. Although depression could not automatically be linked to a specific condition, its symptoms include isolation from others, an inability to see the bigger picture, and a loss of proportion. As Laura Hirshbein notes, depression did not emerge as a "specific disease category" until the 1970s, and it was not included in the *Diagnostic and Statistical Manual of Mental Disorders* as a discrete category until the third edition in 1980, but reports of depression started to appear in magazines in the late 1950s, although it was rarely specifically defined.[124] The psychiatrists Richard and Katherine Gordon distinguished between "sensitizers," "pressurizers," and "precipitators" (see chapter 5), but more often reactive depression (linked to bereavement, divorce, or loss of employment), physiological depression (due to hormonal imbalance, hyperthyroidism, or aging), and existential depression (feelings of entrapment, displacement, or uncertainty) were confused. In the first half of the twentieth century, doctors distinguished between depressive symptoms that manifested themselves as "normal states" linked to periods of stress, nervousness, or melancholia and symptoms that emerged as "disease states requiring treatment" or sometimes invasive forms of somatic therapy.[125] However, medication such as chlorpromazine was administered to both schizophrenic patients and those with depressive symptoms. Even though a new antidepressant in the 1950s, imipramine, was measured for its "social effectiveness," Hirshbein notes that its medical usefulness was open to question.[126] Clinical trials of the drug during the 1960s showed that it improved depressive symptoms, but questions of nomenclature and the effectiveness of drug treatments led to a circular view of depressed patients as "those who could be shown to have responded to antidepressants."[127] Just as neurasthenia was often linked to women's biology at the beginning of the century, so Hirshbein detects an entrenched view of depression as a female condition that often overlooked environmental and structural factors in its diagnosis and treatment.[128] Charlotte Silverman tried to redress this trend in her 1968 study *The Epidemiology of Depression*, which closes with a quotation from Martin Buber about the investigator's need to "gaze beyond the limits" of a single discipline in order to fully understand the many contours of reality.[129]

The medical view was particularly limited because depression was sometimes linked to a range of external and internal factors. In an attempt to redress this oversight, in 1969 a cross-hospital study at the National Institute of Mental Health identified connections between depression and feelings of guilt and worthlessness, hostility, anxiety, "subjective uncertainty," insomnia, "retardation in speech and behavior," "bizarre thoughts and behavior," and "denial of illness," among other factors.[130] The association between depression and female life-cycle experiences (puberty, menstruation, pregnancy, and menopause) ignored statistics such as suicide rates, the overdiagnosis of conditions such as schizophrenia among particular ethnic groups, or the relationship between depression and war neurosis (which might have been a factor, albeit indirectly, in Kennedy's and Johnson's depressions that coincided with the escalation of combat).[131]

A survey published in 1990 indicated that suicide rates were significantly higher for men in the period 1967–1971 than they had been previously. Particularly because cross-cultural studies were rare until the 1970s, this study is important for its inclusion of the categories of race, gender, and age. It identified forty to fifty-four as the peak suicide years for women (perhaps linked to menopause or the onset of middle age), whereas suicides among black men peaked between their early twenties and early thirties, and suicide rates among white men rose significantly after their early thirties.[132] The statistics concerning African American suicide rates confirmed field studies such as Kenneth Clark's *Dark Ghetto: Dilemmas of Social Power* (1965), which examined what Clark called the pathology of the urban ghetto (including suicide and homicide), and cultural representations such as Cross Damon, an angry young black Chicagoan in Richard Wright's novel *The Outsider* (1953), whose suicidal tendencies stem from a nexus of existential dread, economic alienation, racial stigma, periodic drunkenness, and tricky relationships with his mother and girlfriend.[133]

To flesh out these statistics, I want to briefly consider two other African American texts that explore how depression manifests itself, the first leading to suicide and the second to obsessive drinking verging on the psychopathological. The first example dramatizes the downfall of a young black man in the first part of James Baldwin's complex novel *Another Country* (1962). A year earlier, in *The Fire Next Time*, Baldwin had written a letter to his nephew, emphasizing the importance of face-to-face contact and kinship as a bulwark against institutional racism. Baldwin was very interested in faces, as dramatically realized in his debate with the theologian Reinhold Niebuhr in the aftermath of the bombing of the 16th Street Baptist Church in Birmingham, Alabama, in September 1963. Mourning the loss of four innocent girls in the church bombing, Baldwin's emotions ran high during the dialogue, arguing for a "new face" and a "new consciousness" to replace the missing face of Christ from one of the stained glass windows that had been shattered by the bomb.[134] In contrast to the "alabaster face" of Christ that Baldwin linked to the racially motivated crime, the jazz musician Rufus Scott has a dark face (literally and metaphorically) that haunts all the other characters in *Another Country*, following his suicidal jump off the George Washington Bridge at the end of the first chapter. Without money or prospects, having recently experienced a destructive relationship with a white southern woman, and intensely isolated as a young bisexual black man, Scott is groped in a Times Square cinema on the first page of the book. His feelings of dispossession have socioeconomic roots and, possibly, a pathological source, although this is never identified. Instead, Scott's condition is presented in existential terms, linking self-worth to mental health: he is described as "one of the fallen . . . entirely alone, and dying of it, he was part of an unprecedented multitude."[135] This sense of aloneness verges on a prepsychotic state as Scott wanders the streets of Manhattan, facing demons that other young New Yorkers sitting in drugstores hold off with coffee and cigarettes as legiti-mized forms of social medication. With no supportive community or relationship to alleviate his depression, Scott's moment of existential recognition comes when he faces the dark waters of the Hudson River moments before he jumps from the bridge: "He dropped his head as though someone had struck him and looked down at the water. . . . He was black and the water was black."[136] Echoing earlier literary suicidal leaps off the Brooklyn Bridge—including the nameless "bedlamite" in the prelude of Hart Crane's *The Bridge* (1930) and the jobless Bud Korpenning in John Dos Passos's *Manhattan Transfer* (1925)—Scott's jump ends his life before the reader gets to know him, leaving Baldwin's other characters to sift through their own memories and desires in the remainder of the novel.[137]

The second example is Walter Lee Younger in Lorraine Hansberry's *A Raisin in the Sun*, played by Sidney Poitier on stage in 1959 and in the 1961 film version. Walter does not have the kind of brief, tragic end that Scott has, but he teeters on the edge of psychosis through the play (his sister, Beneatha, continually berates him for his crazy behavior), and he sinks into an alcohol-fueled depression when he discovers that his mother has different plans from his for a $10,000 insurance windfall that the family will receive following his father's premature death. Whereas Walter dreams of own-ing a liquor store, his mother, Lena, plans to move the family to a more affluent and largely white neighborhood, Clybourne Park, where they would have more space and light. Although the play veers away from tragedy to suggest that the Younger family might actually thrive away from the "rat-trap" of their South Side apartment (despite the white backlash to their intended move), Walter's psychological damage seems too intense and his behavior too erratic to suggest that all will be well.

Hansberry and Baldwin were less interested in medical diagnosis than in expos-ing the inner torments of young black men living in ghettos, undergoing the "cumu-lative effects of racial oppression and economic marginality."[138] This is partly because *Another Country* predates urban field studies such as Kenneth Clark's *Dark Ghetto* and Lee Rainwater's *Beyond Ghetto Walls* (1970), as well as cross-cultural accounts such as the 1973 volume *Racism and Mental Health*.[139] Although race and sexuality were fundamen-tal categories for Baldwin, he was also interested in conditions that are ontologically prior to accidents of birth. On this level, the experiences of Ellen West in Binswanger's case study, Deborah Blau in *I Never Promised You a Rose Garden*, and Rufus Scott in *Another Country* are all linked to an existential condition that Maslow called "human diminution." This term represented a deliberate attempt on Maslow's part to move away from a medical model that "puts neurosis into the same universe of discourse as ulcers, lesions, bacterial invasions, broken bones, or tumors" in order to consider "loss of meaning," doubt, grief, anger, despair, dislike, "loss of courage or of hope," or "recognition that one's life is being wasted."[140] Maslow arguably failed to identify socio-economic pressures that give rise to such "human diminution," and he did not place as much emphasis on forming meaningful relationships as Rogers and Binswanger did. However, in his 1966 lecture at Duquesne University (quoted in chapter 4), Maslow echoed Fromm's thesis about the postwar fear of freedom and Riesman's idea of the

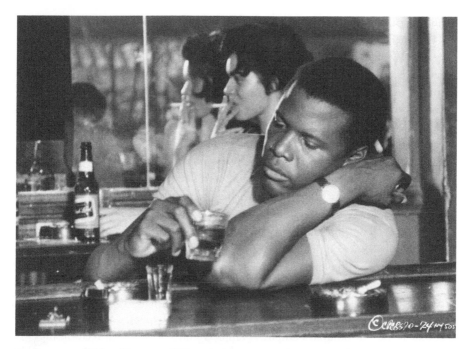

FIGURE 8.1   Walter Younger (Sidney Poitier) tries to overcome his depression with a three-day drinking session. *A Raisin in the Sun* (Daniel Petrie, Columbia, 1961).

other-directed character type. As Maslow notes, to compensate for feelings of emptiness, the existentially depleted individual "guides himself by clocks, rules, calendars, schedules, agendas, and by hints and cues from other people," rather than fashioning a creative life in more meaningful ways.[141] Although two of the examples discussed here—Ellen West and Rufus Scott—end in suicide, the narrative of Deborah Blau's return to health suggests that new life choices can emerge positively from facing existential demons, rather than covering them up with drugs or social palliatives.

To further demonstrate this existential project of reconciling meaningful individualism (being-in-the-world) and authentic relationships (being-in-the-world-with-others), I want to conclude with another healthening narrative that pulls together the themes of this chapter by combining alternative lifestyle choices with a therapeutic movement toward others. Walker Percy's novel *The Last Gentleman* deals with depression, like other literary narratives of the mid-1960s (such as John Updike's 1963 novel *The Centaur*), but with a difference: *The Last Gentleman* was written by a physician. Percy received his MD in 1941 from Columbia University, and as a pathology intern at Bellevue Hospital he was directly involved in autopsies before a three-year bout with tuberculosis during the war cut short his medical career. He was institutionalized in a sanatorium at Saranac Lake, New York, during which time he read existential philosophy (Søren Kierkegaard, Gabriel Marcel, and later Binswanger, to whom Percy refers in a 1961 essay), he joined the Roman Catholic Church, and he contemplated becoming a serious writer.[142] Percy recovered from tuberculosis but never returned to medicine, partly because his previous belief in "the beauty of the scientific method" had been replaced by a broader awareness of the "singular predicament of man in the very world which has been transformed by this science," together with the realization that there was "a huge gap in the scientific view of the world."[143] Percy's engagement with illness was not just experiential and professional. In *The Last Gentleman*, his second novel, Percy grappled with a long-running trend in his Mississippian family going back to the late eighteenth century: in every generation, a male family member committed suicide, including the author's grandfather, and his father in 1929, when Walker was thirteen. In addition, in every generation a female family member had been treated for psychotic behavior, including his mother—who drowned in a car crash in 1931, which may have been an accident or another suicidal act.[144] In *The Last Gentleman*, a young wandering southerner, Will Barrett, suffers profoundly from his father's suicide, contributing to his periodic amnesiac fugue states that lead him to therapy during his stay at the Manhattan YMCA.

Bertram Wyatt-Brown reads the therapy session that the twenty-five-year-old Barrett undergoes at the beginning of *The Last Gentleman* as a reflection of Percy's three-year course of therapy with the Canadian analyst Janet Rioch during Percy's time as a Columbia student. Rioch had been analyzed by Harry Stack Sullivan and was an advocate of Sullivan's empirical emphasis on interpersonal relationships—a theme that weaves throughout Percy's writing.[145] *The Last Gentleman* is not autobiographical, though: for example, Barrett is an engineer by training, and he abandons therapy early in the novel to purchase a telescope through which he thinks he will be better able to see. Robert Coles points out that Barrett is an "underground man," reflecting the protagonist of Percy's debut novel, *The Moviegoer* (1962), and earlier underground characters in existential novels, such as Ralph Ellison's *Invisible Man* and Fyodor Dostoevsky's 1864 protomodernist *Notes from Underground*.[146] Barrett relates his life story to his analyst, and we find out that as a younger man Barrett existed in "a state of pure possibility, not knowing what sort of man he was or what he must do," but this was not an existentially free space due to a "nervous condition" and "spells of amnesia" that contributed to his feeling that he did not "quite know what was what."[147] He develops coping strategies, however: he finds that books on mental hygiene help him to see clearly at times, he reads widely in psychology and religion, he finds museum visits and musical recitals improve his sense of well-being, and he comes to an early conclusion that "it is people who count . . . one's warmth toward and understanding of people."[148] But this range of techniques does not prevent Barrett from leading a largely "unproductive and solitary life," fearing groups, and having fugue states in which he forgets his name and the rest of his identity.

The Last Gentleman can be read as a healthening narrative in that Barrett learns to live with his nervous condition. Indeed, his condition can be seen as enabling at times: he has episodes of déjà vu when "he could see things afresh," he has a "knack of divining persons and situations," and he has a capacity for empathy.[149] This does not prevent him from having amnesiac lapses, experiencing episodes of bewilderment, and alternating between "fits of passion and depression." Barrett is shaped by his environment—his southern past and father's suicide, his ongoing experience of hospitals as patient and visitor, the backdrop of riots in Harlem, and the fear that a Cold War nerve gas attack might contaminate or wipe out New York's residents— but he also finds that relationships and travel help to prevent the cycle of depression and suicide like the one that ended his father's life. Rejecting the surrogate father figure of his analyst, he finds an alternative paternal figure in another displaced south- erner, Mr. Vaught; a friend in Vaught's son, Jamie, who is hospitalized with leukemia; and a new love in Vaught's daughter, Kitty. But rather than being a straightforward narrative that leads to marriage and psychic stability, *The Last Gentleman* follows an elliptical path, with Barrett continuing to wander. He leaves Manhattan to return to the South on a journey simultaneously forward and backward, which leads to fur- ther relationships with Jamie Vaught (a physician with suicidal tendencies) and the "pseudo-Negro" magazine photographer Forney Aiken (who travels through the South in an attempt to document the plight of southern blacks).[150] These complex relationships reveal that Barrett's life is continually remade: it is no longer a horizon of "pure possibility," but neither is it a rigid structure with a settled endpoint. On this level, the novel implies—perhaps taking up Erik Erikson's mantra of "Change, Chance, Choice" (see chapter 6)—that only by forging new experiential patterns can compulsive behavior be checked and inherited tendencies modified. In this way, Percy suggests that relationships, mobility, and insight cannot overcome medical conditions but are ingredients of a creative life.

We saw at the beginning of this chapter how President Johnson's program for a more caring and effective health service would be enacted through the establishment of community action programs rooted in particular spaces and serving particular needs. A broader trend running through the first half of the 1960s, on the levels of ideas and practice, is a profound engagement with the therapeutic potential of inter- personal relationships, as the discussion of *The Last Gentleman* illustrates. Existen- tial and humanistic strains of psychology, psychiatry, and psychoanalysis are crucial to this trend—downplaying, on the one hand, the Freudian concepts of repression and transference and, on the other hand, the scientific belief in eradicating illness in favor of receptive and creative relationships in which the power dynamic between doctor and patient can be reconfigured (as Rogers, Sullivan, and Fromm-Reichmann believed) or dissolved (in the case of Walker Percy's character Will Barrett). Two key examples of 1960s healthening narratives discussed here, *I Never Promised You a Rose Garden* and *The Last Gentleman,* explore the intersection between institutionalization and personal freedom, but their upward trajectories do not ignore darker impulses that lead to depression, schizophrenia, and suicide—attempted in the case of Debo- rah Blau, successfully carried out in the racially charged milieu of Baldwin's *Another Country,* an inherited pattern for Percy's southern family, and an ongoing reality for creative artists into and beyond the late 1960s. Depression continued to be seen as a symptom rather than a condition in its own right through the 1970s and beyond.

9   *Counterculture*

The previous two chapters focused on the growing critique of institutionalized medicine during the 1960s, ranging from the social psychology of Erving Goffman and cultural exposés of mental hospitals in chapter 7 to the humanistic and existential topics of chapter 8. I deliberately included Freud infrequently in these discussions in order to exemplify one of the central arguments of this book: that Freudianism has often been too quickly identified as the privileged postwar discourse. However, although a number of key figures challenged the Freudian emphasis on libido as the primary determining factor of psychological health or neurosis, strains of Freudian thought were undoubtedly strong in the 1960s, particularly when wedded to social theories drawn from Marx or Hegel. Erich Fromm argued, for example, that the development of technocratic society that gives rise to productive individuals often leads to the repression of personal creativity and freedom, and Herbert Marcuse (who argued against the neo-Freudians, including Fromm) critiqued technological progress as a "whole system of domination and coordination" in *Eros and Civilization* (1956) and *One Dimensional Man* (1964).[1] Freudian concepts were often used to critique neo-Victorian values and conservative politics, but, for the likes of Marcuse, Freudian thought needed rescuing from its own inherent conservatism via a thoroughgoing analysis of alienation, labor, and economic relations. Marcuse wanted to combine human rationality with the utopian impulses of Freud's later work on instinct theory, while many other thinkers on the "Freudian Left" (as Paul Robinson called it) were keen to link social theory and depth psychology as part of the broader shift in the social sciences in the mid-1960s away from structures of organization and toward issues of personal value, freedom, and social change.[2]

Mirroring this intellectual shift, in the lead article in the first issue of the *Journal of Transpersonal Psychology* (soon to become the official publication of the Association for Transpersonal Psychology, founded in 1972), Abraham Maslow envisaged a humanistic revolution that would mark a "turn back to human needs" and a renewed faith in therapeutic culture.[3] Privileging human experience over behaviorism or Freudianism (the first and second forces of psychology), Maslow focused on values and emotions, many of which helped to transcend the "geographical limitations of the self" within relationships and communities.[4] Groundedness was important for Maslow, but so was the individual's need for transcendence. The "transpersonal" turn was yet another attempt to move beyond the mode of diagnosis and complaint that marked social criticism in the 1950s and the early 1960s, to focus on values rather than function and to identify new possibilities through heightened (or peak) experiences and "an increased awareness of interpersonal relations."[5] This also marks a shift from the third force of psychology (humanist and existential psychology) to a fourth force rooted in the transpersonal and transhuman, merging an almost mystical understanding of biological connectedness with an awareness of the social and cultural spaces that individuals and communities share. This shift also marked the transition from the *Journal of Humanistic Psychology* (called the *Phoenix* when it was founded in 1961) to the *Journal of Transpersonal Psychology*, launched by Maslow and the quasi-mystical editor Anthony Sutich in the spring of 1969.[6]

Maslow based his vision on shared experience (which was at odds with institutionalized forms of religion, science, and governance), a respectful beholding of the other person (developed from Martin Buber's philosophy), and love (the fusion of eros and agape), in addition to seeing psychological, spiritual, and moral education as prime therapeutic goals. This might seem like a utopian project or at least as excessively optimistic, turning away from socialized forms of knowledge (including science and medicine) toward a romanticized notion of "ultimate values."[7] The view is certainly hopeful, but Maslow insisted that it embodied "realistic possibilities" based on an "empirical vision of something which is in truth a human being and which, therefore, can be actualized," even if this is evident only in "a fraction of one per cent of the population."[8] The alternative is to surrender to insidious social forces: "The bombs and buttons that men control are still waiting. It is possible that they may wipe us all out. Yet, it is also possible that they will not wipe us out."[9]

Three Therapeutic Trends

Although Maslow's interest in transpersonal and self actualizing experiences that move beyond a narrowly conceived conception of human needs struck a chord in the late 1960s, it relied on the critique of organized society that the middle section of this book has traced. Before returning in more detail to institutional critiques and more permissive models of therapy that illustrate the turbulence of the late 1960s, the first section of this final chapter sketches out three interconnected therapeutic trends that favor a diffuse cultural expression of health and illness over a reliance on medicalized language: Herbert Marcuse's criticism of postwar society linked to sublimated sexual energies; Frederick Perls's Gestalt therapy, as an internal critique of both Freudianism and behaviorism; and Timothy Leary's gospel of self-medication and cultural vanguardism. Taken together, these three examples illustrate the widespread attempt to reconceptualize the relationship between health and illness in the second half of the 1960s, thereby demonstrating that Freudian thought was only one part of a much more complex whole.

Marcuse's *One Dimensional Man* is a representative text of 1960s social critique, mainly because he used the abstract categories that characterized postwar sociology ("the organization man," "the man in the gray flannel suit," "the lonely crowd," "the sane society") to promote a more actively engaged stance. Following his thesis in *Eros and Civilization* that modern industrial society was predicated on the repression of erotic potential, in *One Dimensional Man* Marcuse analyzes "the ideology of industrial society" (the subtitle of his book). His central metaphor of one-dimensionality implies a constriction of mental life and a routinized response to stimuli. Although this critique is not framed explicitly in pathological terms, it is clear that Marcuse saw habituated behavior as a mass cultural illness in the face of economic exploitation, accumulated waste, the triumph of technology, and a permanent readiness for war that legitimizes some forms of aggression and criminalizes others.[10] Marcuse did not just want to identify the factors that account for this malaise; rather, he moved toward advocating a new form of rationality that would give rise to "new values, new resources, and new faculties of contestation and reconstruction," as he outlined in 1968, by which time his thought had a sharper and more radical edge.[11]

The fact that Marcuse did not write at length about one-dimensionality in terms of pathology does not weaken his critique, partly because he wanted to see how the "strains and stresses" of postwar society are "grounded in the normal functioning" of the individuals that compose it, rather than focusing exclusively on its "disturbances and diseases." Indeed, a number of critics pushed Marcuse's thought in the direction of pathology. For example, just as he believed that the "ruthlessness, moral indifference, and persistent aggressiveness" demanded by big business confuses "normality" with the "distortion and mutilation of a human being," so the Beat theologian Alan Watts argued that big business often turns employees into "phantoms" and "abstractions," with little to look forward to but "prostate trouble, false teeth, and wrinkled skin" on retirement.[12] Marcuse, Fromm, and Watts all believed that sickness stems from the blind alignment of an individual's values with postwar capitalist ideology, particularly when, as Marcuse argued, basic social institutions and relations "do not permit the use of the available material and intellectual resources for the optimal development and satisfaction of individual needs."[13] This rhetoric was also deployed by the creativity guru and practitioner Buryl Payne in his popular 1973 book *Getting There without Drugs,* which begins: "We have also come, as a culture, to treating people like things—and manipulating them as though they were objects—so many tin soldiers and mechanical clerks— and this subtle and pervasive philosophy of squeezing everything into rational schemes has actually made people more thinglike, more robotized and dehumanized."[14] Payne did not directly refer to Marcuse (his influences were Alfred Korzybski and George Gurdjieff), and he propelled his discussion toward extrasensory perception and mystical experiences rather than the need to radically reorganize social relations. But this quotation demonstrates how Marcuse's critique of Western society had been absorbed into the critical mainstream by the end of the decade.

Marcuse did not advocate a straightforward shift toward Marx at the expense of Freud, but he wanted to explore the potential that Marx left open for consciousness to have a central role in orchestrating social revolution.[15] Thus, in the epilogue to *Eros and Civilization*, Marcuse distanced himself from the neo-Freudians. To his mind, they did not go far enough in their revisionist reading of Freud, and he accused them of abandoning "the instinctual dynamic" and weakening "the social substance of psychoanalysis" in favor of an idealistic conception of the self.[16] Similarly, he thought that Fromm confused sexual desire with a general sense of happiness and sought a form of freedom that "can be practiced even in chains," rather than striving for full-scale social reorganization.[17] Marcuse was wary of the pacifying role that nationalistic culture sometimes plays, serving to deaden the imagination, commodify aesthetics, and close off alternative avenues of expression; he was particularly scathing about the mass media that sells the benefits of "overwhelming efficiency and an increased standard of living" at the expense of "the free development of human needs and faculties."[18] For Marcuse, "new forms of control" organized at political, intellectual, technological, and economic levels had made "unfreedom" palatable to a whole generation of Americans.[19]

Marcuse's discussion here wavers between a bleak assessment of contemporary society and a revolutionary spirit. With the threat of nuclear extinction hanging over *One Dimensional Man*, Marcuse offers only two escapes from this overly rational, scientifically controlled environment. First, he recommends that those incorporated into the system should seek to release their erotic potential and "liberate the imagination" through a politically attuned "art of life"; second, he urges those on the outside ("the outcasts and outsiders, the persecuted of other races and other colors, the unemployed and the unemployable") to collectively demonstrate that political reorganization is possible.[20] Marcuse claimed that to "go out into the streets" in 1964 "without arms, without protection, in order to ask for the most primitive civil rights" is a means of exposing the inherent violence and unfreedom on which the social system is predicated.[21]

Fromm and Marcuse made creative use of Freud, but other thinkers, such as Thomas Szasz, rejected the scientific basis of psychoanalysis, or at least worried that Freudian clichés had weakened Freud's original theories. From a different angle, one of the founding figures of Gestalt therapy, Frederick Perls, wrote in 1969 that "it took us a long time to debunk the whole Freudian crap, and now we are entering a new and more dangerous phase."[22] Perls was critical of Freud's focus on patriarchal structures, which Perls believed made patients feel more neurotic and privileged the analytic couch over creative modes of face-to-face encounter. This is not entirely an accurate assessment of Freud, but Perls's provocative intention was to fill in "the holes in the personality to make the person whole and complete again."[23] In fact, although Perls's criticism targeted a popular Freudian strain dominated by "quacks and con-men," his target was not Norman Vincent Peale's elision of health and a conservative business ethos, but rather the culture of faddism and the quick fix: "We are entering the phase of the turn-onners: turn on to instant cure, instant joy, instant sensory-awareness."[24] Perls did not slide back toward Freud as a reaction to pseudotherapeutic promises, but he mapped out a third alternative that links to his early work on Gestalt therapy with the ideas of Paul Goodman at the beginning of the 1950s: "Between the Scylla of conditioning, and the Charybdis of turning on, there is something—a person that is real, a person who takes a stand."[25] Perls did not have a robust social theory to fully articulate what this "stand" might be, but his emphasis on the hard work of therapy is evident throughout *Gestalt Therapy Verbatim*, largely based on group therapy sessions at the Esalen Institute in Big Sur, California, which specialized in yoga, meditation, muscle message, and group therapy.[26] Perls was living at Esalen between 1964 and 1969, where he made training films such as *Awareness* (1969), in which he stressed that personal growth relies on the patient's self-awareness of a mediating point (a mid-zone or *Mitwelt*) between the self and society, facilitated through encounter groups.

In an author's note to the 1969 edition of *Gestalt Therapy*, Perls worried about individuals having existential holes where their eyes and ears should be, particularly those "who talk and talk and expect the world to listen" and those who "don't listen to the voices of their environment . . . and stay on an empty intellectual level."[27] The search for wisdom, self-awareness, and participation were crucial for Perls and Goodman (and for Watts, another figure linked to Esalen)—a quest that should be activated by the throwing off of selfhood. According to this view, a strong, autonomous ego is not the remedy for neurosis but actually a feature of the neurotic personality. Autonomy is preferable to blind conformity or the continual need for approval, as David Riesman argued (see chapter 4), but often it is linked to rigid boundaries that are erected around an inviolable private world. Such barrier building inhibits the release of the human potential that Perls and Goodman saw as the fundamental ingredient of therapy—potential that can be realized only through the constant negotiation of ego boundaries and receptivity to others.[28] Rather than a discrete entity, Perls saw the individual as part of an ongoing process of exchange: what he calls a series of "unfinished situations—incomplete gestalts" that make up a life.[29] He shared with Goodman, Rogers, and Maslow an expanded concept of self-actualization and fulfillment of potential in dialogue with the environment and others, arguing that individuals habitually function at 5 percent to 15 percent of their capacity.[30]

Perls rarely drew from Freudian concepts, perhaps because Freud had given him little time during their only meeting in 1936. Perls's focus on unfulfilled potential and the therapeutic requirement to find the "impasse" that would allow for personal growth had more in common with the tradition of positive thinking, but with the caveat that personal growth is hard work, involving the continual process of self-examination and receptivity to an ever-changing environment. He avoided medical and psychiatric terms, replacing "neurosis" with "growth disorder" and preferring to draw on educational theory.[31] In this respect his ideas approximated Erik Erikson's developmental model of maturation but paid closer attention to the patient's dream-scape, in line with existential analysts like Ludwig Binswanger. This is not to say that Perls neglected community: indeed, he often saw patients in groups, and he held intensive workshops with around twenty-four patients each at Esalen in the summer of 1968. Although Perls's mode of analysis can be seen as the culmination of the existential and humanistic trends discussed in the previous chapter, it was also a new age trend that was very easy to parody or burlesque, as Paul Mazursky does in his comedy film *Bob & Carol & Ted & Alice* (1969), which combines group and regression therapy with the kind of bourgeois therapeutic lifestyle choices that Perls dismissed as faddism. But it becomes difficult to separate legitimate from faddish practices because the therapeutic community at the beginning of *Bob & Carol & Ted*

& Alice was based loosely on the Esalen Institute and echoed the holistic techniques promoted by the Esalen psychologist William Schutz in his 1967 book *Joy* (both texts are discussed below).

The human potential movement included a wide range of therapeutic and health-related practices in the last third of the 1960s, with serious ideas often interwoven with populist statements. Walter Truett Anderson likened the ideological ferment on the West Coast in the late 1960s to the Great Awakening in New England during the eighteenth century, replacing doctrine with spirituality and accommodating a range of "psychologists and mystics, scientists and artists, professors and poets," who put ideas drawn from the church, academy, and clinic into practice across a broad sweep of culture—or what Linda Sargent Wood (following the environmentalist Rachel Carson) calls a "web of life."[32] Looking back from the early 1980s, Anderson worried that the essence of humanistic psychology was being diluted in "the various Aquarian, estian, and transformational faiths."[33]

This mixture of serious thought and populism can be seen in Perls's rearticulation of Gestalt therapy in his later books, and it was certainly true of Timothy Leary, who channeled his focus on "The Social Dimensions of Personality: Group Structure and Process"—the title of his PhD thesis at the University of California at Berkeley in 1950—toward his adopted role as psychedelic guru and outspoken advocate for the health benefits of LSD in the mid-1960s. In the intervening period, Leary had written a serious study called *Interpersonal Diagnosis of Personality* (1957), which had developed the emphasis on human relationships in Sullivan's and Erikson's work. In this book, Leary acknowledges that the term "interpersonal relations" had "become so popular that, at times, it appears destined to join those ill-fated concepts rendered meaningless by the frequency and pious generality of their usage," but he wanted to combine Sullivan's work on interpersonal behavior and motivation with Erikson's development of "an objective, functional system for predicting the behavior of adult patients in the psychiatric clinic."[34] Although Leary never abandoned this emphasis on interpersonal relationships, his experiments with LSD pushed him toward a mode of do-it-yourself theology and an evangelical advocacy of expanding consciousness via psychedelic drugs. In this guise, Leary promoted a plethora of countercultural trends within an overarching "politics of ecstasy" (to cite the title of his 1968 book) that had the potential to shake the nation out of its complacent one-dimensionality. These trends included the use of natural and manufactured hallucinogens; the performance poetry of the "celestial clown," Allen Ginsberg; the "guerrilla tactics" of Ken Kesey's Merry Pranksters; and the Eastern religion that Watts promoted in his radio and television appearances.[35] Leary believed that the only way to prevent the authorities from using drug warfare against unsuspecting American citizens, soldiers, and patients was for young Americans to self-medicate, grab the initiative, and push the "molecular revolution" toward "fun and love."[36]

Although it is difficult to separate the serious and self-promoting sides of Leary's philosophy in the late 1960s, his interest in "neurological politics" (as he titled the final chapter of *Politics of Ecstasy*, originally presented to the Yippies before the August

1968 Democratic national convention in Chicago) was an effort to ground the "revelatory potentialities of the human nervous system" in a theory of the body.[37] This was
not a systematic scientific study, but his emphasis on "genetic wisdom" and "organic
evolution" (including "the organic duty" of the young "to mutate, to drop out, to
initiate a new social structure" when the "government becomes destructive of life,
liberty, and harmony") places the permanence of biological change at the center of
his therapeutic philosophy.[38] He was later to formalize this as a version of "scientific
humanism—the belief in the rapid evolution of intelligence in the human species and
in the individual human being."[39] For Leary, the "ecstasy of mutation" is not another
version of positive thinking; instead, he claims that the joys and pains of transition
are "equally balanced" but also that "genetic necessity" should compel us to "detach
ourselves from [the] uncaring madness" of "menopausal" authorities.[40] It is not clear
whether "genetic necessity" is wholly beyond the individual's control or whether it
can be reshaped (or re-imprinted) by the brain through transcendental experiences.
But *Politics of Ecstasy* ends with an alternative Declaration of Independence, in which
equality, harmony, and the inalienable rights of "freedom of body, pursuit of joy, and
the expansion of consciousness" means turning our backs on mendacity, hatred, and
armed conflict.[41]

Leary's emphasis on the indivisibility of "flesh and consciousness" is an exaggerated form of the mid-1960s trend of approaching identity and health from a holistic
perspective.[42] This can be seen in the growth of alternative and homeopathic medicine in the 1960s, the popularity of holistic therapy, the search for balance between
different branches of healing, the interest in yoga and posture for purifying the body
and for redressing ailments (embodied in the widely read *Light on Yoga* (1966) by the
Indian educator B.K.S. Iyengar), and the fusion of spiritual and medical categories.
That fusion may best be epitomized by the classicist Norman O. Brown's radical
rereading of Freud in an attempt to bring about a secular "resurrection of the body,"
as the last chapter of Brown's major work, *Life against Death* (1959), is titled.

Brown was fundamentally a religious rather than a scientific or medical thinker,
leading Richard King to comment that his work was "not so much a critique of 'the
organized system' or 'advanced industrial society' or a plea for 'mental health' or
'freer expression' as it is a radical questioning of [deep-rooted] assumptions about
man and culture."[43] The Phi Beta Kappa Oration that Brown gave at Columbia University in May 1960 summarized his agonistic position toward mainstream society
and foreshadowed what was to follow in his more mystical *Love's Body* (1966). In this
speech, Brown identified a problem ("mind at the end of its tether") and a solution
("blessed madness of the maenad and the bacchant"), by which he meant that the
latent power of mysticism should flow into American life as a renewing force that
transcends what can be empirically known by science and what is classified as knowledge in universities.[44] Brown developed a dialectical vision that brought body and
mind together in a "symbolic consciousness" that does not seek transcendental flights
away from worldly matters but "terminates in the body" and "remains faithful to the
earth."[45] Brown and Marcuse disagreed on the terms of this dialectical process, and

Brown veered too far away from medical theories of illness and health for his thought to be central to this chapter, but his expression of a new and potentially revolutionary embodied consciousness was a strong current that runs through a range of cultural responses in the mid- to late 1960s.

Anti-Psychiatry: Conservatives and Rebels

These broad countercultural strains provide a context for the anti-psychiatry movement, which represented an assault on institutionalized medicine and the family unit as complicit parts of the micropolitics of everyday life. Arguably anti-psychiatry was not a movement at all, but a transnational trend that came to public attention when a number of thinkers attacked psychiatry as a meaningful branch of medicine, seeing it as an agent of control that seeks conformity through rhetorical strategies and disciplinary forms of therapy. Szasz was the most outspoken American advocate of the movement (although he did not favor the term "anti-psychiatry"), but it included figures on both sides of the Atlantic in the late 1960s and early 1970s: Thomas Scheff in the United States, R. D. Laing in Britain, Gilles Deleuze and Félix Guattari in France, and Franco Basaglia in Italy.[46] The term "anti-psychiatry" was codified in 1967, when the British psychiatrist David Cooper published *Psychiatry and Anti-Psychiatry*, but it moved in numerous directions, including attempts to dispel myths surrounding mental illness, a challenge to the psychoanalytic repression thesis, a critique of psychiatric nomenclature, and an exposé of the negative mediating role that the family played in a culture of "general social alienation and estrangement."[47] Its critique was bound up with discourses of freedom as codified in the Congress on the Dialectics of Liberation, held in London in the summer of 1967 to discuss "radical innovation" in psychiatry and social thought by bringing together the likes of Laing and Cooper with Marcuse and Goodman.[48]

The lineage of anti-psychiatry can be traced through the 1960s, but it also encompasses the critique of postwar society developed by Fromm and Marcuse. In his essay on "Aggressiveness in Advanced Industrial Society," for example, Marcuse saw social control not as "centralized in any agency" but as "diffused throughout society, exercised by the neighbors, community, peer groups, mass media, corporations, and (perhaps least of all) government."[49] He also sees the social and behavioral sciences (particularly in the guise of industrial sociology and psychology) as coercive and potentially repressive tools, suggesting that "mental health, normality, is not that of the individual but of his society."[50] Marcuse's view was that therapy at the level of the individual is ineffective, and potentially worse than ineffective if it makes individuals feel better about the "mutilated" conditions of their existence. Psychiatry might alternatively "prepare the mental ground for such a struggle—but then psychiatry would be a subversive undertaking" in line with a political "struggle against society."[51] It is this notion of subversive practice that gave anti-psychiatrists leverage to attack psychiatry as a repressive practice that invents diagnostic categories to subdue struggle and dissent.

Cooper was critical of psychiatric nosology and the damaging role played by many families of schizophrenic patients, but he was more concerned with institutional strictures and the tendency for hospitals to place patients diagnosed with psychiatric disorders in wards adjacent to those for patients suffering from brain diseases.[52] Schizophrenia had become a widely accepted but elastic psychiatric label that accounted for many kinds of deviant or disruptive behavior and was often treated with psychotropic drugs or disciplinary forms of therapy. In this respect, Cooper saw the label as involving a "subtle, psychological, mythical, mystical, spiritual violence" exacted on the schizophrenic patient—a diagnosis that he estimates accounted for two-thirds of the beds in mental hospitals by 1967.[53] In *Being Mentally Ill* (1966), Thomas Scheff also discussed the dangers of medical labeling and the consequences of committing patients to institutions on the basis of what he saw as faulty diagnosis. By examining clinical evidence, Scheff concluded that the symptoms of mental illness should be conceptualized not as pathology but as nonconformity resulting from a whole range of stimuli, with organic disease being only one cause. In this respect, Scheff drew on Goffman's theory that social norms police and label symptoms such as "withdrawal, hallucinations, continual muttering, [and] posturing" as "violations" of predefined rules.[54] Social participation on this basis is not codified as an explicit rule, but it sets a horizon of expectation that shapes public roles and contributes to an unattractive picture of the schizophrenic as "a passive, inward-dwelling, remote person who lacks interpersonal and other competences that other members of the society see as necessary to maintain or improve one's status in society."[55] As such, normative social networks serve to pathologize daily life, making it easy for authorities to label rule breaking and nonconformist behavior as types of mental illness. In response, Scheff advocated an expansive sociological approach and criticized psychoanalysis for its neglect of broader "aspects of the social context that are vital for understanding mental disorder"—aspects that Fromm and Marcuse also focused on.[56]

Earlier in the decade—before anti-psychiatry had a name—Szasz attacked psychiatry in *The Myth of Mental Illness* (1961) for being an ineffectual science that masks rhetorical persuasion behind medical respectability. Szasz thought that the root of the problem was the fact that the psychiatric establishment creates problems out of individuals rather than seeking to actually cure illness—an argument that was far removed from calls in the 1940s for psychiatry to emerge from the shadow of medicine and develop its own professional identity and vocabulary. Szasz held a fairly narrow conception of illness: what he later called "a condition of the body" defined "as a structural or functional abnormality of cells, tissues, organs or bodies"—this, for Szasz, is the proper field of medical treatment, whereas psychiatry instead attends to the range of behavioral, interpersonal, and expressive modes.[57] According to Szasz's account, psychiatry is successful when it persuades the patient and community of its ability to diagnose and treat idiosyncratic or deviant behavior, deploying pseudomedical nomenclature that is not rooted deeply enough in organic disease to be a valid focus of professional practice. Indeed, Szasz argued that patients often collude in the myth of mental illness, impersonating sick people to attract attention and deliberately playing the role of "passive patient." This differs from Cooper's view of "invalidation" as a condition usually brought about by coercion ("a person is progressively made to conform to the inert, passive identity of invalid or patient"), which, in turn, is linked to Scheff's view of the deleterious effects of labeling and of unstated normative rules.[58]

Although he did most of his work in the United Kingdom, R. D. Laing offers a more obvious link to the counterculture than Szasz, particularly as Laing met with Ginsberg and Leary in 1964 and attracted a student readership with the Penguin reissue of *The Divided Self* in 1965, followed by his manifesto, *The Politics of Experience*, two years later.[59] Laing had experimented with LSD during his private practice in London in the early 1960s and had conducted research into the relationship between schizophrenia and hallucinogens, following his work in the late 1950s with borderline psychotics at the Tavistock Clinic in London (where he was trained by D. W. Winnicott). Although Laing was critical of the schizophrenogenic forces within family units that can lead to a son or daughter to be labeled as schizophrenic, his work was less combative and counter-conspiratorial than Szasz's project to dismantle the whole historical apparatus of psychiatry.[60] Whereas Szasz criticized psychiatry for "bootlegging" humanistic values (his actual focus was on psychiatric-related abortions), Laing developed his interests in existential philosophy (he read Harry Stack Sullivan in the early 1950s and wrote a paper on Paul Tillich in 1957) to better locate patients within their intersecting personal and social worlds.[61] Although Laing saw himself as a "conservative revolutionary" and spoke out against repressive institutions, he did not fully condemn psychiatry as a patriarchal and authoritarian practice that historically imprisoned forces of "unreason," as Michel Foucault called them in *Folie et déraison* (1961), translated in an abridged form as *Madness and Civilization* in a series edited by Laing.[62] Instead, Laing's clinical work in London paralleled the kind of detailed family research conducted by the US National Institute of Mental Health in the late 1950s and early 1960s. For Laing, the family dynamic was a mediating structure between the clinic and patient—a structure that, by the mid-1960s, was starting to show signs of strain, leading Cooper to title his 1970 book *The Death of the Family*.

Laing was more interested than Szasz in forming intellectual links with existential and psychiatric figures, as well as with Foucault's critique of networks of power and Goffman's work on stigma.[63] Although Goffman collaborated with Szasz on the formation in 1970 of the American Association for the Abolition of Involuntary Mental Hospitalization (see the conclusion of this book for a discussion of that association), Goffman did not agree that mental illness was a myth, seeing it instead as a form of social deviation based on offenses to "the frontiers of bourgeois order," as Foucault called them.[64] Goffman argued that the regulation of behavior was diffused across a range of social practices and was particularly acute for patients suffering from, or diagnosed with, mental illness. In mild cases of schizophrenia, the patient may evade the stigma of the "blemish," which might be exacerbated by the loss of a limb, physical disfigurement, or a congenital condition such as Down syndrome. However, as Goffman discussed in a 1969 article called "The Insanity of Place," hospitalized patients must find their own survival techniques in the face of disciplinary practices (as outlined in *Asylums*), but in the outside world each of the many forms of "social organization in which the patient participates has its special set of offenses" that help to codify mental illness.[65] In an attempt to maintain organizational order, the family might conceal certain neuropsychological disorders from the patient, thinking it is in his or her best interests. However, Goffman argues that mania, hallucinations, and paranoid delusions can disturb the daily practices of a family unit and result in the patient's inability or refusal to abide "by the standards that form the common ground of all those to whom [he or she is] closely related."[66]

The result is that the individual is watched by other members of the household—a regime that is "disguised lest the patient suspect he is under constant surveillance."[67] Goffman thought that this "secret management" might spread to friends, employers, other "potential sources of aid," and, in extreme cases, even to the court, making these groups complicit in the management of the patient. Goffman argued that this is based on a conspiratorial model that might be benignly initiated in the individual's best interest, but the conspiracy can soon spread: "The patient finds himself in a world that has only the appearance of innocence . . . at home, when his glance suddenly shifts in a conversation, he may find naked evidence of collusive teamwork against him." This potentially dystopian scenario is unlikely to do the individual any good, leading to a paranoid culture in which a network of surveillance usurps a caring environment; the family unit becomes "a no-man's land," and the home a place where wounds are "inflicted" rather than assuaged.[68] Based on this evidence, it is not surprising that many young Americans rejected the family as a nurturing environment in the mid-1960s and viewed organized society as sick or pathological in its disproportionate reactions to social change.

The paranoid environment that Goffman discusses in "The Insanity of Place," and that Richard Hofstadter had identified earlier in the decade within political discourse, by no means tells the whole story about where therapy was moving in the late 1960s, but it helps to explain why anti-psychiatry promoted a deep mistrust for institutionalized care, with equal attention given to the hospital and the home. It also links the story of the suffering individual to structures of family, schools, clinics, and courts in an ever-widening net from which there seemed to be no escape, particularly in the disaffected climate of 1968 following the assassination of two public figures of hope: Martin Luther King Jr. and Robert Kennedy. This conforms to a standard periodization of the late 1960s: if 1965–1967 saw the affirmative flowering of the counterculture, particularly on the West Coast, then 1968–1969 gave rise to a disillusioned sense that lasting social reorganization was impossible and that health and illness were managed (or possibly even manufactured) through collusion. These discourses even invaded presidential politics. Just as President Lyndon Johnson's progressive domestic plans foundered over his paranoid foreign policy in Vietnam, he was succeeded in the White House by the archetypal postwar paranoid figure: Richard Nixon.

Paranoia: Drugs, War, and Rage

The previous two chapters discussed the first two presidents of the 1960s, both in terms of health reform and as individuals who suffered from deep-rooted maladies before and during their terms in office. We have also seen the role that Nixon played as Dwight Eisenhower's vice president and as a presidential candidate in 1960 within the arena of health and illness, including speculation that he was consulting a psychiatrist in the mid-1950s and leftist suspicion that he was a paranoid narcissist. It is tricky, in hindsight, to disentangle these rumors from the discredited figure that emerged from Watergate, but they marked Nixon's 1968 presidential campaign and his first few years as president almost as much as his impeachment marked his second term. For cultural commentators on the left and center left, Nixon was an anti-therapeutic figure. This view was crystallized in Garry Wills's biography *Nixon Agonistes* (1970), which portrays Nixon as a haunted and lonely figure struggling against "illness, sleeplessness, fatigue," a disengaged, "plastic man" at odds with himself, "losing and gaining control in halts and jerks."[69] Nixon embodied some interesting paradoxes, however. Herblock, one of his fiercest critics, noted that he was both an immovable object ("an endless succession of 'new' Nixons kept to turning out to be the same Nixon as before") and a mercurial figure ("in some cartoons there were several masks—sometimes with several Nixons behind them").[70]

There were earlier signs of these conflicting characteristics. For example, William Costello ended his unauthorized biography of 1960, *The Facts about Nixon*, with these lines: "In his lexicon, despite every effort at candor, the dark threat is always implicit. The unspoken warning lingers, a shadowy source of anxiety and fear." Jules Witcover, writing in 1970, likened hearing the bitter concession speech that Nixon made in November 1962 (when Nixon failed in his bid to become governor of California) to "stumbling unannounced into a man's monologue to his analyst." And Arthur Schlesinger Jr. described Nixon's successful 1968 presidential campaign as one of "banality and evasion," which rested on Nixon's limiting his public appearances (much as Eisenhower had done in 1956) to avoid the weariness that had hampered his 1960 campaign.[71] Unlike the recently assassinated Robert Kennedy—whom Schlesinger saw as the only candidate who could identify "with the victims and casualties of our society" and who was capable "of bridging these gaps and unifying the country"—Nixon avoided hard questions of race and poverty, and although he claimed to be in touch with the young, it was clear to Schlesinger and Wills that he did not know them at all.[72] Not only was Nixon a throwback, for Schlesinger, to the "rootless, sectionless, classless, mobile 'new men' who inhabit . . . the 'technostructure'" that thinkers had critiqued since the mid-1950s, but Nixon also embodied a paranoid style of politics: he was "extremely uptight under his blandness, desperately aware of his own vulnerability to tension and fatigue," prone to compulsive actions, and fearful of conspiracies.[73] The facts that Nixon tried to "tranquilize public opinion" in 1969 (as one journalist described it) through a series of small strategic withdrawals from Vietnam (but without delivering on his election promise of wholesale withdrawal) and that he had a tendency to "get caught up in his subject," such as when he accused Charles Manson of being guilty of eight murders in August 1970 (before Manson had even gone to trial), suggests that Nixon could at times be as hot-headed as he could be disengaged at others.[74]

However, Nixon was a more interesting president than his caricatures suggest. In his first inaugural address, on 20 January 1969, he foresaw "an era of negotiation" that would follow a year of "confrontation" in which the Vietnam War had worsened abroad and assassinations and race riots had taken place at home. Detecting that the nation was "rich in goods, but ragged in spirit," Nixon sought openness on a global scale, which, linked to his record on Cold War détente and his quest to place the nation's "international commitments on a sustainable long-term basis," was among his strongest legacies.[75] However, his emphasis on technology positions him squarely within a Cold War context that loops back to his two terms as Eisenhower's vice president, and his record on welfare was shaky: he tried to tackle poverty by giving the Office of Economic Opportunity a renewed role in 1969, and he made pollution and environmental damage a priority in 1970, but his early years in the White House were dogged by concerns about the cost of welfare and the criticism leveled at him by black leaders that he was failing to uphold civil rights commitments. It actually took until 1972 for Nixon to scale back Johnson's welfare reforms, but it was clear from the outset that he favored the businessman rather than the pluralistic cultures that helped to shape the identity politics of the mid-1960s.

With this in mind, it is worth looking more closely at the discourse of paranoia before moving back to discuss an emerging sector of American culture—alternative therapeutic communities—that countered the more cynical view that the culture of the late 1960s was disorganized and in need of strong conservative leadership. These alternative communities did not really register on Nixon's radar, except for his condemnation of Timothy Leary and his dislike of hippies and left-wing intellectuals. Richard Hofstadter had defined paranoid style in his 1964 essay "The Paranoid Style in American Politics" as a mind-set of "heated exaggeration, suspiciousness, and conspiratorial fantasy" that could be most easily identified in the right-wing populism of Senator Joseph McCarthy, but for which a claim could be made across much of the political spectrum.[76] Although Nixon embodied the paranoid style (perhaps fueled by the media's harsh treatment of him), Hofstadter did not mention him explicitly in his 1964 essay; nevertheless, Nixon's long-standing right-wing suspicion of intellectuals and Jews was a key element in the conspiracy theories that Hofstadter outlined.[77] Hofstadter made it clear that he was not "using the expression 'paranoid style' . . . in a clinical sense" and that his interest lay in "the use of paranoid modes of expression by more or less normal people," particularly those involved in national politics.[78] This version of paranoia differs markedly from Freud's by placing private neuroses within the public sphere, but both versions involve an overactive mind that applies logic in an extreme way and makes connections between potentially disconnected events or objects.[79] These broader discourses of paranoia were in step with a growing interest in normal psychopathology, in contrast to the previous focus on institutionalized cases of schizophrenia and psychosis.

Just as Norman O. Brown's embodied mysticism provided a keynote for the mid-1960s, so the paranoid style described by Hofstadter also had strong cultural resonances, running through Philip K. Dick's fiction (and Dick's interest in anti-psychiatry in his 1964 novel, *Clans of the Alphane Moon*); William Burroughs's experimental novels such as *The Soft Machine* (1966; first published in Paris in 1961), which explores the ways in which human bodies are socially controlled and manipulated; and Kurt Vonnegut's borderline psychotic characters Eliot Rosewater and Billy Pilgrim in *Slaughterhouse-Five* (1969). The paranoid style also arose in many facets of public life, from the reemergence of Cold War hostilities in the early 1960s to President Johnson's anxious foreign policy during 1966–1968 that compromised his health and convinced him not to seek reelection. Paranoia is also related to the growing drug culture as a psychosomatic response to a variety of hallucinogens, narcotics, and prescription drugs, particularly when linked to long-term use and dependency. If countercultural thinkers were arguing that anxiety should be embraced as an existentially authentic counterpoint to one-dimensional white-collar life, then (on a medical level) anxiety could easily turn into debilitating neurosis or paranoia, in which real and imagined conspiracies push the individual into thinking that he or she is a victim of the military-industrial-medical complex.

Arguments about the liberating role of drugs were diametrically opposed to the hard line taken on marijuana and heroin by authorities, fueling concerns among parents, educators, and doctors—particularly when evidence of "panic and fear, depersonalization, gross confusion and disorientation, depression and paranoia" came to public attention.[80] LSD was, of course, the most high profile drug of the time, provoking mixed messages about its dangers and potential benefits. Although the history of LSD in the United States goes back to military experiments with it as a "truth drug" in World War II and the Korean War, it was touted in the 1960s as a therapeutic and consciousness-expanding drug by a range of public figures, including Aldous Huxley, Timothy Leary, Ken Kesey, Cary Grant, the Beatles, and the self-proclaimed hippie leader Stephen Gaskin, both before and after LSD was criminalized in October 1968. In the belief that LSD might bring distinct scientific benefits and that "numerous mysteries of human nature, of sanity and madness, or prevention and cure, would shortly yield to the onslaughts of modern science," a conference on hallucinations was sponsored by the American Psychiatric Association and the American Association for the Advancement of Science in late 1958. Four years later, LSD was tested on a bull elephant in Oklahoma City as a possible means for controlling aggression (the experiment failed), and TV shows such as a CBS Reports program in 1966 explored the effects of LSD on volunteers under scientific supervision.[81] Roger Corman's countercultural film *The Trip* (1967) uses surrealist techniques to explore the psychic dangers of LSD, but it also mines deeper psychological and social truths as the tripper (Peter Fonda) and the guide (Bruce Dern) provide a different therapeutic model to that of the patient and doctor. Although Leary, Kesey, and Gaskin continued to promote such therapeutic and cultural benefits with missionary zeal into the late 1960s, the portrayal of LSD in the media became less favorable in 1967, when reports emerged about psychological disturbances and "genetic disruptions" caused prolonged use, and antidrug books like Buryl Payne's *Getting There without Drugs* argued that hallucinogens serve only to amplify "personality defects" and precipitate feelings of being "overwhelmed or overloaded."[82]

Drug use among young Americans was at a high by the end of the decade, leading to a symposium on drugs and youth at Rutgers University in 1968, a handbook for parents by the Parents League of Houston, and a number of high-profile articles on drugs in schools and colleges collected in *Drugs and Youth* by the National Council for Social Studies in 1971.[83] Nixon was also concerned with the rise of drug use among people under twenty-one: he announced to Congress on 14 July 1969 that such use had become "a serious national threat to the personal health and safety of millions of Americans."[84] The president focused on strengthening legislation banning the sale and importation of drugs, and he asked the Department of Health, Education, and Welfare to research the effectiveness of rehabilitation programs and to focus public education on drugs. Although Nixon worried that no "American parent can send a son or daughter to college today without exposing the young man or woman to drug abuse," one area on which he did not comment was narcotic use among soldiers stationed in Vietnam.[85] The US Army claimed that less than 2 percent of soldiers were using narcotics, but other estimates were that between 10 percent and 25 percent of US forces in Vietnam were regularly using heroin and that up to 75 percent smoked marijuana, as reported by John Steinbeck IV, son of the famous author, who was

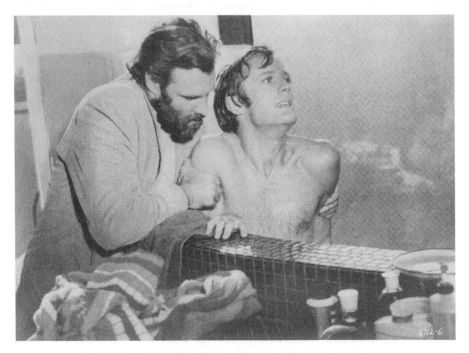

FIGURE 9.1   Paul Groves (Peter Fonda) is guided by John (Bruce Dern) during his LSD experience. *The Trip* (Roger Corman, American International Pictures, 1967).

based there in 1965 and returned to Vietnam in 1968 as a journalist and broadcaster, publishing his candid memoir, *In Touch*, in 1969.[86]

World War II and the Korean War gave rise to feelings of worthlessness and victimhood among many wounded or disabled veterans. But for soldiers in Vietnam, the psychosocial stakes were much higher—particularly after 1966, when the public protests against the war started to filter through to troops stationed overseas. Paranoia was prevalent in this period, partly linked to clashes with authorities but also because drugs played an increasingly large role. Cocaine and heroin were particularly popular among the troops (who most often smoked during patrol), but so were amphetamines (popularly known as pep pills) and a headache remedy called Binoctal, which were given freely by medics to soldiers, as well as opium, which was widely available in South Vietnam.[87] Marijuana was a sociable drug that often led to a sense of "calm, perceiving detachment" among soldiers and was tolerated as long as the soldier continued to "follow orders and perform the job."[88] But heroin was a different matter. And the fact that many soldiers, or "GI Junkies," continued to use drugs after leaving the armed forces was a "source of annoyance and embarrassment to the Nixon Administration," particularly by 1971, when *Newsweek* reported that drug addiction was the third most important national problem.[89]

An essay published in 1972 called "Drug Abuse in Combat" divided military troops into three groups: an older group of "juicers," people who tended to drink heavily; younger troops who drank but also smoked marijuana; and a third group of "heads," who regularly used heroin, hallucinogenic drugs, and amphetamines.[90] All three groups tended to use alcohol or drugs "to block out psychic pain . . . and feelings of personal inadequacy and alienation," with some discharged soldiers claiming that their drug use started at the time they first encountered antiwar literature or when they came to realize the futility of the war.[91] Instead of the euphoric feelings brought on by marijuana described by Steinbeck, common among troops were feelings of depression and helplessness, a paranoid sense of having been cheated, and suicidal impulses. It was not clear whether these feelings were exacerbated by narcotics, or whether drug use was an attempt to alleviate deep-seated fears. Either way, the authors of "Drug Abuse in Combat" conclude that recreational drug use among soldiers might be considered "therapy in disguise," a form of self-medication to alleviate the horrors of war.[92]

Chapter 1 discussed the return of GIs from World War II and the social vacuum that awaited many of them. For soldiers who went absent without leave or returned with injuries from Vietnam, this sense of emptiness was exacerbated, particularly following the mass slaughter of the Tet Offensive in early 1968. The estimate in the early 1970s was that 18 percent of returning veterans were unemployed, with a much higher rate for younger recruits and those from ethnic minority groups. Together with the drug problems among US troops in Vietnam, this lack of social opportunity created what the authors of "Drug Abuse in Combat" somewhat apocalyptically described as "a permanent population of estranged, alienated, second-class citizens who will swell the ranks of the unemployed street drifters and add substantially to America's already epidemic drug abuse problem."[93]

Widespread drug use in Vietnam might be read as a symptom of social disorganization, particularly in 1968, when the assassinations of King and Kennedy led to national mourning and revolutionary fervor. The paranoid style was not merely linked to right-wing politics or drug use in Vietnam; it was also connected to intense feelings of dispossession and alienation among minority groups, particularly African Americans. This was reflected in the use of the symbol of a black Trojan horse by the radical African American leader Eldridge Cleaver in his essay, "The Black Man's Stake in Vietnam" (1968). Cleaver linked the experience of African American soldiers in Vietnam (who made up 16 percent of the troops stationed there) and racial oppression at home, arguing that the Trojan horse was "deplorably disorganized" and in need of radical unification to "guarantee the safe future" of African Americans.[94] As one of the founders of the Black Panther Party, its self-proclaimed Health, Information, and Intelligence Minister, and a fringe presidential candidate in 1968, Cleaver advocated criminal activities to tackle white supremacy and to aid the poor. However, his motives were often mixed. For example, after being involved in Panther shootings in Oakland, he fled to Algeria in 1970, where he welcomed Timothy Leary, another exile, to his house. They took acid and smoked marijuana together, but Cleaver then placed Leary under arrest by the Panthers on the suspicion that Leary was a counter-revolutionary. Soon afterward, Cleaver said that he was through with "the whole silly psychedelic drug culture quasi-political movement," although in the 1980s he became addicted to crack cocaine.[95]

There were other, more plausible, attempts to gauge the social factors that shaped the use of drugs within black communities. In *Dark Ghetto*, Kenneth Clark examined economics and class in relation to drug addiction in Harlem (which was ten times higher there between 1955 and 1961 than elsewhere in Manhattan), while Steinbeck pointed out that racially integrated troops might be one reason for the culture of marijuana in Vietnam—a drug that, along with heroin, was common in ghettos and often central to the gang wars documented in *Dark Ghetto*.[96] Although, as Daniel Matlin discusses, Clark overgeneralized certain aspects of ghetto life, he saw signs of healthy defiance in the social unrest of Harlem and strong therapeutic benefits in developing grass-roots community programs to promote "exposure, prevention, and control of the drug traffic and detoxification and intensive aftercare treatment for young addicts."[97] But Clark noted that drug use and addiction among black communities has a complex etiology and cannot simply be identified as a "ghetto" problem, as is evident in James Baldwin's short story "Sonny's Blues" (1957), which echoes the lives of the jazz musicians Charlie Parker, Ella Fitzgerald, and Billie Holiday in linking heroin use to creativity.[98]

Prolonged oppression, victimization, and low social status were just some of the factors identified by Kenneth Clark and Frantz Fanon that provided a socio-psychological context for the race riots of 1968. More recent commentators, such as the sociologist James Summerville, have read both the protests against the Vietnam War and the race riots as a "rebellion against the overorganization of society," particularly the kind of "turgid and bureaucratic" institutions that contributed to poor self-esteem within African American communities and prolonged the discourse of damage psychology.[99] Although it is easy to overstate this anti-institutional trend, Summerville offers positive examples of progressive institutions that supported local communities. He mentions the Harlem Neighborhoods Association, which worked closely with Kenneth Clark in identifying a program for social change, and Meharry Medical College following the Nashville riots of April 1967 (the African American activist Stokely Carmichael was blamed for causing the riots by his speech the week before at Tennessee State University)—Meharry's staff members were eager to work closely with Nashville's diverse communities and to apply holistic medical models to real-life situations, as discussed in the previous chapter.[100]

The clearest statement linking mental health issues to black identity politics was the 1968 mass-market book *Black Rage*, written by two black doctors, William Grier and Price Cobbs. The cultural politics of the white counterculture tended to revolve around issues of freedom, alternative lifestyles, and the expansion of horizons, often linked to drug use. However, *Black Rage* (which was first conceived of in 1966, before King's assassination) attempted to offset any notion that psychotherapy should be used as a form of social control and to promote a positive direction for black mental health among the "smoldering racial tensions" that had continued despite *Brown* and the passage of the Civil Rights Act.[101] *Black Rage* echoed the anger embedded in Richard Wright's 1940 novel, *Native Son*, but Grier and Cobbs paralleled Fanon's attack on institutional racism and moved beyond discourses of victimization and inadequacy to embrace agency. In so doing, *Black Rage* formed part of what Daryl Michael Scott calls the "radical assault on damage imagery" in the late 1960s.[102] It also foreshadowed more-pointed attacks on racism in the medical profession, as evidenced by Stokely Carmichael's contribution to the Congress on the Dialectics of Liberation in July 1967 and a panel on "Black Power: An Identity Crisis," organized by Louis West under the auspices of the American Psychiatric Association. In Boston in May 1968, the panelists (including the African American activist and psychiatrist Charles Pinderhughes) examined racial psychodynamics and accused the National Institution of Mental Health of continued racism. This laid the conceptual ground for a potential split between black and white psychiatrists in 1969, followed by a number of demands that African American psychiatrists made of the association in the name of racial equality.[103] Similarly, although *Black Rage* contains progressive elements (Cobbs was involved in a number of interracial workshops at the Esalen Institute from 1965 to 1968), after King's assassination Grier and Cobbs found it difficult to sustain the optimism of the human potential movement or to look beyond deep-rooted aggression among African Americans that "grows out of oppression" and cannot be rerouted without wholesale changes to social structures.[104]

Focusing on the cultural roots of oppression and bemoaning the dearth of black psychiatrists in the 1960s, the authors—perhaps deliberately—do not mention drugs but concentrate instead on the need for clinicians to distinguish "unconscious depression from conscious despair, paranoia from adaptive wariness, and . . . the difference between a sick man and a sick nation."[105] The kind of paranoia displayed by one of Grier and Cobbs's case studies (Miss Y) arose from feelings of persecution from her family, friends, and co-workers, and it led the authors to suggest that "the development of a 'healthy' cultural paranoia" (free from drugs, either used for self-medication or prescribed) is to be encouraged in the black community.[106] They were eager to distinguish paranoid psychosis from "cultural paranoia," which they saw as a survival mechanism and an adaptive response to what they called "the Black Norm."[107] It is no easy task to subtract this "Black Norm" from clinical psychosis, but the authors argued that eliding the two confuses the "proper subject" of therapy with a web of cultural patterns and prejudices that further damages patients.[108]

If one goal of the counterculture was to seek alternative psychological states through drug use, then another seeks to avoid cultural myopia and—as Grier and Cobbs saw it, in the wake of King's assassination—to exist in the "tidal wave of fury and rage" guided by self-reliance and, where it can be trusted, solidarity within a community.[109] It is to this subject of therapeutic communities that the final part of this chapter turns, particularly to two grass-roots initiatives that came to prominence amid the revolutionary fervor of the mid-1960s.

Therapeutic Communities

The first line of Goodman's New Reformation: Notes of a Neolithic Conservative (1970) echoes Marcuse in its description of the dehumanizing pull of postwar society. There is a sense that the turbulence of 1968 and 1969 had exaggerated and quickened the alienation that Goodman had discussed at the beginning of the decade in Growing Up Absurd, leading to the crumbling of the social reorganization that Presidents Kennedy and Johnson had tried to facilitate. However, Goodman's New Reformation is not a jeremiad or a diatribe against the "mass man," and he quickly shifts to reflecting on those he sees on the streets, whom he thinks are no "less human, less people" than when he was a boy fifty years earlier. Rather than one-dimensional robots with "glazed eyes," he saw young Americans at the end of the 1960s as simply "sadder, more harassed, more anxious."[110] Goodman maintained that prolonged social dehumanization can lead to full-blown psychosis, but he did not take an anti-psychiatry line on the rhetorical construction of mental illness, seeing in the new youth movement the potential to help reorganize social relations. This combination of anxiety and hope echoes the ideas of the alternative therapeutic communities that emerged in the 1960s.

The utopianism of the late 1960s has been widely celebrated and reviled, but it is worth exploring here, both to offset the bleak and distrustful social outlook explored above and to assess how therapeutic communities applied humanistic philosophy in the direction of interpersonal and group relationships. This view veers away from the cynicism of anti-psychiatrists toward affirmative models of self-development within a group context broadly in line with Philip Rieff's notion of a therapy of commitment. I want to discuss two models in this final section. The first is the free clinic model, which arose largely on the West Coast from the mid-1960s to the early 1970s and combined idealism with a hard-nosed realism in terms of drug abuse and drug-related disease. The second is the fusion of therapy, mysticism, and physical renewal that has a longer genealogy, but that found its most famous expression in the Esalen Institute on the Pacific Coast in central California, which was a center for countercultural ideals and alternative therapies. These therapies flourished on the West Coast in the context of a wave of cutbacks for state psychiatric hospitals when California's new governor, Ronald Reagan, slashed the budget for the state's Department of Mental Hygiene in 1967—only to reinstate some funding two years later, when it became clear that a large number of fragile patients had been released prematurely.[111]

The first of these grass-roots models is closely related to communal living, which found its freest expressions around San Francisco and Santa Cruz, beginning in the middle of the decade. The free clinic model was linked in spirit to President Johnson's Community Action Program, but the clinics functioned at a local level, rather than as part of a federal or state initiative. The free clinic movement adopted what Louis West, the chair of the psychology department at the University of California at Los Angeles (and one of the scientists in the LSD elephant experiment of 1962), called the "green rebellion" against the "sterile family and community lifestyle of the suburbs," epitomized by the urban commune and extending through the neighborhood free clinic.[112] The first free clinic was established in the heart of the Haight-Ashbury neighborhood in San Francisco in June 1967, but it survived well beyond the so-called Summer of Love, when media attention on the city encouraged a "wave of homeless and jobless refugees" to move there only a few months later, some of them having been prematurely released from state mental hospitals.[113] The emergence of the Haight-Ashbury Free Medical Clinic marked a cultural moment when the community-action group the Diggers were distributing free food in the Golden Gate Park area, but it was also an anti-establishment institution that quickly learned the hard realities of what a free medical service meant—particularly as hepatitis, venereal disease, and drug-related squalor were common in "crashpad communes."[114]

The number of free clinics quickly rose to 61 by 1969 and 135 by 1972 (11 of the original clinics had closed by 1970), most of them operating with an open-door policy and welcoming clients whatever their condition. The National Free Clinic Council (NFCC) chair David E. Smith described this philosophy as involving "no probing questions, no 'morality trips,' no red tape, no files, no labelling or judging, no 'put downs,'" and having a "respect for personhood."[115] Most of these clinics were established on the West Coast, such as the Open Door Clinic in Seattle, the Black Man's Free Clinic in the Fillmore district of San Francisco, and the Berkeley Free Clinic on Telegraph Avenue in Oakland. However, there were also clinics in Tucson, Arizona; two in Boston; five in Canada; and one in the basement of a church in Austin, Texas, that opened near the University of Texas in April 1970, providing services for one night a week and run by a team of volunteer medical and lay staff members.[116] The primary work of the Haight-Ashbury Free Clinic related to drug use, but across the country clinics experienced a range of medical and psychological issues, often linked to feelings of alienation and isolation among their young clients.

The NFCC ran a symposium on neighborhood medical facilities at the San Francisco Medical Center in early 1970 as a way to chart the flourishing of free clinics, which—in Smith's words—were "the one viable alternative to our moribund, bureaucratized health care and delivery system [providing] badly needed services where there are none."[117] Reacting against the perception that official medicine was fragmenting into subspecialties and losing sight of general healthcare, the NFCC's mission was to promote healthcare as a priority that "transcends clinical medicine," based on the "fulfillment of basic human needs, both physical and mental . . . within a context of total health—individual, community, and social health. Total health care implies adequate personnel and facilities, full access to services, and a major new emphasis on preventive medicine via public education."[118] Within this context, the NFCC was eager to improve quality and pursued five objectives: (1) to provide a focal point for the "sociomedical momentum" of free clinics; (2) to disseminate information on healthcare; (3) to distribute national funding between free clinics; (4) to sponsor a regular symposium; and (5) to provide consultation on improving services and establishing new clinics.[119]

The NFCC was idealistic in its goals of treating "a variety of ills under one roof," its emphasis on "free" treatment (the clinics were funded by modest donations), its use of an open-door policy at the heart of a community, and its philosophy of the whole person. But it was realistic in terms of the medical problems with which the clinics commonly dealt: drug use, sexually transmitted diseases, birth control, malnutrition, and dental health, as well as psychological problems linked to the use of LSD or heroin, abortions, and diffuse forms of neurosis. The Haight-Ashbury Free Clinic illustrates this mixture of idealism and realism, linked to the growth of bohemian culture near Golden Gate Park between 1963 and 1967, but extending its work well beyond Haight-Ashbury's white, middle-class residents. By 1970 the clinic was seeing 150,000 clients a year and providing a service unavailable elsewhere in the city, although San Francisco was touted as one of the best-equipped cities for hospitals (it had twenty-six hospitals in 1960). After opening in 1968, the Black Man's Free Clinic, in the Fillmore area of San Francisco, had a more modest clientele of about 8,500 people a year (70 percent of whom were black), while the People's Community Clinic in Austin saw over 3,000 clients per year (1 percent of Austin's population) in 5,500 separate visits, most of which were from the young, transients, and migrants.

On a more realistic level, the Haight-Ashbury Free Clinic dealt mostly with health and crime-related problems associated with inner-city ghettos, particularly those of residents in communal housing, draft dodgers, squatters, the homeless, "hoodies," and "unwanted people."[120] The director of psychiatry at the Clinic, Ernest Dernberg (a refugee from Nazi Germany), successfully treated some clients, but staff members tended to refer clients with serious and complicated medical problems to institutions such as the Planned Parenthood and Venereal Disease Clinic or for free out-of-hours treatment at San Francisco General Hospital. This contrasts with 90 percent of clients treated at the Austin clinic, whose problems included respiratory infections, hepatitis, skin disorders, and immunizations. And the Black Man's Free Clinic saw regular cases of chronic and acute psychological disturbances, fewer of which were linked to drug use than was the case at the Haight-Ashbury Free Clinic.[121] The San Francisco and Austin clinics were frequented by hippies, leading one commentator to describe the Austin clinic as follows:

> The first impression one has on entering the clinic is overwhelming. Young people with long hair are everywhere, sitting on the floor, on chairs and benches, or standing in line to be registered. Frequently a tape deck is playing music is the waiting area. . . . Other than their youth and hair, a striking feature of the clinic patients is their courtesy and patience while waiting to be seen.[122]

At the 1970 symposium, the NFCC tried to counter the "square" view that hippies—many of whom had middle-class backgrounds and had chosen a communal lifestyle—"have forfeited whatever right they might have had to conventional medical services."[123] The general dislike of hippies (and the bias in their favor of the free clinic movement) was emphasized when the NFCC unsuccessfully applied for a National Institute of Mental Health grant to research a project led by the criminologist Roger Smith called "The Hippies—Studies of a Drug Based Culture." The project was later funded, but under a different title: "Psycho-Social Factors in Drug Abuse."[124]

David Smith specialized in drug use, and he published a number of books on the consequences of using heroin, marijuana, amphetamines, and tranquilizers. Anxiety and paranoia were common characteristics of the clients of the Haight-Ashbury Free Clinic who used drugs, and many of them saw the world as "a frightening, empty and hostile place rather than a natural repository which can be reclaimed through a new sense of fraternity."[125] Smith did not promote drug use, even though he smoked marijuana partly as a means to help dissolve the conventional institutional relationship between doctor and patient. In fact, Smith demystified drugs. The book he coedited with George Gay was titled *It's So Good, Don't Even Try It Once: Heroin in Perspective* (1972), and a year later—with Donald Wesson—he edited another book, *Uppers and Downers*, with the intention of heightening the reader's awareness of the "relatively unknown aspect of the drug problem—the abuse of stimulants and depressants" and counteracting "inefficient government programs, and naive statements by public officials concerning drug abuse."[126] Free clinic workers often met clients who were openly using LSD and heroin, although Smith noted an increasing trend for "poly-drug abuse."[127] Some clinics, such as the one in Austin, referred clients experiencing bad acid trips to a lay clinic, Middle Earth, located at the YMCA at the University of Texas, and referred heroin users to the local mental health center.[128] Smith discussed the realities of drug use in the passionate account of the Haight-Ashbury Free Clinic, *Love Needs Care* (1971), including a dramatic scene in the Episcopal Peace Center—which, beginning in the autumn of 1968, formed an annex around the corner from the main clinic. Intended as a "tranquil refuge," the annex was full of patients "in every imaginable form of dress and undress. Some of the young people were wrapped in blankets, their anguished faces barely visible behind blood-soaked bandages. Others . . . were huddled together, trying to stay warm."[129]

Rather than a heroic picture of peace-loving hippies, this account reveals "hopelessness" among the clientele and a steep learning curve for the clinic's interns and volunteers. Some psychiatric and counseling work was possible, but in cases of severe or long-term drug use, physicians were obliged to administer sedatives and tranquilizers to "pacify acutely toxic people" and to counter "the paranoia and hallucinosis characteristic of chronic toxicity."[130] In the account of the clients housed in the clinic's annex in the autumn of 1968, Smith and his coauthor John Luce mention a girl who tried to jump out of the window suffering from paranoid fright, a young man who pulled a gun in pursuit of a pusher whom he claimed had sold him contaminated drugs, and another young man who existed in "a chemically induced state of well-being" that he called "Terminal Euphoria" and who liked to boast about how much heroin he could inject.[131] The cases worsened through 1968 and 1969, particularly when the Manson murders of August 1969 caused anxiety among young people in San Francisco and Los Angeles (Manson had lived in Berkeley in 1967, and he had homes in Topanga Canyon and Death Valley in 1968–1969). Ripples of distress throughout the West Coast were linked to the fact that Manson based his distorted philosophy of Helter Skelter on popular music (particularly the Beatles' White Album), and the Manson Family was composed of what would in other circumstances just be regular hippie youths. But "the complex intermeshing of highly unlikely and bizarre circumstances" had turned one of Manson's followers into "a psychologically loaded gun," as a prison psychiatrist described Leslie Van Houten, a member of the family and an accomplice in the murder of Sharon Tate.[132]

Not all the anxieties experienced by clients of the free clinics could be linked to elements of the national scene, including the disillusionment with the Vietnam War, dismay at the assassinations of 1968, or the shock of the Manson murders in 1969. Nevertheless, Roger Smith tried to unearth the complex social factors that influenced the behavior of many drug users who visited the Haight-Ashbury Free Clinic as part of his National Institute of Mental Health project. Smith had worked as a community organizer and probation officer before volunteering to work at the clinic in the spring of 1968 (where he counseled Manson and members of his family); he brought patients for observation and shelter to his Tiburon home; and he developed a detoxification zone in the clinic's annex. A second example of the interface between the work of free clinics and broader social factors is the case of the Berkeley Free Clinic, which opened in the spring of 1969 at the time of the People's Park crisis in Oakland, when it became clear that the establishment could no longer be trusted to care for the young. The crisis emerged from a conflict over the rightful use of the People's Park. On 15 May 1969, organized student protests took place in the park, leading to retaliation from an overly aggressive police force that led to 128 hospitalizations and one death. The Berkeley Free Clinic buffered such social conflict by opening a rap center for group sessions that demanded that young participants make varying degrees of commitment to attend regular sessions, as well as initiating a drug information project in 1969 and consultations with high schools, often involving the acting out of scenarios in which teachers were used as amateur actors.[133]

The sense that things were changing in 1968–1969 was also linked to the disappearance of the hippie philosophy that had given impetus to the Haight-Ashbury Free Medical Clinic in 1967. Only a year later, the chair of the NFCC concluded that the bohemians and hippies who once inhabited the Haight neighborhood had been replaced by speed freaks, drug dealers, and "rip-off artists" who had shattered an already fragile bohemian community lacking the cohesion and flexibility to last in the long run.[134] In response to this shift in clientele, the clinic opened a heroin section in November 1969 to deal with the rise of "new junkies" who had "entered the heroin scene during the demise of the hippie movement and at a time of general disillusionment in the counterculture."[135] By 1972 this new breed of heroin and multidrug users represented over 57 percent of the addicts seen at the clinic.

There were lighter representations of the free clinic—notably Elvis Presley's final film, *Change of Habit* (1969), set in an urban ghetto on the West Coast—but this ambivalent attitude toward drugs brings me to the second of my examples of new therapeutic communities: the Esalen Institute. The free clinic movement balanced the idealism of free healthcare and the realism of dealing with drug use among fragmenting communities, but the Esalen Institute, located thirty-five miles south of Monterey, offered a very different model of collective therapy. This chapter has already discussed the role of Frederick Perls, who was involved in Gestalt therapy in the early 1950s and the rise of alternative therapeutic practices in the mid-1960s. Perls was only one charismatic (and not wholly liked) example of the many kinds of therapists who practiced at the Esalen Institute, which also offered meditation, yoga, group encounters, visualization, psychodramatic practices, spa therapy, and other somatic disciplines. The institute was founded in 1962 by two Stanford University graduates, Michael Murphy and Richard Price. As a student, Murphy had converted to Hinduism (after listening to Frederic Spiegelberg's lectures on contemporary religion at Stanford), and he saw the institute as a place "where Western and Eastern thinkers and practitioners could meet in order to fuse the best of both cultural visions and create a new way of being (or indeed becoming) human." In contrast, Price had experienced invasive forms of therapy as treatment for assumed psychosis during military service in the late 1950s, and he saw Esalen as "a place of healing, as a refuge from the cruelties of Western culture."[136] This balance between alternate worldviews, "education for transcendence" (the title of Murphy's article in the first issue of the *Journal of Transpersonal Psychology*), and a retreat from medical officialdom, marked the institute as a sacred place for Murphy and Price, and for its broad sweep of practitioners and many clients during the 1960s and beyond.[137] Esalen was, and still is, a very private place. Many rumors circulate about famous writers and musicians who went to the institute in the 1960s and 1970s, including Henry Miller, Hunter S. Thompson, George Harrison, Susan Sontag, Joan Baez, and John Denver. According to other rumors, Nixon's administration blamed Esalen for indoctrinating Charles Manson and, therefore, considered the institute partly responsible for the Manson murders.[138]

Murphy and Price were no strangers to psychedelic drugs. They were friends of Timothy Leary in the mid-1960s; Price used psychedelics "in his own person

voyaging"; and Murphy remembers eight trips on peyote and LSD during the early
years of Esalen, although he stopped in 1966 when the trips became more "painful."[139]
They claimed that the period 1966–1970 "was the most tumultuous, out-of-control
time," when drugs were rife throughout that stretch of the California coast (there
were three drug-related suicides at Esalen), but they did not plan the institute to be a
"psychedelic initiation center," and they banned the sale of drugs at the institute and
their use in seminars.[140] Just as Murphy and Price steered away from medical drugs
in favor of meditation and yoga, so Murphy (more than Price) was a strong advocate
of a "non-drug route" to personal enlightenment.[141] This is related to the fact that
Esalen's natural hot springs, on land purchased by Murphy's grandfather, made it perfect for a health spa, and to the statement by George Leonard, Esalen's vice president
and the editor of Look, that the institute was devised to "help, not the few, but the
many toward a vastly expanded capacity to learn, to love, to feel deeply, to create" by
rejecting "the tired dualism" of body and mind in which "the joys of the senses" are
neglected or downgraded.[142] Although Esalen's coastal location and philosophy made
the institute very different from the free clinics in West Coast urban centers, both ventures promoted holistic philosophies. Esalen operated as a nonprofit organization,
with a mission to develop therapeutic techniques in other localities—such as a San
Francisco center that was more closely linked to the everyday realities of urban and
suburban life. Esalen also acted as a training hub for psychologists, social workers,
educators, and psychotherapists (an estimated seven hundred had visited the institute
by 1967). It was also a health center for around four thousand clients per year in the
mid-1960s, who paid between $60 for weekend seminars to $160 for five-day workshops and $3,000 for a nine-month residential fellow course.[143]

Numerous sectors of the public were interested in Esalen, and not just in the Bay
Area, where there was a wave of interest in popular courses on meditation and yoga
in the late 1960s.[144] This interest stemmed partly from publicity about Frederick Perls
and Alan Watts as gurus of alternative therapy in the mid-1960s, but also from interest
in Maslow, who launched the San Francisco branch of Esalen in January 1966; Joy, the
widely read book by the Esalen therapist William Schutz; a December 1967 article in
the New York Times by the journalist Leo Litwak about his revelatory visit to Esalen
in the summer of that year (the article was reprinted in 1968 in a collection of best
magazine articles); Paul Masursky's box office success, Bob & Carol & Ted & Alice; and
Murphy's visit to London in the summer of 1970 to meet members of the Association
for Humanistic Psychology and take the Esalen message to Britain.[145]

Schutz's popular Joy is the arguably the best expression of the Esalen experience
and the human potential movement. The book presents "joy methods" in nontechni-
cal language; it encourages the reader to explore his or her "unused potential"; and
it advocates a "wide variety of approaches," many of which can be practiced outside
of an institution, and steers away from drugs.[146] Schutz does not offer panaceas but a
renewed awareness of the body and techniques that combine the verbal and the nonverbal and balance self-exploration with personal interaction. The book is broadly in
line with Maslow's theory of self-actualization and promotes exercise to overcome

neurosis and bodily debilitation. Schutz makes forays into addressing social repression, but he concentrates on the benefits of encounter groups, psychodrama, physical release, and meditation as techniques that can help to recenter the self in its relation to others. This is to be achieved through a threefold theory of interpersonal behavior that Schutz had outlined in the late 1950s: inclusion ("the need to be with people and to be alone"), control (a combination of self-determination and receptivity to others), and affection (steering a course between "emotional entanglement" and a "bleak, sterile life without love, warmth, tenderness, and someone to confide in").[147] "Openness and honesty" are the driving forces of *Joy*, but the book also presents a fear that the moment will soon pass unless human potential is grasped.[148] Schutz ends his prologue by reflecting on his son and the future—"The future is exciting. The pursuit of joy is exciting. The time is now. We'd better hurry. The culture is already getting to him—Ethan looks as if he is beginning to feel frightened and guilty"—and he closes the book with the renewal of possibility, as Ethan looks out and reaches toward the night sky.[149]

This engagement with the "now" of the late 1960s as a therapeutic moment has its most popular expression in Paul Mazursky's 1969 film *Bob & Carol & Ted & Alice*, with which this chapter closes. Mazursky had recently become a devotee of Esalen; visiting the institute for a weekend with his wife had given him the impetus to coauthor the first twenty pages of the *Bob & Carol & Ted & Alice* screenplay, and he was pleased that the film did not compromise self-expression and the feelings of openness that Esalen had awakened in him.[150] This is developed through the film's use of method acting, but only to a degree. The long opening sequence of the film is accompanied by Handel's "Hallelujah Chorus" and depicts expansive views of the Big Sur coast, intercut with shots of the spa, nude meditation, tai chi, and scream therapy at sunrise (a shot that includes Mazursky in silhouette), which all emphasize the special qualities of Esalen. The opening introduces Bob (Robert Culp), a documentary filmmaker, and his wife, Carol (Natalie Wood), as they arrive at "the Institute" for a weekend residency course. We then cut to a twenty-four-hour group therapy session that includes candid introductions from the residents, the therapist's nondirective encouragement, disconcerting close-ups of the residents as they "try to learn something about the other person" without speaking, and a group session in which Carol's openness to others is contrasted with Bob's disengagement and deep-seated anxiety, which surfaces during lengthy group therapy. The opening section teeters between documentary realism, a sensitive representation of the residents learning to be emotionally open with each other (including a tender scene between Bob and Carol), and uncomfortable satire as an indulgent group hug ends the Esalen sequence.

The remainder of the film veers toward a comedy of social manners as Bob and Carol test out their Esalen experience on their friends Ted (Elliott Gould) and Alice (Dyan Cannon), a more conventional couple whose growing interest in new experiences serves to challenge the boundaries between "hip" and "square" (Cannon started going to Esalen after making the film, perhaps as a response to her divorce from Cary Grant in 1968, after he reputedly forced her to take LSD).[151] Bob and Carol's

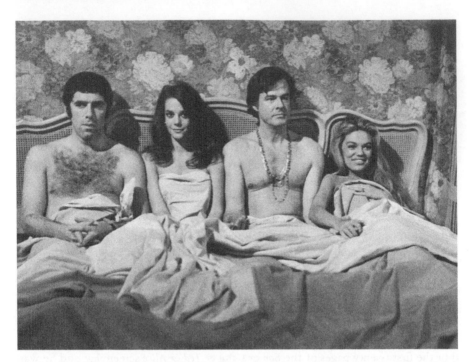

FIGURE 9.2   Elliot Gould, Natalie Wood, Robert Culp, and Dyan Cannon (left to right) self-administer group therapy after a visit to The Institute. *Bob & Carol & Ted & Alice* (Paul Mazursky, Columbia, 1969).

new age pretentions are exposed through group situations and conversations that lead to admissions of affairs, a marijuana session, Alice's visit to a psychiatrist, and a planned foursome—all of which leaves the Esalen experience behind for a fairly light-hearted poke at late 1960s bourgeois manners. If this is a representation of "normal neurosis," then the engagement with discourses of health and illness is fairly thin. Mazursky's stated aim was to be both funny and touching, but what begins as the potential for group therapy to break through neurotic barriers dissolves into social comedy akin to Woody Allen's films of the late 1960s and 1970s, rather than the complex sexuality that Philip Roth explored in his psychoanalytic novel of 1969, *Portnoy's Complaint*—in which sexual release is rarely wholly liberating. Group therapy was not always portrayed in such a positive light: in the 1967 novel and 1970 film *Diary of a Mad Housewife*, for example, the group session proves useless for Tina Balser, and her psychiatrist shows himself to be insensitive to her domestic frustrations. Neverthe-less, *Bob & Carol & Ted & Alice* marks an optimistic moment for the human potential movement, as is evident when Bob encourages Ted to grasp the liberating spirit of the Institute. However, given that the film was shot during Richard Nixon's victorious presidential campaign, perhaps Mazursky recognized that the human potential move-ment was already passing into history.

Although Mazursky believed that the Esalen experience actually worked for these two couples, the closing nighttime scene of the film marks this ambivalence about the substance of the human potential movement. The final scene mirrors the opening sequence by depicting a ritual procession of couples (including gay, lesbian, African American, and American Indian couples) mingling on a Las Vegas hotel forecourt, swapping the dramatic Big Sur coastline and the Esalen retreat for the practice of encounter therapy in everyday life. As the couples congregate outside the hotel, individuals break away to stare silently and intently into other faces, and we hear the sentimental (and potentially nostalgic) strains of Burt Bacharach and Hal David's 1965 song, "What the World Needs Now Is Love." The film ends with a rapturous shot of the two lead couples reunited on the forecourt, suggesting that their neuroses have been magically overcome through sexualized joy. In this way, *Bob & Carol & Ted & Alice* engages with the popular face of therapy, but in so doing it diffuses the revolutionary potential of the therapeutic community and, arguably, weakens the searching social critique promoted by many of the thinkers featured in this chapter.

Conclusion

BEYOND THE TWO CULTURES?

The third section of this book has explored the ways in which realism and idealism are tightly woven into discourses of American healthcare after World War II. We have seen how developments in humanist, transpersonal, and group therapy during the 1960s challenged the normative model of medical science that prevailed during the early Cold War period. We have also seen, however, that although institutional critiques accelerated the transition from large state-run hospitals at mid-century toward more integrated therapeutic structures, this shift did not completely shake the foundations of regulatory medical practice, which persisted into and beyond the 1970s. Gerald Grob has pointed out the attendant dangers of this shift toward a community-based system (he argues that "many chronically and severely mental ill persons . . . were often cast adrift in communities without access to support services or the basic necessities of life"), but this is to conflate the practical difficulties that community healthcare faced in the 1970s with its philosophical challenge to the structures of organized medicine.[1]

Following Thomas Kuhn's 1962 book *The Structure of Scientific Revolutions*, it is tempting to suggest that, starting in the late 1950s and increasing in force and range in the 1960s, there was a revolution, or paradigm shift, away from conventional (what Kuhn would call "normal") medical and psychiatric practice. In a postscript to the book's second edition, Kuhn claims that a "paradigm" is both "the entire constellation of beliefs, values, techniques . . . shared by the members of a given community" and a "puzzle-solution" to questions that conventional science is unable to resolve.[2] Kuhn argues that a revolution need not be "a large change" and is not always predicated on crisis, although crises are "the usual prelude," providing "a self-correcting mechanism which ensures that the rigidity of normal science will not forever go unchallenged."[3] From this perspective, I would argue that the revolutionary shift charted in this book was precipitated by a crisis in patient care, in which supreme confidence in medical authority was replaced by a broad reconceptualization of selfhood and intersubjectivity. This chimes with Kuhn's view that revolutionary change might be brought about through tacit awareness of problems that normal science cannot address. Kuhn warned against applying his theory of scientific paradigms wholesale to all spheres of thought and practice, but he ends his postscript by indicating the need for comparative studies in related fields that have different epistemological and historical trajectories.

Kuhn's reading is instructive for thinking about postwar shifts in scientific practice, although his conception of change is quite different from that of thinkers like Herbert Marcuse, who advocated cultural upheaval as an engine for social reorganization.

However, rather than a complete paradigm shift, I have argued throughout this book that revolutions in medical knowledge and practice bind two opposing trends in a tight knot: the one trend reasserting the authority of medical science and the other positioning medicine as a healing art that upholds the needs and rights of the patient. Kuhn would see the growth of holistic practice as a paradigm shift that led to a new therapeutic language—one focused on the patient—but in his view, such a wholesale shift away from medical authority would be to ignore the ways in which these paradigms continued to inform each other. In fact, I would argue that this rhythm of opposition and synergy is embedded in the dialectic pattern that structures the three sections of this book. Rather than a radical paradigm shift, then, the pattern of fragmentation, organization, and reorganization emphasizes the ways in which discourses continued to combine and clash.

I proposed in the introduction that medical humanities can be positioned in a middle ground between the two cultures of the arts and sciences in the postwar period, but this remained an uncomfortable terrain into the 1960s, beset by conceptual problems and disagreements similar to those of a decade earlier. Thus, the dichotomies of the two cultures persisted, albeit with moments of recognition that these oppositions were unhelpful for both practitioner and patient. One example of this was a 1973 essay written by the psychologist Carl Pitts, in which he discerned that behaviorists and humanists deliberately misread one another: "The humanists seem to view the behaviorists as manipulative, depersonalizing, and controlling slaves to scientism, concerned with forcing men into submission, conformity, and docility. The behaviorists view humanists as soft-headed, non-scientific, vague, sentimental, and hopelessly caught up in nonoperational meaningless values."[4] Reflecting on Kuhn's "paradigm clash" and Pitts's own education (he was drawn to Rogerian humanist psychology but also appreciated the laboratory), this essay tried to erode dichotomies that ossify around these perceived oppositions. Suggesting that the divisions are, in fact, more "a matter of style than intent," Pitts concluded by proposing that professional psychology should be interested in objective underlying factors but should also attend closely to personal motivation.[5] In his brief response to Pitts's article, Carl Rogers acknowledged that behaviorists had actually "come a long way" since the mid-1950s (when he held a debate with B. F. Skinner) in recognizing that individuals have a "capacity for choice and decision and subjective appraisal," rather than being wholly determined by external (social, economic, cultural) or internal (biological, psychological, instinctive) factors.[6]

Another key change was an emerging recognition of the importance of narrative for understanding identity, health, and sickness. Although narrative modes in the medical humanities did not really come to the fore until the late 1970s and the 1980s, there were some early signs of their arrival, both in the existential emphasis that selfhood needs to be continually remade and in sociological accounts of role-playing and the complex interactions within and beyond the family structure. Erving Goffman's theory of "face work" (as discussed in chapter 8) is important in this second regard, but with some qualifications that link social roles to a more personalized state of identity formation promoted by the likes of Rogers and Rollo May. This oscillation between personal identity and role-playing characterizes a number of studies written in the 1960s, but it was often accompanied by an awareness of the limits that mental and physical illness impose on social participation, such as those explored in Jerry Schatzberg's film *Puzzle of a Downfall Child* (1970), in which the psychological breakdown of fashion model Lou Sand is dramatized by the split image of Faye Dunaway on the movie poster, with one half of her face beautifully composed and the other haunted and disheveled.

Despite the persistence of such oppositions, it is clear that the two-cultures model that dominated the 1950s was too simplistic for those thinkers who had started to recognize that health and illness are not abstractions in need of diagnosis, but lived realities bound up in personal, social, and historical narratives that implicate family, community, region, and nation. This might suggest a progressive outlook in which polar opposites dissolve within a more creative middle space—a version of what Karl Menninger called a "vital balance" in his 1963 book of that name, playing off Arthur Schlesinger Jr.'s earlier conception of a "vital center."[7] However, this middle space was not necessarily therapeutic or immune to the vagaries of national politics, as explored in a special issue of the *American Journal of Psychotherapy* on "Psychiatry and Its Relationship to Political Behavior," in October 1970.

It is worth returning briefly to the topic of politics to map out this more complex terrain, particularly because President Richard Nixon took healthcare policy at the end of the 1960s in a different direction from that of his two Democratic predecessors. In his first State of the Union address—in January 1970, in the heat of the Vietnam War and with the attack on Cambodia only three months away—Nixon looked ahead to the bicentennial of 1976 and foretold a peaceful country that would have "abolished hunger," could offer a "minimum income" for all American families, and would have "made enormous progress in providing better housing, faster transportation, improved health, and superior education."[8] Nixon called for a renewal of the nation's "driving dream," but he had his eye on scaling back President Lyndon Johnson's welfare system, which he called "a colossal failure" in his first domestic address as president in August 1969 and which he would later accuse of being "a monstrous, consuming outrage."[9] With unrest among African American communities and a wave of student demonstrations (including the Kent State shootings of 4 May, provoked by a demonstration against the invasion of Cambodia), 1970 was a year of turbulent transition from the liberal promises of the early and mid-1960s to a more fractious and fragmented phase of cultural opposition to government, based on what Nixon described as a "chasm of misunderstanding" separating "old and young."[10]

On the positive side, Nixon promised that "no American family will be prevented from obtaining basic medical care by inability to pay" (but his Family Health Insurance Plan was stalled by Congress until 1972); in his second State of the Union Address, he pledged new funding for preventive medicine (in search of a cure for cancer); and three months earlier he had signed into law the Developmental Disabilities Services and Facilities Construction Act, to mark a "new phase in the Federal

Government's efforts to provide a better life for all mentally retarded and other developmentally disabled citizens", which now included people with cerebral palsy and epilepsy.[11] However, despite a steady level of activity on healthcare matters across Nixon's six years in the White House, his administration arguably lacked the social commitment of the previous two.[12] This explains why, at the end of the 1960s, many medical trends were moving further away from national initiatives, as evidenced by the rise of alternative and homeopathic medicine and the beginnings of the disability rights movement, in the form of New York's Disabled in Action organization and the Physically Disabled Students Program at the University of California at Berkeley. The emergence of disability activism and identity politics based on gender, race, and sexuality were key social changes at the beginning of the 1970s, and they indicate that medicine, psychiatry, and healthcare had become a more diffuse field than the two-cultures model credited.

Seven Trajectories

If we take a snapshot of medical, psychiatric, and psychoanalytic studies published in 1970, we can identify seven broad trajectories with different therapeutic arcs that give a much more variegated picture than Nixon's heathcare agenda does. Although the three dominant themes of this book—fragmentation, organization, and reorganization—suggest that the dialectic sequence might have played itself out by 1970, we can see evidence of all three patterns within these seven trajectories. But that does not mean that thinkers and practitioners in 1970 were circling around exactly the same issues as their predecessors in 1945, with a heightened awareness of increasingly pluralistic cultural currents; the realization that normal psychopathology is present in everyday life rather than confined to specialist institutions; more flexibility in the understanding of family psychodynamics; heightened public awareness of mental health issues; and a perceived crisis in patient care.

The first of these seven trajectories was the growing interest in medical and psychological affinities with aesthetics, including new essays on literary writers, collections such as Frederick Crews's *Psychoanalysis and the Literary Process* (1970), and a renewed emphasis on creativity in Judith Groch's *The Right to Create* (1969), in which Groch is as scathing about mind control and "organized persuasion" as she is passionate about the need to expand "personal creative resources" to ward off the emphasis on technology and automation.[13] The second trajectory was an emerging focus on ethnic groups and cross-cultural studies of other cultures (albeit often filtered through essentialist categories) such as *The African Mind in Health and Disease*, commissioned by the World Health Organization, and Jean Briggs's anthropological study *Never in Anger: Portrait of an Eskimo Family*, based on detailed fieldwork in the Canadian Northwest Territories in the mid-1960s that was partly funded by the National Institute of Mental Health, which examined both social and psychological structures in and beyond the Eskimo family.[14]

Third was a renewed interest in aggression and violence in the wake of the "chronic day-to-day quiet violence against the human spirit" that Kenneth Clark had observed in 1964 in response to the Harlem riots.[15] The renewed violence at the end of the decade perturbed Nixon, particularly when linked to campus demonstrations, Black Power, and the emergence of the Weathermen (the militant faction of the student movement). This trend was often inflected by political activism, such as Hannah Arendt's 1970 study *On Violence* (which made use of Frantz Fanon's psychiatric vocabulary), the RAND report titled *Rebellion and Authority* (1970), and the volume *Conflict: Violence and Nonviolence* (1971).[16] Studies of violence often addressed psychological and psychiatric issues, as is the case with *Violence and the Struggle for Existence* (1970) produced by the Department of Psychiatry at Stanford University, and the close attention to the complex psychosocial causes of violence was symbolized by an open letter from psychologist Saul Rosenzweig in 1970, in which he called for the establishment of an International Society for the Study of Aggression.[17] Also dovetailing with this trend were further studies on stress among soldiers in Vietnam, including a five-year study (from the escalation of conflict in mid-1965 to de-escalation in mid-1970), featured in the *Bulletin of the Menninger Clinic* in November 1970, and two studies by Peter Bourne of the Walter Reed Army Institute of Research, *The Psychology and Physiology of Stress* (1969) and *Men, Stress, and Vietnam* (1970). Combining field studies of military personnel and civilians in South Vietnam, Bourne observed many cases of aggression among troops, as well as frustration born out of "constant uncertainty."[18]

The fourth trajectory combined ongoing clinical accounts of schizophrenia, new clinical studies of autistic children, and a growing focus on depression, often linked to suicidal tendencies.[19] Some projects looked outward to the psychodynamics of family life or to the language of development and education, but other studies remained squarely focused on psychobiology. An example of the latter is a conference on depressive illnesses sponsored by the Department of Health, Education, and Welfare and held at the College of William and Mary in the spring of 1969. The conference focused on biochemistry, physiology, endocrinology, and the psychopathology of depression rather than broader factors of status, poverty, race, and gender. Nonetheless, looking to the future, the conference organizers thought that there was more to learn about "the effects of physiological and psychological stress, especially chronic stress" brought on by war experiences, and the effects of drugs on the chemical balance of the brain and thyroid.[20]

This leads onto the fifth trajectory: a topical interest in drugs that can be divided into three divergent currents. First, new studies on the healing power of recreational drugs (such as three studies in 1970, Erich Goode's *The Marijuana Smokers*, Barbara Lewis's *The Sexual Power of Marijuana*, and David Smith's *The New Social Drug*) jostled with advertisements for a range of prescription drugs, such as Ritalin (for chronic fatigue), Serax (for anxiety), Eskalith (for mania), Sinequan (an antidepressant and tranquilizer all in one), and Stelazine (purported to relieve "delusions, hallucination, and confused, irrational thoughts that so often torment paranoid schizophrenics")—all of which indicates, as Andrew Scull argues, that the "transformative effects of the drugs revolution on the psychiatric profession" were accelerating at the end of the 1960s (Grob notes that 60 percent of psychoanalysts were prescribing medications by 1976).[21] Second, chiming with President Nixon's fears about drugs and social decline was the view that the dramatic increase in the use of narcotics could lead to a wave of dependency and new forms of illness, as discussed by an American Psychoanalytic Association panel titled "Psychoanalytic Evaluation of Addiction and Habituation" in May 1969 and in a report published in the *Bulletin of the Menninger Clinic* in July 1970.[22] And third was the growing trend of avoiding drugs, either within a course of therapy or through the use of natural remedies, popularized by Buryl Payne in *Getting There without Drugs* (1973).

The sixth trajectory was a stronger emphasis on the relatedness between biology and psychology, which was often framed in holistic terms. Alexander Lowen and Arthur Janov were two therapists in this camp whose theories proved popular in the 1970s, with John Lennon and Yoko Ono becoming two of Janov's high-profile clients at the time of the Beatles' breakup in 1970. Lowen set up his own center in New York in 1956, as did Janov in Santa Monica in 1968, as a means of developing practical theories that could do justice to the entire human organism. A former student of Wilhelm Reich's, Lowen set out his theory of bioenergetics in *The Language of the Body* (1958) and *The Betrayal of the Body* (1967) and he saw mind and body as parts of a continuum: a theory that he extended into the realm of creativity in *Pleasure* (1970). Janov was potentially more revolutionary in tackling the roots of primal trauma, moving beyond the talking cure—which he felt targeted cognition at the expense of emotional and visceral responses. His 1970 manifesto, *The Primal Scream*, set out his somatosensory theory, in which repression manifests itself in "muscular rigidity," as if Janov was projecting a critique of rigid social organization onto the human organism itself.[23] He went much further than simply promoting yogic and movement exercises, tapping into deeper layers of pain that he argued start to accrete from the child's initial months. Janov's manifesto was insistent: "What we need is something total—a joining together at *once* of the body and mind" in order to retrieve "fragmented feelings from the symptomatic spillways and piece them back together into one complete and clear feeling."[24] Nevertheless, primal therapy produced some mixed therapeutic results and proved dangerous for some patients, even though Janov steered away from advocating the use of hallucinogenic drugs because they "artificially open up individuals to more reality than they can tolerate" and are liable to dissolve the "integrity of the organism."[25]

A different manifestation of this trend to fuse biology and psychology is the volume *Anorexia and Obesity* (1970), which collected pioneering work on eating disorders, such as the German-born psychoanalyst Hilde Bruch's study of fifty-one anorexic patients (mostly women) between the early 1940s and late 1960s. Bruch noted that anorexia was on the increase between the ages of eleven and twenty-eight as "a disorder involving extensive disturbances in personality development" and a concerted attempt for the individual to gain self-control.[26] Following her 1952 advice book *Don't Be Afraid of Your Child: A Guide for Perplexed Parents* (and having offered advice to Frieda-Fromm Reichmann on the treatment of the teenage patient Deborah Blau, as discussed in chapter 8), Bruch examined family context, signs of depression, and problems of diagnosis and therapy, outlining the sensitive approach needed by psychiatrists toward complex eating disorders. She encouraged patients to be "active participants" in therapy, in the hope that they will "learn to apply this participation to real life situations" by discovering the "capacity for initiative" rather than perpetuating the compulsive cycle of gorging or fasting.[27] Bruch critiqued directive models of psychotherapy that reinforced "underlying pathological factors," but she failed to look to the cultural sphere, where a study of the mass media or literary representation in, say, Sylvia Plath's *The Bell Jar* might have revealed wider influences on the development of teenage anorexia.

The seventh trajectory was arguably the most pronounced at the end of the 1960s: the politicization of illness that radically affected views of medical treatment and patients' rights. This trend was perhaps most visible in terms of consciousness raising within the women's movement, extending beyond the founding of the National Organization for Women in 1965 to focus on reproductive rights, increased awareness of birth control, the decriminalization of abortion, and a critique of the masculinist bias of organized medicine, which Alice Wolfson called a "zealously guarded monopoly."[28] Evidence for this trend can be seen in the emergence of women's clinics in the 1970s based on the community health model; political advocacy for women's rights at local, state, and federal levels; and the publication of the landmark volume *Our Bodies, Ourselves* (originally titled *Women and Their Bodies: A Course*) by the Boston Women's Health Book Collective in 1970.[29] This project grew out of a course focusing on women's health, sexuality, and motherhood, placing women's experiences at the center of healthcare by identifying narrative connections between individual experiences and the social and medical conditions that shape them.[30] Although the Boston group was limited in terms of ethnicity (all its members were white), age (between twenty-four and forty) and socioeconomic background (middle-class with a college education), the members self-consciously discussed "womanhood from the inside out" and consulted widely with other women's groups, aiming to cross "over the socially created barriers of race, color, income and class, and to feel a sense of identity with all women in the experience of being female."[31]

Susan Wells argues that the Boston project helped to educate readers and politicized women's medical experiences, linking stories that confront the medicalization of women's lives with healthening narratives of "self-formation," particularly as the book grew in scope and texture during the mid-1970s and early 1980s.[32] The politicized, grass-roots, and collective dimensions of the project are central for recognizing this as a breakthrough moment in health literature, and women's healthcare in particular. Balancing personal experience, informed debate, and awareness of the limitations of published studies on women's health, the group attempted to share "knowledge and power" by raising awareness and developing new support networks.[33] However, the emphasis is almost exclusively on the body in the early editions of *Our Bodies, Ourselves*, positioned at the intersection of biology and society. Discussions of psychiatry and counseling were limited to commentaries on anger, emotional reactions to masturbation and menstruation, the impact of abortion and rape, and issues of well-being during child rearing and menopause. "Body education" was seen as vital for tackling "ignorance, uncertainty—even, at worst, shame—about our physical selves," a homology, perhaps, to the social stigma that Goffman had discussed a decade earlier. But the project also aligns neatly with three broader trends: the importance of sexuality for the counterculture; the community healthcare initiatives discussed in chapters 8 and 9; and "untapped energies" that might allow readers to become "more confident, more autonomous, stronger, and more whole."[34] *Our Bodies, Ourselves* did not adopt the militant stance of the radical feminist Shulamith Firestone, who—in *The Dialectic of Sex*, published the same year—called for women to transcend the biological and psychological oppression of pregnancy and motherhood and looked toward a cybernetic solution to reproduction. Firestone criticized the National Organization for Women for dealing only with "the more superficial symptoms of sexism"; attacked Freudian thought for subsuming the feminist agenda; and adapted Reich's theories in her attempt to release sexuality from normative structures.[35] In contrast, the Boston group focused on women's awareness of their changing bodies and promoted self-knowledge and self-respect across the whole life cycle, from childhood to old age.

Emerging Patterns and Polemics

We might see this new attentiveness to particular conditions and local communities as a shift from a mid-century paradigm toward heightened awareness of what Gregory Bateson, at a 1968 conference on "Effects of Conscious Purpose on Human Adaptation," described as an integrated pattern that he believed was essential for promulgating health. Rather than the rigid organizational logic of the 1950s, Bateson looked to a healthy "single system of environment" in which "civilization" and "environment" mesh in synergistic ways—an approach that Buckminster Fuller was exploring in his futuristic architecture at the end of the 1960s.[36] This conception of an "ongoing complex system" provided a way of overcoming what the German sociologist Max Weber had called the separate spheres of modernity, in which distinct arenas of human activity became divided off from each other in the early twentieth century, closely linked to the professionalization of academic disciplines.[37] Bateson later developed this idea in *Mind and Nature: A Necessary Unity* (1979) by emphasizing adaptability and respect for difference, but he had started to explore these terms in an October 1970 presentation to urban planners, "Ecology and Flexibility in Urban Civilization." In this talk he stressed the importance of "social flexibility" as the precondition for a "healthy system" that can "be compared to an acrobat on a high wire [who] must be free to move from one position of instability to another. . . . If his arms are fixed or paralyzed (isolated from communication), he must fall."[38] In contrast to health as an "uncommitted potentiality for change," Bateson saw pathology as the "eating up" of flexibility by rigid forms of organization.[39] He did not offer a prescriptive model of health; rather, he looked toward a broader cultural and social horizon against which health might be measured. This view may appear to be value free, but we should note that Bateson tacitly evoked a moral and existential commitment to embrace change and flexibility, which some medical conditions might prohibit.

The openness and receptivity promoted by Abraham Maslow, Rogers, and those involved in the encounter group practices on the West Coast in the second half of the 1960s are testament to the importance of Bateson's insights. Published the same year as Rogers's *Encounter Groups*, the edited volume *Encounter* (1970), for example, emphasized "honesty, openness, and responsibility" and a willingness to embrace experience in order to search out "answers to existence."[40] This swings the pendulum away from scientific authority to interpersonal experience, in which the individual is no longer seen as a "patient" but finds a balance between active autonomy and surrendering to the group. Although encounter groups were sometimes taken as a model for communal living, this, in itself, is not a guarantor for health, although it can offer a support structure for ailing or anxious individuals. A good example is provided by Erving Polster, from the Gestalt Institute in Cleveland, Ohio, who tested out this model on a local coffee-shop community over nine months in 1967–1968. Polster attempted to put into practice the insights of B. F. Skinner in his thought-experiment novel *Walden II* (1948), which imagined a communal version of Henry David Thoreau's *Walden* where social problems (including health issues) are solved with the help of scientific technology. Echoing the spirit of *Walden II*—but without fully adopting Skinner's technocractic and behaviorist emphasis, and also ignoring Noam Chomsky's published criticism in 1959 that Skinner's communal version of Walden was in fact a dystopia[41] Polster's coffee-shop experiment pointed toward a more endemic change in community structures:

> The small group is too small a world to live in. In society, since interconnectedness and interdependence are unavoidable, there must be some way of relating to the larger community. Otherwise we invite secrecy . . . or we become esoteric, spreading bewilderment. . . . In experiencing the largeness of the community, there is a contagion of spirit which stretches beyond the exclusive workings of the now familiar intimate smallness of the encounter group.[42]

Interpersonal issues of conflict and dissent emerged in the course of Polster's experiment, but so did the realization that aggression can be channeled without resorting to destructive violence. Polster shared Skinner's view that studies of heterogeneous social formations and the impact of mass culture would demand different and more flexible strategies. However, in the healthening climate of the encounter group, Polster believed that it is possible to work through an individual's anxieties within the group experience without resorting to invasive therapeutic techniques or reasserting the medical authority of the doctor.

Gerald Grob has argued that in 1970 it became difficult to define "a clear and unambiguous mental health policy."[43] However, these examples suggest that 1970 was, in many ways, a progressive moment in the medical and social sciences, in which prescriptive authority and diagnostic rigidity had given way to a perspective that was both panoramic and sensitive to individual and group circumstance—or what Polster calls the attempt to "put Utopia back on the map."[44] Far from utopian, but imbued with optimism for the future, Rosalynn Carter's work on mental health (as discussed in the preface) also stems from this moment, galvanized by a fresh exposé of dire conditions at the Central State Hospital in Milledgeville, Georgia, where one of Jimmy Carter's cousins was a long-term inpatient.[45] Six years before entering the White House, the Carters demonstrated that, together, grass-roots activism and politically sponsored action can make a difference at local and regional levels: Rosalynn Carter worked with drug addicts, volunteered at the Atlanta Regional Hospital, and promoted community services for psychiatric patients and children's summer camps; while Jimmy Carter, as governor of Georgia, approved substantial funds to help "mentally retarded" children and invited Eunice Kennedy Shriver to hold the Special Olympics in Georgia in 1970.[46]

Nevertheless, others felt that rather than working with the medical establishment, an oppositional stance was needed in order to prevent medicine from being further integrated into the military-industrial complex. As evidence of this, a number of grass-roots groups and publications emerged in 1970. The Insane Liberation Front was formed in Portland, Oregon, as a branch of the emerging disability rights movement that was linked to the San Francisco–based magazine Madness Network News, beginning in 1972. In late 1969 the Radical Therapist Collective was formed in Minot, North Dakota; the group launched its journal, the Radical Therapist, the following spring with an emphasis on countering what the collective believed were exploitative orthodox therapies. And in Syracuse, New York, Thomas Szasz, George Alexander, and Erving Goffman established the American Association for the Abolition of Involuntary Mental Hospitalization (AAAIMH), followed in 1971 by the group's newsletter, the Abolitionist, and an annual conference (both of which ran until 1979). The AAAIMH argued that institutionalized psychiatry, in particular, served only to subjugate the patient and that treatment and facilities for patients at the end of the 1960s—particularly the poor and other vulnerable groups—had changed little over the last twenty-five years.

Szasz was the most vocal spokesman of the AAAIMH, following up his 1961 treatise The Myth of Mental Illness with two books in 1970: the first a collection of 1960s essays, Ideology and Insanity, and the second his provocative study The Manufacture of Madness, which set out the argument that not only is "the concept of mental illness . . . erroneous and misleading," but also "the ethical convictions and social arrangements based on this concept constitute an immoral ideology of intolerance."[47] Szasz argued that psychiatry destroys the patient's rights, and that any attempt to reject treatment or a refusal "to submit to psychiatric authority" is often interpreted "as a further sign of [the patient's] illness."[48] Szasz's study polemically (and rather reductively) positions institutional psychiatry and the mental health movement within a long history of persecution of social deviants, but he elides far too many historical moments and social trends in constructing a vast international conspiracy on behalf of psychiatrists to promulgate the "myth of mental illness" as a means of subjugating patients. Szasz continued to produce passionate polemics into the 1980s and 1990s, and he worked with the Church of Scientology to create a museum, Psychiatry: An Industry of Death, in Los Angeles, which opened in 2005 with a focus on human rights violations during the long history of psychiatry. Despite his tendency to draw fanciful connections, Szasz's anger was real and needs to be placed alongside more affirmative currents that suggest "individual liberty, human diversity, and respect for persons" (all of which Szasz upholds) were widely practiced by 1970.[49]

We might argue that Szasz's polemic, the formation of the AAAIMH, and the consciousness-raising of activist groups in the late 1960s were successful in bringing to the public's attention issues that had previously been largely the domain of clinical medicine and psychiatry. However, as this book has demonstrated, this moment of public awareness was not new, with films, fiction, autobiography, and the mass media providing multiple channels for discussions of health and illness through the postwar period. For example, a six-part NBC series, *The Psychiatrist*, ran in 1971, in the wake of the December 1970 TV film *The Psychiatrist: God Bless the Children*.

As the preface of this book outlined, the stigma debates of the 1990s suggest that public awareness of mental health issues—particularly medical conditions in which it is difficult to differentiate between physical and mental health—still have a long way to go. The use of stigmatizing phrases like "injury," "damage," and "lack" to describe mental illness or congenital conditions decreased during the 1970s, but they persisted in some forms of literary fiction, where they were often linked to explorations of a "sick society"[50]—a term adopted by the radical vanguard of the Students for a Democratic Society to describe the harm the nation was exacting on its citizens.[51] A brief closing example of this trend is Saul Bellow's 1970 novel, *Mr. Sammler's Planet*, in which the seventy-year-old protagonist Artur Sammler tries to cling to his health in the face of accelerating social change and a very different climate than the one he remembers from his youth. For Sammler, in the current world neither federal planning nor cultural revolution provide satisfactory answers to social ills. He feels that he is physically and psychologically "breaking up" (he has only one good eye, and "irregular big fragments inside were melting, sparkling with pain, floating off"), implying that he cannot keep pace with the realities of the early 1970s.[52] Although his mind remains sharp, in his beleaguered and myopic state Sammler would, most likely, have been blind to the ways in which a combination of federal and local forces had started to positively shape the understanding and treatment of health and illness, leading, a few years later, to a renewed attention to mental health during Jimmy Carter's presidency and gradual improvement of public facilities through the efforts of the disability rights movement, symbolized by periodic amendments to the Developmental Disabilities Act between 1975 and 2000, and by the Americans with Disabilities Act of 1990.

This book has shown that the longer history of healthcare in the United States is shot through with moments of optimism and instances of deep pessimism, in which it is often hard to separate out progressive from realist perspectives and where the politics of therapy are always open to debate. Nevertheless, within the post–World War II revolutions in American healthcare, the trends outlined in this conclusion suggest that by 1970, medicine, psychiatry, and their cultural articulations were closer than ever before. Thus, Gregory Bateson's proposal of an integrated pattern provides us with a more useful metaphor than the two-cultures model for exploring these complex interconnections.

Notes

PREFACE

1. Hillary Rodham Clinton, "Working for a Healthier America," remarks at the White House Conference on Mental Health, Howard University, Washington, DC, 7 June 1999, clinton4.nara.gov/WH/EOP/First_Lady/html/generalspeeches/1999/19990607.html.

2. Donna E. Shalala, "Message," in US Department of Health and Human Services, *Mental Health: A Report of the Surgeon General* (Rockville, MD: US Department of Health and Human Services, 1999, profiles.nlm.nih.gov/ps/access/NNBBHS.pdf). This public discussion coincided with a wave of scholarly interest in stigma, particularly under the auspices of the Chicago Consortium for Stigma Research. See, for example, Patrick W. Corrigan, "The Impact of Stigma on Severe Mental Illness," *Cognitive and Behavioral Practice* 5, no. 2 (1998): 201–222; and Patrick W. Corrigan and Amy C. Watson, "Understanding the Impact of Stigma on People with Mental Illness," *World Psychiatry* 1, no. 1 (2002): 16–20.

3. Ian Dowbiggin makes a similar point in *The Quest for Mental Health: A Tale of Science, Medicine, Scandal, Sorrow, and Mass Society* (Cambridge: Cambridge University Press, 2011), 1–7.

4. Cited in Theda Skocpol, *Boomerang: Health Care Reform and the Turn against Government*, paperback ed. (New York: Norton, 1997), 5.

5. Ibid., 189.

6. Michael F. Hogan, "Achieving the Promise: Transforming Mental Health Care in America" (July 2003, mentalhealth.about.com/library/free/blCoverLetter.htm).

7. Erving Goffman, *Stigma: Notes on the Management of Spoiled Identity* (Englewood Cliffs, NJ: Prentice-Hall, 1963).

8. Rosalynn Carter with Susan K. Golant, *Helping Someone with Mental Illness* (New York: Random House, 1998), 149–150.

9. US Department of Health and Human Services, *Mental Health*, 1; Monroe Lerner and Odin W. Anderson, *Health Progress in the United States: 1900–1960* (Chicago: University of Chicago Press, 1963), 161.

10. US Department of Health and Human Services, *Mental Health*, 3–4. The 1963 figures, given in terms of "disability-adjusted life years," are: cardiovascular conditions, 18.6; mental illness (including suicide), 15.4; malignant diseases, including cancer, 15.0; respiratory conditions, 4.8; alcohol use 4.7; infectious and parasitic diseases, 2.8; drug use 1.5.

11. Ibid., 5.

12. Anne Harrington, *The Cure Within: A History of Mind-Body Medicine* (New York: Norton, 2008), 17; Charles R. Rosenberg, *Our Present Complaint: American Medicine, Then and Now* (Baltimore: Johns Hopkins University Press, 2007), 70–71.

13. Rosenberg, *Our Present Complaint*, 139.

INTRODUCTION

1. Quoted in James P. Mitchell, *How American Buying Habits Change* (Washington, DC: US Department of Labor, 1959), 176.

2. See Abraham Maslow, "Neurosis as a Failure of Personal Growth," lecture at the Institute of Man Symposium, Duquesne University, 18 November 1966 (Maslow Papers, M111, Archives of the History of American Psychology, University of Akron, Akron, OH).

3. Morris J. Vogel and Charles E. Rosenberg, eds., *The Therapeutic Revolution: Essays in the Social History of American Medicine* (Philadelphia: University of Pennsylvania Press, 1979), 4; Leon Chertok and Raymond de Saussure, *The Therapeutic Revolution, from Mesmer to Freud*, trans. R. H. Ahrenfeldt (New York: Brunner/Mazel, 1979), xii. For American mental health care in the early twentieth century, see Joel T. Braslow, *Mental Ills and Bodily Cures: Psychiatric Treatment in the First Half of the Twentieth Century* (Berkeley: University of California Press, 1997); Eric Caplan, *Mind Games: American Culture and the Birth of Psychotherap*, paperback ed. (Berkeley: University of California Press, 2001).

4. Charles E. Rosenberg, "The Therapeutic Revolution: Medicine, Meaning, Social Change in Nineteenth-Century America," in *The Therapeutic Revolution*, ed. Vogel and Rosenberg, 18.

5. John Harley Warner, *The Therapeutic Perspective: Medical Practice, Knowledge, and Identity in America, 1820–1885* (Cambridge, MA: Harvard University Press, 1986), 87.

6. Quoted in Paul Starr, *The Social Transformation of American Medicine* (New York: Basic, 1982), 101.

7. Chertok and de Saussure, *The Therapeutic Revolution*, xii. See also Andrew Cunningham and Perry Williams, ed., *The Laboratory Revolution in Medicine* (Cambridge: Cambridge University Press, 1992).

8. Andrew M. Fearnley reminds us that the 1920s and 1930s witnessed a retreat from European ideas among many American psychiatrists, before another shift in response to émigré intellectuals occurred in the mid-1940s and 1950s. But he also warns us not to generalize about seeing something monolithically "American" or "European" among such a great variety of thought and practice ("Methods to Madness: Race, Knowledge, and American Psychiatry, 1880–2000" [PhD diss., University of Cambridge, 2012], 11–13).

9. James H. Capshew, *Psychologists on the March: Science, Practice, and Professional Identity in America, 1929–1969* (Cambridge: Cambridge University Press, 1999).

10. See Gail A. Hornstein, "The Return of the Repressed: Psychology's Problematic Relations with Psychoanalysis, 1909–1960," *American Psychology* 47, no. 2 (1992): 254–263.

11. For a discussion of the growing membership of the American Psychiatric Association, see Melvin Sabshin, *Changing American Psychiatry: A Personal Perspective* (Washington, DC: American Psychiatric Publishing, 2008).

12. Sidney Hook, "Summary of the Symposium," in *The Health Care Issues of the 1960s* (New York: Group Health Insurance, 1963), 183.

13. Ibid., 192.

14. For debates about democratic health in mid-nineteenth-century America, see Michael E. Staub, *Madness Is Civilization: When the Diagnosis Was Social, 1948–1980* (Chicago: University of Chicago Press, 2011), 23–35. For debates in the United Kingdom, see Mathew Thomson, *Psychological Subjects: Identity, Culture, and Health in Twentieth-Century Britain* (Oxford: Oxford University Press, 2006), 209–249.

15. Philip Rieff, *The Triumph of the Therapeutic: Uses of Faith after Freud* (Chicago: University of Chicago Press, [1966] 1987).

16. Frederick S. Perls et al., *Gestalt Therapy: Excitement and Growth in the Human Personality* (London: Penguin, [1951] 1973), 14.

17. Eli Ginzberg noted that national healthcare costs had risen from $43 billion in 1950 (adjusted for inflation) to $75 billion in 1969. He considered Nixon's warning that these costs were destabilizing the economy as "premature and exaggerated" but later projected that healthcare costs would exceed $2 trillion by the year 2000 (*Medical Gridlock and Health Reform* [Boulder, CO: Westview, 1994], 4–5). Ginzberg was not far wrong in his projection: US healthcare cost $2.3 trillion (16 percent of the gross domestic product) in 2007 and the projected figures from the Centers for Medicare and Medicaid Services for 2020 are $4.6 trillion and 19.8 percent (https://www.cms.gov/Research-Statistics-Data-and-Systems/Statistics-Trends-and-Reports/NationalHealthExpendData/downloads/proj2010.pdf).

18. For a similar point, see David Pingitore, "Family Medicine: American Culture in American Medicine," *Science as Culture* 4, no. 2 (1993): 167.

19. Hugo Münsterberg, *Psychology and Industrial Efficiency* (Boston: Houghton Mifflin, 1913), 13.

20. Monique Wittig, "The Straight Mind," *Feminist Issues* 1, no. 1 (1980): 106.

21. Bert Hansen, *Picturing Medical Progress from Pasteur to Polio: A History of Mass Media Images and Popular Attitudes in America* (New Brunswick, NJ: Rutgers University Press, 2009), 10. See also John C. Burnham, "American Medicine's Golden Age: What Happened to It," *Science* 215 (19 March 1982): 1474–1479.

22. "American Life and Times 1900–1950," *Life*, 2 January 1950, 34–35; Vannevar Bush, *Science—The Endless Frontier* (Washington, DC: National Science Foundation, [1945] 1960).

23. Paul Haun, "Psychiatry and the Ancillary Services," *American Journal of Psychiatry* 107, no. 2 (1950): 102.

24. Earl Lomon Koos, *The Health of Regionville: What the People Thought and Did about It* (New York: Columbia University Press, 1954), 4.

25. See also Andrew Scull, "The Mental Health Sector and the Social Sciences in Post–World War II USA," *History of Psychiatry* 22, no. 1 (2011): 3–19, and no. 3 (2011): 268–284; Catherine Fussinger, "'Therapeutic Community,' Psychiatry's Reformers and Antipsychiatrists: Reconsidering Changes in the Field of Psychiatry after World War II," *History of Psychiatry* 22, no. 2 (2011): 146–163; José Brunner and Orna Ophir, "'In Good Times and In Bad': Boundary Relations of Psychoanalysis in Post-War USA," *History of Psychiatry* 22, no. 2 (2011): 215–231.

26. C. P. Snow, *The Two Cultures and the Scientific Revolution* (New York: Cambridge University Press, 1959).

27. See Lionel Trilling, "The Leavis-Snow Controversy," in Lionel Trilling, *Beyond Culture: Essays on Literature and Learning* (New York: Viking, 1965), 145–177.

28. Archibald MacLeish, "To Face the Real Crisis: Man Himself," *New York Times*, 25 December 1960.

29. Lewis Mumford, *The Human Way Out* (Wallingford, PA: Pendle Hill, 1958), 3; Paul Engle, "Poetry Is Ordinary Language Raised to the Nth Power," *New York Times Book Review*, 17 February 1957.

30. Jacob Bronowksi, *The Common Sense of Science* (New York: Vintage, 1951), 5.

31. Ibid.

32. Daniel Cordle, *Postmodern Postures: Literature, Science and the Two Cultures Debate* (Brookfield, VT: Ashgate, 1999), 43.

33. Paul Ricoeur, *Freud and Philosophy: An Essay on Interpretation*, trans. Denis Savage (New Haven: Yale University Press, 1970).

34. Bronowski, *The Common Sense of Science*, 11.

35. J.A.V. Butler, *Science and Human Life* (New York: Basic, 1957), 6.

36. Ibid.

37. Richard H. King, *Race, Culture, and the Intellectuals, 1940–1970* (Baltimore: Johns Hopkins University Press, 2004).

38. R. Buckminster Fuller, "The Prospects for Humanity," *Saturday Review*, 29 August 1964, 4.

39. Buckminster Fuller, untitled talk at the 15th Conference of Psychology Program Directors and Consultants in State, Federal and Territorial Mental Health Programs, Chicago, IL, 1-2 September 1965.

40. Rieff, *The Triumph of the Therapeutic*, 76–78.

41. Cordle, *Postmodern Postures*, 51.

CHAPTER 1 — GOING HOME

1. Harry S. Truman, "National Health Program," 79th Congress, 1st Session, 19 November 1945 (Washington: Government Printing Office, 1945), 1.

2. Irvin L. Child and Marjorie van de Water, eds., *Psychology for the Returning Serviceman* (New York: Penguin, 1945).

3. Alfred Schutz, *Collected Papers*, vol. 2, *Studies in Social Theory*, ed. Arvid Brodersen (The Hague: Martinus Nijhoff, 1964), 116.

4. Nolan D. C. Lewis, "What the Wars' Experiences Have Taught Us in Psychiatry," in New York Academy of Medicine, *Medicine in the Postwar World* (New York: Columbia University Press, 1948), 54–68.

5. Howard L. Holley, *A History of Medicine in Alabama* (Birmingham: University of Alabama School of Medicine, 1982), 342–343. For a broader discussion of Truman's health care proposals, see Monte M. Poen, *Harry S. Truman versus the Medical Lobby: The Genesis of Medicare* (Columbia: University of Missouri Press, 1979).

6. Robert Fyne, *The Hollywood Propaganda of World War II* (Metuchen, NJ: Scarecrow, 1994), 121.

7. Frank J. Sladen, ed., *Psychiatry and the War* (Springfield, IL: Charles C. Thomas, 1943), 296.

8. Norman Q. Brill and Gilbert W. Beebe, *A Follow-Up Study of War Neuroses* (Washington: National Research Council, 1955), 138–139.

9. David A. Gerber, "Heroes and Misfits: The Troubled Social Reintegration of Disabled Veterans in *The Best Years of Our Lives*," *American Quarterly* 46, no. 4 (1994): 545.

10. Willard Waller, *The Veteran Comes Back* (New York: Dryden, 1944), 186.

11. Ibid., 56.

12. Ibid., 186.

13. It was not until 1950 that the federal government financially supported "totally and permanently disabled" citizens (excluding those with mental disorders), and even then each state was left to determine its own definition of "totally and permanently" (Hazel Kyrk, *The Family in the American Economy* [Chicago: University of Chicago Press, 1953], 224–225).

14. Gerber, "Heroes and Misfits," 545.

15. Carl I. Hovland et al., *Experiments on Mass Communication*, vol. 3 of *Studies in Social Psychology in World War II* (Princeton: Princeton University Press, 1949), 15.

16. Dana B. Polan, "Blind Insights and Dark Passages: The Problem of Placement in Forties Film," *Velvet Light Trap* 20 (Summer 1983): 28.

17. John Huston, *An Open Book* (New York: Knopf, 1980), 125.

18. The War Department argued that the censorship of *Let There Be Light* was to protect the confidentiality of the patients and in 1947 endorsed a fictional remake of the film, titled *Shades of Grey*. See Gary Edgerton, "Revisiting the Recordings of Wars Past: Remembering the Documentary Trilogy of John Huston," in *Reflections in a Male Eye: John Huston and the American Experience*, ed. Gaylyn Studlar and David Desser (Washington: Smithsonian Institution Press, 1993), 51–57; C. A. Morgan III, "From *Let There Be Light* to *Shades of Grey*: The Construction of Authoritative Knowledge about Combat Fatigue (1945–48)," in *Signs of Life: Medicine and Cinema*, ed. Graeme Harper and Andrew Moor (London: Wallflower, 2005), 132–152.

19. See George H. Roeder Jr., *The Censored War: American Visual Experience during World War II* (New Haven: Yale University Press, 1993), 13–14.

20. Peter Roffman and Jim Purdy, *The Hollywood Social Problem Film: Madness, Despair and Politics from the Depression to the Fifties* (Bloomington: Indiana University Press, 1981), 228.

21. Bernard F. Dick, *The Star-Spangled Screen: The American World War II Film*, rev. ed. (Lexington: University Press of Kentucky, 1996), 213.

22. William Menninger, *Psychiatry in a Troubled World* (New York: Macmillan, 1948), 558.

23. Nathan G. Hale Jr., *The Rise and Crisis of Psychoanalysis in the United States: Freud and the Americans, 1917–1985* (New York: Oxford University Press, 1995), 13. See also Millais Culpin, *Psychoneuroses of War and Peace* (Cambridge: Cambridge University Press, 1920), 1.

24. Eva Moskowitz, *In Therapy We Trust* (Baltimore: Johns Hopkins University Press, 2001), 131–148. See also Ellen Herman, *The Romance of American Psychology: Political Culture in the Age of Experts*, paperback ed. (Berkeley: University of California Press, 1996), 82–123.

25. Menninger, *Psychiatry in a Troubled World*, 7. The Menninger Clinic ran seminars in June 1941 on the relationship between psychiatry and national defense, dealing with the selective service draft; detecting "psychoneurotic," "psychopathic," and "feebleminded" recruits; and the importance of psychiatry for civilians during times of war. See *Bulletin of the Menninger Clinic* 5, no. 5 (1941).

26. Leonard D. Heaton, ed., *Neuropsychiatry in World War II* (Washington: Department of the Army, 1966), 1:20–22; Albert Deutsch, "Military Psychiatry: World War II, 1941–1943," in *One Hundred Years of American Psychiatry*, ed. J. K. Hall et al. (New York: Columbia University Press, 1944), 423–424.

27. Albert E. Cowdrey, *Fighting for Life: American Military Medicine in World War II* (New York: Free Press, 1994), 25.

28. *The History of the Medical Department of the United States Navy in World War II* (Washington: Government Printing Office, 1953), 1:v.

29. These conditions are outlined among 1,200 cases in Roy Grinker and John Spiegel, *War Neuroses* (Philadelphia: Blakiston, 1945), 78–105.

30. This figure of 40–50 percent of all war veterans suffering from combat exhaustion is debatable. The later film *Let There Be Light*, for example, estimated the figure at 20 percent.

31. Quoted in Cowdrey, *Fighting for Life*, 137–138.

32. Hale, *The Rise and Crisis of Psychoanalysis in the United States*, 189. Hale notes that not only was this psychiatrist, Martin Berezin, unable to deal with all the psychiatric casualties at Guadalcanal, but the commanding general also ordered these soldiers to be court-martialed as a disgrace to the outfit.

33. Sladen, *Psychiatry and the War*, 277.

34. Ibid., 240.

35. Ibid., 246.

36. Ibid., 254.

37. Ibid., 251.

38. Ibid., 275.

39. See Douglass W. Orr, "Objectives of the Selective Service Psychiatric Classification," *Bulletin of the Menninger Clinic* 5, no. 5 (1941): 131–133.

40. Heaton, *Neuropsychiatry in World War II*, 1:xiii.

41. Established in 1938, the William Alanson White Psychiatric Foundation was the first organization to promote the use of psychiatry in the armed forces.

42. Deutsch, "Military Psychiatry," 426. Heaton, *Neuropsychiatry in World War II*, 1:166.

43. Heaton, Neuropsychiatry in World War II, 230.

44. See Paul Fussell, *Wartime: Understanding and Behavior in the Second World War* (Oxford: Oxford University Press, 1989), 152.

45. Sladen, *Psychiatry and the War*, 337.

46. See Willard Waller, *The Veteran Comes Back* (New York: Dryden, 1944); Charles Bolté, *The New Veteran* (New York: Reynal and Hitchcock, 1945).

47. "Federal Aid Urged for War-Blinded," *New York Times*, 10 September 1942.

48. Waller, *The Veteran Comes Back*, 259.

49. Ibid., 305.

50. Howard A. Rusk, "Rehabilitation," *New York Times*, 29 September 1946.

51. "Veterans Get Jolt on Business Hopes," *New York Times*, 29 April 1945.

52. Quoted in "Wants Film Shown Free," *New York Times*, 3 September 1945.

53. Truman, "National Health Program," 11.

54. Eric Wittkower, "The War-Disabled: Their Emotional, Social, and Occupational Situation," *British Medical Journal* (28 April 1945): 587–90.

55. Bosley Crowther, "Clarity through Films," *New York Times*, 15 April 1945.

56. David A. Gerber, "Introduction: Finding Disabled Veterans in History," in *Disabled Veterans in History*, ed. David A. Gerber (Ann Arbor: University of Michigan Press, 2000), 2.

57. Kaja Silverman, *Male Subjectivity at the Margins* (New York: Routledge, 1992), 53.

58. Bosley Crowther, "Films about Marines," *New York Times*, 2 September 1945.

59. MacKinlay Kantor, *Glory for Me* (New York: Coward-McCann, 1945). Kantor is little remembered today, and Paul Fussell criticizes him alongside other popular wartime American writers for their "laying aside of all normal standards of art and intellect" (*Wartime*, 175).

60. Kantor, *Glory for Me*, 3.

61. Ibid., 13.

62. Ibid., 17.

63. Gerber, "Heroes and Misfits," 556.

64. Quoted in Heaton, *Neuropsychiatry in World War II*, 1:231.

65. Silverman, *Male Subjectivity at the Margins*, 86.

66. The infantilization of Homer in this scene was obviously contrived. William Wyler, the director, commented in 1947 on the "delicate problems of bringing a boy and a girl to a bedroom at night, with the boy getting into his pajama top, revealing his leather harness . . . and taking the harness off. . . . We solved the problems without the slightest suggestion of indelicacy, and without presenting Homer's hooks in a shocking or horrifying manner" (quoted in Jan Herman, *A Talent for Trouble: The Life of Hollywood's Most Acclaimed Director, William Wyler* [New York: Putnam, 1995], 284).

67. A postwar study on amputation noted that occupational therapy for bilateral amputees is one of the trickiest challenges for the health profession and that the "therapist's ability to help is in direct relation to the patient's courage and intelligence" (Phyllis Lyttleton, *Occupational Therapy for the Limbless* [London: H. K. Lewis, 1946], 11).

68. Douglas Noble et al., "Psychiatric Disturbances Following Amputation," *American Journal of Psychiatry* 110, no. 8 (1954): 613.

69. Gerber, "Heroes and Misfits: The Troubled Social Reintegration of Disabled Veterans in *The Best Years of Our Lives*," in *Disabled Veterans in History*, ed. Gerber, 85–86.

70. Silverman, *Male Subjectivity at the Margins*, 86.

71. Hale, *The Rise and Crisis of Psychoanalysis in the United States*, 193.

72. *War Blinded Veterans in a Postwar Society: A Social Work Follow Up of Rehabilitations Measures for Blinded Veterans with Service-Connected Disabilities* (Washington: Veterans Administration, 1953), n. p.

73. Robert Bridges, "To the United States of America," in *A Treasury of War Poetry*, ed. George Herbert Clarke (Boston: Houghton Mifflin, 1917), 3. Sargent's painting *Gassed* was discussed by Virginia Woolf in the 1920s and more recently by Santanu Das in *Touch and Intimacy in First World War Literature* (Cambridge: Cambridge University Press, 2006).

74. Culpin, *Psychoneuroses of War and Peace*, 4.

75. Ibid., 47.

76. Frances A. Koestler, *The Unseen Minority: A Social History of Blindness in the United States* (New York: D. McKay, 1976), 261.

77. Herbert C. Yahraes, *What Do You Know about Blindness?* (New York: Public Affairs Committee, 1947), 2.

78. Ibid., 17–18.

79. *The History of the Medical Department of the United States Navy in World War II*, 1:249.

80. Ibid., 1:362. See also Walter R. Miles and Detlev W. Bronk, "Visual Problems," in *Advances in Military Medicine*, ed. E. C. Andrus et al. (Boston: Little, Brown, 1948), 1:261–277.

81. Polan, "Blind Insights and Dark Passages."

82. Roger Butterfield, *Al Schmid, Marine* (New York: Norton, 1944), 13.

83. Ibid., 20.

84. Ibid., 103.

85. Ibid., 107.

86. Ibid., 47.

87. Albert A. Rosner, "Neuropsychiatric Casualties from Guadalcanal," *American Journal of Medical Science* 207 (June 1944): 770.

88. Polan, "Blind Insights and Dark Passages," 29.

89. Sladen, *Psychiatry and the War*, 285. At a Minneapolis conference in 1947, the Committee on Psychiatric Social Work called for more social workers in psychiatric hospitals. The committee believed that only with a significant improvement in the current ratio of one trained psychiatric social worker to a hundred hospital admissions could patient care be improved and the average length of stay reduced (*Bulletin of the Menninger Clinic* 11, no. 6 [1947]: 188–197).

90. Dick notes that Maltz asked that in *Pride of the Marines* "an American Indian and a Jew be in the bunker with Schmid when the grenade explodes because it would 'show America in its best sense and . . . answer the wolfish malice by which some people scorn each other on a racist basis'" (Dick, *The Star-Spangled Screen*, 222).

91. Just as *Pride of the Marines* involved an important World War II battle, so *Lights Out* and *Bright Victory* focus initially on the North Africa campaign, during which significant numbers of psychiatric casualties were sent to US base hospitals suffering from combat exhaustion. Many of the men were returned to combat within forty-eight hours. For a fuller discussion of North African casualties, see Edgar Jones and Simon Wessely, *Shell Shock to PTSD: Military Psychiatry from 1900 to the Gulf War* (Hove, Sussex: Psychology, 2005), 86–88.

92. Koestler, *The Unseen Minority*, 261.

93. Baynard Kendrick, *Bright Victory* (New York: Bantam, 1951), 8.

94. Ibid., 3.

95. Louis Cholden, "Some Psychiatric Problems in the Rehabilitation of the Blind," *Bulletin of the Menninger Clinic* 18, no. 3 (1954): 107.

96. Yahraes, *What Do You Know about Blindness?*, 29.

CHAPTER 2 — IN THE NOIR MIRROR

1. Quoted in Brian Neve, *Film and Politics in America: A Social Tradition* (London: Routledge, 1992), 112–113.

2. Quoted in "The Pursuit of Happiness," *Life*, 12 July 1948, 102.

3. Jonathan Shay, *Achilles in Vietnam: Combat Trauma and the Undoing of Character* (New York: Touchstone, 1994), 4.

4. Sheri Chinen Biesen, *Blackout: World War II and the Origins of Film Noir* (Baltimore: Johns Hopkins University Press, 2005), 59–95.

5. Ray Pratt, *Projecting Paranoia: Conspiratorial Visions in American Film* (Lawrence: University Press of Kansas, 2001), 48.

6. Despite its French name, the noir sensibility arguably appeared in the United States before it did in Europe. It did not emerge in Paris until 1946, when Boris Vian's published translations of two racially charged American novels—Richard Wright's *Native Son* and William Faulkner's *Sanctuary*—led to the emergence of the *série noire* (James Naremore, *More Than Night: Film Noir in its Contexts*, rev. ed. [Berkeley: University of California Press, 2008], 12).

7. Irvin L. Child and Marjorie van de Water, eds., *Psychology for the Returning Serviceman* (New York: Penguin, 1945), 127.

8. See S. Kirson Weinberg, "The Combat Neuroses," *American Journal of Sociology* 51, no. 5 (1946): 465–471.

9. William Menninger, *Psychiatry in a Troubled World* (New York: Macmillan, 1948), 20.

10. Roy R. Grinker and John P. Spiegel, *Men under Stress* (Philadelphia: Blakiston, 1945); Eli Ginzberg, *Breakdown and Recovery* (New York: Columbia University Press, 1959). Research on aggression in Canada and England was also underway in the late 1940s. See Peter McKellar, "The Emotion of Anger in the Expression of Human Aggressiveness," *British Journal of Psychology* 39, no. 3 (1949): 148–155.

11. Ginzberg, *Breakdown and Recovery*, xiii. For an outline of the Conservation of Human Resources Project, see Eli Ginzberg, *Human Resources: The Wealth of a Nation* (New York: Simon and Schuster, 1958).

12. Ginzberg, *Breakdown and Recovery*, 269.

13. Ibid., 275.

14. "The Neuropsychiatric Program," *Journal of the American Medical Association* 130, no. 1 (1946): 36.

15. Albert Deutsch, *The Shame of the States* (New York: Harcourt Brace, 1948).

16. James Dawson, *Aggression and Population* (London: Rockliff, 1946), 10.

17. Ibid., 15.

18. Alix Strachey, *The Unconscious Motives of War: A Psycho-Analytical Contribution* (London: Allen and Unwin, 1957), 21.

19. Dawson, *Aggression and Population*, 54.

20. Vannevar Bush, *Science—The Endless Frontier* (Washington: National Science Foundation, [1945] 1960). The claims about science are from Raymond Fosdick, president of the Rockefeller Foundation, cited in Gregg Mitman, "Dominance, Leadership, and Aggression: Animal Behavior Studies during the Second World War," *Journal of the History of the Behavioral Sciences* 26, no. 1 (1990): 5.

21. Dawson, *Aggression and Population*, 71.

22. J. D. Salinger, "A Perfect Day for Bananafish," *New Yorker*, 31 January 1948, 21–25.

23. John Dollard et al., *Frustration and Aggression* (New Haven: Yale University Press, 1939), 10.

24. Salinger, "A Perfect Day for Bananafish," 25.

25. Robert P. Knight, "The Successful Treatment of a Case of Chronic 'War Neurosis' by the Psychoanalytic Method," *Bulletin of the Menninger Clinic* 6, no. 5 (1942): 153.

26. Karen Horney, *The Neurotic Personality of Our Time* (London: Kegan Paul, Trench, Trubner, [1937] 1947), 39; and Karen Horney, *Neurosis and Human Growth: The Struggle Toward Self-Realization* (New York: Norton, [1950] 1991), 206.

27. Robert Eisler, *Man into Wolf: An Anthropological Interpretation of Sadism, Masochism and Lycanthropy* (New York: Greenwood, [1948] 1969), 51.

28. See Mitman, "Dominance, Leadership, and Aggression," 5.

29. Karen DeMeester, "Trauma and Recovery in Modern Post-War Fiction," PhD diss., Florida State University at Tallahassee, 2000, 17.

30. Frederick M. Allen, "Shock and Refrigeration," *Journal of the American Medical Association* 130, no. 4 (1946): 188–189.

31. Sigmund Freud, "Thoughts for the Times on War and Death," in *The Standard Edition of the Complete Psychological Works of Sigmund Freud*, trans. and ed. James Strachey (London: Hogarth, 1981), 14:279.

32. Shay, *Achilles in Vietnam*, 193.

33. Sigmund Freud, "Our Attitude Towards Death," in The *Standard Edition of the Complete Psychological Works of Sigmund Freud*, 14:289.

34. Karl A. Menninger, *Man against Himself* (London: Harvest, 1938), 408. See also Anthony Sampson, "Freud on the State, Violence, and War," *Diacritics* 35, no. 3 (2005): 90.

35. *Medicine in the Postwar World* (New York: Columbia University Press, 1948), 67–68.

36. Many critics—including Freudians such as Franz Alexander, the director of the Chicago Institute of Psychoanalysis in 1932—worried about the "mythological" nature of Freud's dual instinct theory, which fluctuates between constructive and destructive forces. See Franz Alexander, review of *A New Series of Introductory Lectures on Psychoanalysis* by Sigmund Freud, *Psychoanalytic Review* 21, no. 3 (1934): 340.

37. Gregory Zilboorg, *Mind, Medicine and Man* (New York: Harcourt, Brace, 1943), 229.

38. Ibid., 233.

39. Dollard et al., *Frustration and Aggression*, 47.

40. Philip Wylie, "Winter Novels," *New York Times*, 30 January 1944.

41. The National Committee for Education on Alcoholism, formed in October 1944, claimed that there were six million excessive drinkers nationally and another 600,000 alcoholics.

42. John W. Crowley, *The White Logic: Alcoholism and Gender in American Modernist Fiction* (Amherst: University of Massachusetts Press, 1994), 150.

43. "The Motion Picture Production Code of 1930," www.artsreformation.com/a001/hays-code.html.

44. By 1950 drug treatment for chronic alcoholism in Scandinavia, including the use of the drug Antabuse, was showing success in helping patients abstain from drinking for long periods. See S. Eugene Barrera et al., "The Use of Antabuse in Chronic Alcoholics," *American Journal of Psychiatry* 107, no. 1 (1950): 8–13.

45. Wylie, "Winter Novels."

46. Jacqueline Foertsch, *American Culture in the 1940s* (Edinburgh: Edinburgh University Press, 2008), 129; Erin Redfern, "The Neurosis of Narrative: American Literature and Psychoanalytic Psychiatry during World War II," PhD diss., Northwestern University, 2003, 76–77. For a comparison of the depiction of alcoholism in *The Lost Weekend* and the 1958 television and 1962 film productions of *The Days of Wine and Roses*, see Glen O. Gabbard and Krin Gabbard, *Psychiatry and the Cinema*, 2nd ed. (New York: American Psychiatric Press, 1999), 104–105.

47. Robert P. Knight, "The Dynamics and Treatment of Chronic Alcohol Addiction," *Bulletin of the Menninger Clinic* 1, no. 7 (1937): 233–250. Techniques such as hypnotherapy began to be used to treat alcoholism in the late 1930s, but they had mixed results. See Aaron Paley, "Hypnotherapy in the Treatment of Alcoholism," *Bulletin of the Menninger Clinic* 16, no. 1 (1952): 14–20.

48. G. M. Scott, "Alcoholism and Criminal Behaviour," in *Mental Abnormality and Crime*, ed. L. Radzinowicz and J.W.C. Turner (London: Macmillan, 1944), 163–176.

49. Tom Dardis, *The Thirsty Muse: Alcohol and the American Writer* (New York: Ticknor and Fields, 1989); John W. Crowley, *The White Logic: Alcoholism and Gender in American Modernist Fiction* (Amherst: University of Massachusetts Press, 1994). One psychiatrist noted that "of the seven Americans who were awarded the Nobel Prize for literature" before 1970, four "were alcoholics and a fifth drank heavily" (Donald W. Goodwin, "The Alcoholism of F. Scott Fitzgerald," *Journal of the American Studies Association* 212, no. 1 [1970]: 86).

50. Robert V. Seliger and Victoria Cranford, "Psychiatric Orientation of the Alcoholic Criminal," *Journal of the American Medical Association* 129, no. 6 (1945): 424.

51. Ibid.

52. Ibid. In the early 1950s the Department of Psychiatry at Cornell University ran a number of scientific experiments on chronic alcoholics to examine the relationship between bodily responses and anxiety. See M. Friele Fleetwood and Oskar Diethelm, "Emotions and Biochemical Findings in Alcoholism," *American Journal of Psychiatry* 108, no. 6 (1951): 433–437.

53. Jean-Paul Sartre, *Being and Nothingness: An Essay on Phenomenological Ontology*, trans. Hazel E. Barnes, 2nd ed. (London: Routledge, [1943] 2003), 386–400.

54. Edward J. Kempf, *Psychopathology* (St. Louis: C. V. Mosby, 1920).

55. Paul Fussell, *Wartime: Understanding and Behavior in the Second World War* (Oxford: Oxford University Press, 1989), 273.

56. Ibid., 274.

57. See Andrew Spicer, *Film Noir* (London: Longman, 2002), table 2.1.

58. Bosley Crowther, "Rough Stuff," *New York Times*, 12 May 1946.

59. David Spiegel, "War, Peace and Posttraumatic Stress Disorder," in *American Psychiatry after World War II, 1944–1994*, ed. Roy W. Menninger and John C. Nemiah (Washington: American Psychiatric Press, 2000), 37.

60. For an interesting discussion of visuality in *Murder, My Sweet*, see J. P. Telotte, *Voices in the Dark: The Narrative Patterns of Film Noir* (Urbana: University of Illinois Press, 1989), 88–102.

61. Theodor Adorno, *Minima Moralia*, trans. E. F. N. Jephcott (London: Verso, [1951] 1984), 40.

62. Vincent J. Daly, *Understanding Mental Illness: A Patient's Manual for Group Therapy* (Whitfield: Mississippi State Hospital, 1950), 24.

63. Child and van de Water, *Psychology for the Returning Serviceman*, 187.

64. Edward Dimendberg, *Film Noir and the Spaces of Modernity* (Cambridge: Harvard University Press, 2004), 4.

65. Ibid., 18.

66. Maurice Merleau-Ponty, *The Phenomenology of Perception*, trans. Donald A. Landes (New York: Routledge, [1945] 2012).

67. Erich Fromm, *Escape from Freedom* (New York: Henry Holt, [1941] 1994), 178.

68. Ibid., 182.

69. The major intellectual biography of Fromm is Lawrence J. Friedman, *The Lives of Erich Fromm: Love's Prophet* (New York: Columbia University Press, 2013).

70. "Psychological Medicine," *Bulletin of War Medicine* 6, no. 1 (1945): 42.

71. Ibid., 43.

72. Ibid., 46.

73. Jonathan Freedman, "Alfred Hitchcock and Therapeutic Culture in America," in *Hitchcock's America*, ed. Jonathan Freedman and Richard Millington (New York: Oxford University Press, 1999), 87.

74. Pratt, *Projecting Paranoia*, 57.

75. Ibid..

76. Letter from Joseph Mankiewicz to Karl Menninger, 13 July 1944, in *The Selected Correspondence of Karl A. Menninger, 1919–1945*, ed. Howard J. Faulkner and Virginia D. Pruitt (New Haven: Yale University Press, 1988), 402.

77. Quoted in Pratt, *Projecting Paranoia*, 81.

78. A 1946 article by a criminal psychopathology expert at Columbia University, attacked the deceitful masks worn by postwar women that make them "a product of deception and disguise" (Ralph S. Banay, "The Trouble with Women," *Collier's*, 7 December 1946, 74).

79. Quoted in Crowley, *The White Logic*, 149.

80. Mankiewicz to Menninger, The *Selected Correspondence of Karl A. Menninger*, 402.

81. Letter from Karl Menninger to David O. Selznick, 7 August 1944, *The Selected Correspondence of Karl A. Menninger,* 404.

82. Freedman, "Alfred Hitchcock and Therapeutic Culture," 83–84.

83. Mankiewicz to Menninger, 13 July 1944, *The Selected Correspondence of Karl A. Menninger,* 402.

84. Freedman, "Alfred Hitchcock and Therapeutic Culture," 80.

85. Ibid., 79.

86. Selznick quoted these lines in his letter to Menninger, 22 September 1944, *The Selected Correspondence of Karl A. Menninger,* 406.

87. The importance of doors in *Spellbound* is emphasized by the planned trailer for the film (on which May Romm consulted), in which Hitchcock would claim that the film "deals with methods by which the individual is forced to open these closed doors . . . all of them" in the face of murder and intrigue (quoted in Dan Aulier, *Hitchcock's Secret Notebooks* [London: Bloomsbury, 1999], 558).

88. Karl Menninger, *Man against Himself,* 412.

89. Ralph S. Banay, "Psychopath or Sociopath," in *The Encyclopedia of Mental Health,* ed. Albert Deutsch (New York: Franklin Watts, 1963), 5:1640.

90. Ibid., 5:1640–1641.

91. Ibid., 5:1641–1642.

92. Bosley Crowther, "Straight to the Point," *New York Times,* 27 July 1947.

93. Adrian Scott, "Some of My Worse Friends," *Screen Writer,* October 1947, 4.

94. David Abrahamsen, *Crime and the Human Mind* (London: Chapman and Hall, 1944), vii.

95. Benjamin Karpman, *Case Studies in the Psychopathology of Crime* (Washington: Medical Science, 1948), 3:xxix.

96. Daniel E. Schneider, *The Psychoanalyst and the Artist* (New York: Mentor, 1950), 64. For a discussion on the policing of homosexuality, see Jennifer Terry, *An American Obsession: Science, Medicine, and Homosexuality in Modern Society* (Chicago: University of Chicago Press, 1999), 271.

97. Hervey M. Cleckley, *The Mask of Sanity* (New York: New American Library, [1941] 1982), 226. See also Hervey M. Cleckley, "The Psychopath Viewed Practically," in *The Handbook of Correctional Psychology,* ed. Robert M. Lindner and Robert V. Seliger (New York: Philosophical Library, 1947), 395–412. For an overview of the postwar typology of psychopathology, see Matthew Howard et al., "Promises and Perils of a Psychopathology of Crime: The Troubling Case of Juvenile Delinquency," *Journal of Law and Policy* 14 (2004): 441–483.

98. In the third edition of *The Mask of Sanity* (1955), Cleckley revised his original nomenclature, using "sociopathic" personality, even though (as he noted in 1964) the "older informal term *psychopath* persists" (Hervey M. Cleckley, *The Mask of Sanity* [St. Louis: C. B. Mosby, (1941) 1964], 8).

99. Gregory Zilboorg, *Sigmund Freud: His Exploration of the Mind of Man* (New York: Scribner's, 1951), 8.

100. Walter Bromberg, "The Treatability of the Psychopath," *American Journal of Psychiatry* 110, no. 8 (1954): 608. See also Janet Colaizzi, *Homicidal Insanity, 1800–1985* (Tuscaloosa: University of Alabama Press, 1989), 109.

101. Banay, "Psychopath or Sociopath," in *The Encyclopedia of Mental Health*, ed. Deutsch, 5:1634.

102. Ibid.

103. See Richard Noll, *American Madness: The Rise and Fall of Dementia Praecox* (Cambridge: Harvard University Press, 2011), 243–244; Kempf, *Psychopathology*, 477–515. See also Benjamin Karpman, "Mediate Psychotherapy and the Acute Homosexual Panic (Kempf's Disease)," *Journal of Nervous and Mental Disease* 98, no. 5 (1941): 493–506. For a perceptive reading of this subject, see Matthew T. Helmers, "Homosexual Panic: Unlivable Lives and the Temporality of Sexuality in Literature, Psychiatry and the Law," PhD diss., University of Manchester, 2011, 121–135.

104. For Walker's treatment in Topeka, see Beverly Linet, *Star Crossed: The Story of Robert Walker and Jennifer Jones* (New York: Putnam's, 1986), 229–238.

105. See Michele Morales, "Persistent Pathologies: The Odd Coupling of Alcoholism and Homosexuality in the Discourses of Twentieth Century Science," PhD diss., University of Michigan, 2006, 63–108.

106. David Sievers, *Freud on Broadway: A History of Psychoanalysis and the American Drama* (New York: Hermitage House, 1955), 400–437.

107. H. Warren Dunham, *Sociological Theory and Mental Disorder* (Detroit: Wayne State University Press, 1959), 209–238.

CHAPTER 3 — GROUND ZERO

1. Tom Engelhardt, *The End of Victory Culture: Cold War America and the Disillusioning of a Generation*, rev. ed. (Amherst: University of Massachusetts Press, 2007), 9.

2. For a discussion of civil defense, see Tracy C. Davis, *Stages of Emergency: Cold War Nuclear Civil Defense* (Durham, NC: Duke University Press, 2007).

3. "Film on Atom War Bad for Children," *New York Times*, 21 November 1952. For further discussion of the committee, see Daniel Cordle, *States of Suspense: The Nuclear Age, Postmodernism and United States Fiction and Prose* (Manchester, UK: Manchester University Press, 2008), 48–49.

4. Georgina Feldberg, et al., "Comparative Perspectives on Canadian and American Women's Health Care since 1945," in *Women, Health, and Nation: Canada and the United States since 1945*, ed. Georgina Feldberg et al. (Montreal: McGill-Queen's University Press, 2003), 22. See Herbert Block, *The Herblock Book* (Boston: Beacon, 1952), 112–113.

5. One of the best studies on this subject is Ron Robin, *The Making of the Cold War Enemy: Culture and Politics in the Military-Industrial Complex* (Princeton: Princeton University Press, 2003).

6. Dwight Eisenhower, "Atoms for Peace," 8 December 1953, www.eisenhower.archives
.gov/all_about_ike/speeches/atoms_for_peace.pdf.

7. Ellen Leopold, *Under the Radar: Cancer and the Cold War* (New Brunswick, NJ: Rutgers University Press, 2009), 18–29. For a discussion of the transformation of the military-
industrial complex into the "medical-industrial complex," see Arnold S. Relman, "The New
Medical-Industrial Complex," *New England Journal of Medicine* 303, no. 17 (1980): 963–970. And
for a broader discussion of psychology between 1945 and the early 1960s, see Ellen Herman,
The Romance of American Psychology: Political Culture in the Age of Experts (University of California Press, 1996), 124–162.

8. Bryant Wedge, "The Anticommunist Complex," *American Journal of Psychotherapy* 24,
no. 4 (1970): 561.

9. Paul Starr, *The Social Transformation of American Medicine* (New York: Basic, 1982), 284.

10. Quoted in Monte M. Poen, *Harry S. Truman versus the Medical Lobby: The Genesis of
Medicare* (Columbia: University of Missouri Press, 1979), 130. See also J. Edgar Hoover, *Masters of Deceit* (New York: Henry Holt, 1958), 168.

11. Harold D. Lasswell, *Psychopathology and Politics* (Chicago: University of Chicago Press,
1930), 240–267; Edward Glover, *War, Sadism, and Pacifism* (London: Allen and Unwin, [1933] 1947).

12. Gregory Zilboorg, "Out of Fear and Anguish," *New York Times*, 6 May 1951.

13. Leo Bartemeier et al., "Psychiatric Aspects of the Prevention of Nuclear War," in
Psychiatry and Public Affairs: Group for the Advancement of Psychiatry, ed. Leo H. Bartemeier
(Chicago: Aldane, 1966), 377–378.

14. Ibid., 397.

15. Ibid., 394–396.

16. Erich Fromm, *Escape from Freedom* (New York: Henry Holt, [1941] 1994), 239–255.

17. See Poen, *Harry S. Truman versus the Medical Lobby*, 137, 174–209.

18. Albert Deutsch, *The Shame of the States* (New York: Harcourt, Brace, 1948), 166.

19. Eileen Welsome, *The Plutonium Files: America's Secret Experiments in the Cold War*
(New York: Random House, 1999). For burn research, see Susan E. Lederer, "Darkened by
the Shadow of the Atom: Burn Research in 1950s America," in *Man, Medicine, and the State:
The Human Body as an Object of Government Sponsored Medical Research in the 20th Century*, ed.
Wolfgang U. Eckart (Stuttgart: Steiner, 2006), 263–278.

20. Oliver Cope, "The Burn Problem," in *Advances in Military Medicine*, ed. E. C. Andrus
et al. (Boston: Little, Brown, 1948), 1:149–158.

21. See Leonard H. Glantz, "The Influence of the Nuremberg Code on U.S. Statutes and
Regulations," in *The Nazi Doctors and the Nuremberg Code: Human Rights in Human Experimentation*,
ed. George J. Annas and Michael A. Grodin (New York: Oxford University Press, 1992), 183–200.

22. Lederer, "Darkened by the Shadow of the Atom," 273. Lederer points out that the
RKO film *Experiment Alcatraz* (1950) emphasized the voluntary nature of the radiation experiments that were carried out on prisoners in return for their freedom.

23. George J. Annas, "The Nuremberg Code in U.S. Courts: Ethics versus Expediency," in *The Nazi Doctors and the Nuremberg Code*, ed. Annas and Grodin, 204. As Lederer notes, Hollywood representations of experiments on human subjects were rare after World War II, following a number of such representations in the 1930s that medical societies objected to. See Susan E. Lederer, "Hollywood and Human Experimentation: Representing Research in Popular Film," in *Medicine's Moving Pictures: Medicine, Health, and Bodies in American Film and Television*, ed. Leslie J. Regan et al. (Rochester, NY: Rochester University Press, 2007), 282–306.

24. John C. Flanagan, "Psychology in the World Emergency," in *Psychology in the World Emergency*, ed. John C. Flanagan et al. (Pittsburgh: University of Pittsburgh Press, 1952), 5.

25. See Jonathan D. Moreno, "'The Only Feasible Means': The Pentagon's Ambivalent Relationship with the Nuremberg Code," *Hastings Center Report* 26, no. 5 (1996): 11. See also Jonathan Moreno, *Undue Risk: Secret State Experiments on Humans* (New York: Routledge, 2001), 53–86.

26. Flanagan, "Psychology in the World Emergency," 14.

27. Sidney Shalett Washington, "Mammoth Cave, Washington, D.C.," *New York Times*, 27 June 1943.

28. George F. Kennan, "The Sources of Soviet Conduct," *Foreign Affairs*, July 1947, 566–582; Walter Lippmann, *The Cold War: A Study of U.S. Foreign Policy* (New York: Harper, [1947] 1972).

29. Lori Lyn Bogle, *The Pentagon's Battle for the American Mind: The Early Cold War* (College Station: Texas A&M University Press, 2004), 94.

30. See Michael Nelson, *War of the Black Heavens: The Battles of Western Broadcasting in the Cold War* (Syracuse, NY: Syracuse University Press, 1997).

31. Robert T. Holt and Robert W. van de Velde, *Strategic Psychological Operations and American Foreign Policy* (Chicago: University of Chicago Press, 1960), v.

32. Cited in Christopher Simpson, *Science of Coercion: Communication Research and Psychological Warfare, 1945–1960* (New York: Oxford University Press, 1994), 12. See also Murray Dyer, *The Weapon on the Wall: Rethinking Psychological Warfare* (Baltimore: Johns Hopkins University Press, 1959).

33. Simpson, *Science of Coercion*, 13.

34. Carol Rutz, *A Nation Betrayed: Secret Cold War Experiments Performed on Our Children and Other Innocent People* (Grass Lake, MI: Fidelity, 2001), xiii–xv; Gerald Kutcher, "Cancer Therapy and Military Cold-War Research: Crossing Epistemological and Ethical Boundaries," *History Workshop Journal* 56, no. 1 (2003): 105–130; Gerald Kutcher, *Contested Medicine: Cancer Research and the Military* (Chicago: University of Chicago Press, 2009); Gretchen Krueger, *Hope and Suffering: Children, Cancer and the Paradox of Experimental Medicine* (Baltimore: Johns Hopkins University Press, 2008).

35. Nuclear experimentation was conducted widely in the 1950s. This included work at the Chemical Defence Experimental Station at Porton Down, in Dorset, England, in which

volunteers were exposed to nerve gas in the name of strengthening national defense; many subjects suffered long-term health problems but received no reparation. See Robert Bud and Philip Gummett, eds, *Cold War, Hot Science: Applied Research in Britain's Defence Laboratories, 1945–1990* (London: Routledge, 1999), 297–298; Kevin Brown, *Fighting Fit: Health, Medicine and War in the Twentieth Century* (Stroud, Gloucestershire: History, 2008), 194.

36. See Moreno, "'The Only Feasible Means.'"

37. Lewis Mumford, *The Pentagon of Power* (New York: Harcourt Brace Jovanovich, 1970), 268.

38. Ibid., 294.

39. Norman Mailer, *Armies of the Night* (New York: Plume, [1968] 1994), 135, 125.

40. New York Academy of Medicine, *Medicine in the Postwar World* (New York: Columbia University Press, 1948), v.

41. Arthur K. Solomon, "The Atom in Medicine," in *Medicine in the Postwar World*, 26–27.

42. Ibid., 33, 36.

43. "To Our Readers," *New Yorker*, 31 August 1946, 15.

44. John Hersey, "A Reporter at Large: Hiroshima," *New Yorker*, 31 August 1946, 17–18.

45. Quoted in Francis V. O'Connor, *Jackson Pollock* (New York: Museum of Modern Art, 1967), 79.

46. Paul Boyer, *By the Bomb's Early Light: American Thought and Culture at the Dawn of the Atomic Age,* with a new preface (Chapel Hill: University of North Carolina Press, 1994), 208.

47. Diana Preston, *Before the Fallout: From Marie Curie to Hiroshima* (New York: Walker, 2005), 5.

48. Adolph Gottlieb and Mark Rothko, "Radio Script, 'The Portrait and the Modern Artist,' 1943", in *Abstract Expressionism: Creators and Critics: An Anthology*, ed. Clifford Ross (New York: Harry N. Abrams, 1990), 212.

49. Boyer, *By the Bomb's Early Light*, 65.

50. Quoted in Preston, *Before the Fallout*, 312.

51. Boyer, *By the Bomb's Early Light*, 205.

52. *The Effect of Bombing on Health and Medical Care in Germany* (Washington: War Department, 30 October 1945), 1.

53. *The Atomic Bomb Casualty Commission, 1947–1975: A General Report on the ABBC-JNIH Joint Research Program* (Hiroshima: Atomic Bomb Casualty Commission, 1978), 17.

54. National Research Council, "Genetic Effects of the Atomic Bombs in Hiroshima and Nagasaki," *Science* 106, no. 2754 (1947): 331, reprinted in James V. Neel and William J. Schull, *The Children of Atomic Bomb Survivors: A Genetic Study* (Washington: National Academy Press, 1991), 9. See also Ernest J. Sternglass, *Secret Fallout: Low-Level Radiation from Hiroshima to Three-Mile Island*, paperback ed. (New York: McGraw Hill, 1981), 47–53.

55. James V. Neel et al., "The Children of Parents Exposed to Atomic Bombs: Estimates of the Genetic Doubling Dose of Radiation for Humans," *American Journal of Human Genetics* 46, no. 6 (1990): 1053.

56. Neel and Schull, *The Children of Atomic Bomb Survivors*, 2.

57. Shigeru Nakayama, *Science, Technology and Society in Postwar Japan* (London: Kegan Paul International, 1991), 14–22.

58. Kutcher, "Cancer Therapy and Military Cold-War Research"; *Medical Aspects of Nuclear Energy* (Washington: Armed Forces Special Weapons Project, 1949). A copy of the second item is at the National Library of Medicine.

59. The Committee for the Compilation of Materials on Damage Caused by the Atomic Bombs in Hiroshima and Nagasaki, *Hiroshima and Nagasaki: The Physical, Medical, and Social Effects of the Atomic Bombings*, trans. Eisei Ishikawa and David L. Swain (New York: Basic, [1979] 1981), 5.

60. Ibid., 13–14.

61. Robert Jay Lifton, "Psychological Effects of the Atomic Bomb in Hiroshima: The Theme of Death," *Daedalus* 92, no. 3 (1963): 489.

62. Robert Jay Lifton, *Life in Death: Survivors of Hiroshima* (New York: Random House, 1967), 23; Barnett Newman, "The Sublime Is Now," *Tiger's Eye*, December 1948, 51–53.

63. Quoted in John H. Popham, "Atom Held 'Feeble' in Light of Science," *New York Times*, 11 October 1949.

64. E. C. Andrus et al., *Advances in Military Medicine*, 1:liii.

65. Quoted in "Truman Gives Aim," *New York Times*, 1 December 1950.

66. William Faulkner, "Banquet Speech," 10 December 1950, www.nobelprize.org/nobel _prizes/literature/laureates/1949/faulkner-speech.html.

67. Lifton, *Life in Death*, 165.

68. Ibid., 333–335.

69. Ibid., 354.

70. Michihiko Hachiya, *Hiroshima Diary: The Journal of a Japanese Physician August 6– September 30, 1945*, trans. Warner Wells, rev. ed. (Chapel Hill: University of North Carolina Press, 1995); Yoko Ota, *City of Corpses*, in *Hiroshima: Three Witnesses*, ed. and trans. Richard H. Minear (Princeton: Princeton University Press, 1990), 115–273. For discussion of these texts, see John Wittier Treat, *Writing Ground Zero: Japanese Literature and the Atomic Bomb* (Chicago: University of Chicago Press, 1996).

71. "Mental Health and Atomic Energy," *Science* 127, no. 3290 (1958): 140.

72. Mark Jancovich, *Rational Fears: American Horror in the 1950s* (Manchester, UK: Manchester University Press, 1996), 163. See also Richard Matheson, *The Shrinking Man* (London: Sphere, [1956] 1988), 216.

73. For a helpful discussion of the figure of the physicist, see Cyndy Hendershot, "The Atomic Scientist, Science Fiction Films, and Paranoia: *The Day the Earth Stood Still, This Island Earth* and *Killers from Space*," *Journal of American Culture* 20, no. 1 (1997): 31–41.

74. John F. Kennedy, "Address to the Nation on the Nuclear Test Ban Treaty," 26 July 1963, www.jfklibrary.org/Asset-Viewer/ZNO049DpRUa-kMetjWmSyg.aspx.

75. Quoted in F. Lincoln Grahlfs, *Voices from Ground Zero: Recollections and Feelings of Nuclear Test Veterans* (Lanham, MD: University Press of America, 1996), 38.

76. Howard Ball, *Justice Downwind: America's Atomic Testing Program in the 1950s* (New York: Oxford University Press, 1986), 89.

77. Philip L. Fradkin, *Fallout: An American Nuclear Tragedy* (Boulder, CO: Johnson, [1989] 2004), 1–26.

78. Carole Gallagher, *American Ground Zero: The Secret Nuclear War* (Cambridge: MIT Press, 1993), xiii.

79. Philip Rieff has written a good treatment of the relationship between Cold War science and politics. See his "The Case of Dr. Oppenheimer," in *On Intellectuals: Theoretical Studies, Case Studies*, ed. Philip Rieff (New York: Doubleday, 1969), 314–40.

80. J. Robert Oppenheimer, interview by Edward R. Murrow, *See It Now*, CBS, 4 January 1955.

81. Ibid. For a reading of the Oppenheimer and Murrow interview, see Kai Bird and Martin J. Sherwin, *American Prometheus: The Triumph and Tragedy of J. Robert Oppenheimer* (New York: Vintage, 2006), 556–557.

82. Sternglass, *Secret Fallout*, 4.

83. Oppenheimer, interview by Murrow.

84. Archibald MacLeish, "To Face the Real Crisis," *New York Times*, 25 December 1960.

85. Oppenheimer, interview by Murrow.

86. Albert J. Glass, "Principles of Combat Psychiatry," *Military Medicine* 117, no. 1 (1955): 33. See also Harold M. Voth, "Psychiatric Screening in the Armed Forces," *American Journal of Psychiatry* 110, no. 10 (1954): 748–53.

87. Glass, "Principles of Combat Psychiatry," 33.

88. Stanley Weintraub, *War in the Wards: Korea's Unknown Battle in a Prisoner-of-War Hospital Camp* (San Rafael, CA: Presidio, 1976); John Benton, *Should Be Soldiers: An Army Combat Battalion Medical Aid Station during the Korean War* (Bloomington, IN: 1st Books, 2004).

89. Howard A. Rusk, "Drama of Medicine at Front a Highlight of War in Korea," *New York Times*, 23 August 1953.

90. Brown, *Fighting Fit*, 196–197.

91. George Barrett, "Portrait of the Korean Veteran," *New York Times*, 9 August 1952.

92. William Childress, "The Long March," in William Childress, *Burning the Years and Lobo: Poems 1962–1975* (St. Louis: Essai Seay, 1986), 62.

93. Stephen Endicott and Edward Hagerman, *The United States and Biological Warfare: Secrets from the Early Cold War and Korea* (Bloomington: Indiana University Press, 1998). See also G. Cameron Hurst III, "Biological Weapons: The United States and the Korean War," in *Dark Medicine: Rationalizing Unethical Medical Research*, ed. William R. LaFleur (Bloomington: Indiana University Press, 2007), 105–120.

94. Istavan Rusznyak, "Comments and Communications," *Science* 115, no. 2991 (1952): 472.

95. Detlev Bronk, "Comments and Communications," *Science* 115, no. 2991 (1952): 472–473.

96. Istavan Rusznyak, "Comments and Communications," *Science* 116, no. 3017 (1952): 461.

97. "Comments and Communications," *Science* 116, no. 3017 (1952): 461–462.

98. Endicott and Hagerman, *The United States and Biological Warfare*, ix.

99. Ibid., x.

100. William M. Creasy, "Biological Warfare," *Armed Forces Chemical Journal* 5 (January 1952): 16–18. See also Endicott and Hagerman, *The United States and Biological Warfare*, 64.

101. For the Pentagon response to the Nuremberg Code, see Jonathan Moreno, "Stumbling toward Bioethics: Human Experiments Policy and the Early Cold War," in *Dark Medicine*, ed. LaFleur, 143–144.

102. Edward Hunter, *Brainwashing in Red China: The Calculated Destruction of Men's Minds* (New York: Vanguard, 1951). See also Joost Meerloo, "Pavlov's Dog and Communist Brainwashers," *New York Times Magazine*, 9 May 1954, 33; Harvey M. Weinstein, *Psychiatry and the CIA: Victims of Mind Control* (Washington: American Psychiatric Press, 1990).

103. Henry A. Segal, "Initial Psychiatric Findings of Recently Repatriated Prisoners of War," *American Journal of Psychiatry* 111, no. 5 (1954): 358.

104. Edgar H. Schein, "The Chinese Indoctrination Program for Prisoners of War: A Study of Attempted 'Brainwashing,'" *Psychiatry* 19, no. 2 (1956): 149–172.

105. Segal, "Initial Psychiatric Findings," 359–360.

106. Ibid., 363. The view that Chinese brainwashing practices were fairly ineffective is supported by William C. Bradbury, Samuel M. Meyers, and Albert D. Biderman, the editors of *Mass Behavior in Battle and Captivity: The Communist Soldier in the Korean War* (Chicago: University of Chicago Press, 1968).

107. Murray Illson, "Reds' Psychiatry for P.O.W.'s Bared," *New York Times*, 8 May 1954.

108. Robert Jay Lifton, "Home by Ship: Reaction Patterns of American Prisoners of War Repatriated from North Korea," *American Journal of Psychiatry* 110, no. 10 (1954): 732–739.

109. Robert Jay Lifton, *Thought Reform and the Psychology of Totalism: A Study of "Brainwashing" in China* (New York: Norton, 1961), 5.

110. Ibid.

111. See Albert D. Biderman, *March to Calumny: The Story of American POWs in the Korean War* (New York: Macmillan, 1963).

112. Bogle, *The Pentagon's Battle for the American Mind*, 119–126.

113. Lifton, *Thought Reform and the Psychology of Totalism*, 447–448. See also Philip Rieff, *The Triumph of the Therapeutic* (Chicago: University of Chicago Press, [1966] 1987), 66–78.

114. Lifton, *Thought Reform and the Psychology of Totalism*, 458.

115. Bartemeier et al., "Psychiatric Aspects of the Prevention of Nuclear War," 398.

116. Harold D. Lasswell, *National Security and Individual Freedom* (New York: McGraw-Hill, 1951), 1. For the CIA's mind-control projects, see John Marks, *The Search for the "Manchurian Candidate": The CIA and Mind Control* (New York: Norton, [1979] 1991), 21–33.

117. Lifton, *Thought Reform and the Psychology of Totalism*, 459.

118. Norman Mailer, "The White Negro," in Norman Mailer, *Advertisements for Myself* (London: Flamingo, [1959] 1994), 282.

CHAPTER 4 — ORGANIZATION MEN

1. Vannevar Bush, *Science—The Endless Frontier* (Washington: National Science Foundation, [1945] 1960), 23.

2. Quoted in Robert Griffith, "Dwight D. Eisenhower and the Corporate Commonwealth," *American Historical Review* 87, no. 1 (1982): 90.

3. "Mobilization: The Man at the Wheel," *Time*, 19 February 1951, 22.

4. Charles E. Wilson, "More Defense for Every Dollar," *Nation's Business*, January 1956, 31. See also E. Bruce Geelhoed, *Charles E. Wilson and Controversy at the Pentagon, 1953 to 1957* (Detroit: Wayne State University Press, 1979).

5. Peter F. Drucker, *The Practice of Management* (New York: Harper and Row, 1954), 5.

6. C. Wright Mills, *White Collar: The American Middle Classes*, fiftieth anniversary ed. (Oxford: Oxford University Press, 2002), 208; Drucker, *The Practice of Management*.

7. Mills, *White Collar*, 297. See also Steve Joshua Heims, *Constructing a Social Science for Postwar America: The Cybernetics Group 1946–1953* (Cambridge: MIT Press, 1991), 127.

8. Heims, Constructing a Social Science for Postwar America, 2.

9. Erich Fromm, *The Sane Society* (New York: Holt, 1955), 113.

10. Ibid., 114.

11. Fromm later developed these ideas further. See, for example, his 1968 "Humanistic Planning," in Erich Fromm, *The Crisis of Psychoanalysis* (New York: Holt, 1970), 59–68.

12. In 1970 Robert Townsend codified the growing skepticism toward business organization, describing organization charts as "rigor mortis" and suggesting that reorganization should be done only "as often as major surgery" (*Up the Organization* [London: Coronet, 1970], 123, 150).

13. Abraham Maslow, "Neurosis as a Failure of Personal Growth," paper presented at the Institute of Man Symposium, Duquesne University, Pittsburgh, PA, 18 November 1966, 2.

14. Ibid., 11.

15. David Riesman, *The Lonely Crowd*, rev. ed. (New Haven: Yale University Press, [1950] 2001).

16. John Kenneth Galbraith, *The Affluent Society* (Boston: Houghton Mifflin, 1958), 7.

17. Riesman, *The Lonely Crowd*, xxvi.

18. Ibid., 8.

19. Ibid., 111.

20. Ibid., 114.

21. Margaret Mead, "National Character and the Science of Anthropology," in *Culture and Character: The Work of David Riesman Reviewed*, ed. Seymour Martin Lipset and Leo Lowenthal (Glencoe, IL: Free Press, 1961), 26.

22. Todd Gitlin, preface to Riesman, *The Lonely Crowd*, xi–xix; Joseph Galbo, "From *The Lonely Crowd* to *The Cultural Contradictions of Capitalism* and Beyond: The Shifting Ground of Liberal Narratives," *Journal of the History of the Behavioral Sciences* 40, no. 1 (2004): 47–76.

23. Arthur J. Brodbeck, "Values in *The Lonely Crowd*: Ascent or Descent of Man?," in *Culture and Character*, ed. Lipset and Lowenthal, 43.

24. Wilfred M. McClay, *The Masterless: Self and Society in Modern America* (Chapel Hill: University of North Carolina Press, 1994), 254.

25. Vance Packard, *The Hidden Persuaders* (New York: McKay, 1957).

26. Galbo, "From *The Lonely Crowd* to *The Cultural Contradictions of Capitalism* and Beyond," 60.

27. David Riesman, *Faces in the Crowd: Individual Studies in Character and Politics* (New Haven: Yale University Press, 1952).

28. Alan T. Waterman, introduction to Bush, *Science—The Endless Frontier*, xii.

29. Cited in *Industrial Health and Medical Programs*, ed. Margaret C. Klem et al. (Washington: Public Health Service Division of Industrial Hygiene, 1950). Andrew F. Henry and James F. Short Jr.'s study of the business cycle included a comparison of black and white employees (*Suicide and Homicide: Some Economic, Sociological and Psychological Aspects of Aggression* [New York: Free Press, 1954]).

30. Riesman, *The Lonely Crowd*, 111.

31. Department of Labor, *How American Buying Habits Change* (Washington: Department of Labor, 1959), 3.

32. See Daniel Lee Kleinman, *Politics on the Endless Frontier: Postwar Research Policy in the United States* (Durham, NC: Duke University Press, 1995), 108–109.

33. See Clair Brown, *American Standards of Living 1918–1988* (Oxford: Blackwell, 1994), 188.

34. Department of Labor, *How American Buying Habits Change*, 20.

35. Ibid., 160.

36. Ibid., 165; Brown, *American Standards of Living*, 235.

37. Department of Labor, *How American Buying Habits Change*, 174.

38. Paul Brodeur, *Expendable Americans* (New York: Viking, 1973), 8.

39. Peter F. Drucker, *Technology, Management, and Society* (New York: Harper and Row, 1959), 47.

40. Hugo Münsterberg, *Psychology and Industrial Efficiency* (Boston: Houghton Mifflin, 1913), 307.

41. European Productivity Agency, *Fitting the Job to the Worker* (Paris: European Productivity Agency, 1958), 14.

42. Edwin E. Ghiselli and Clarence W. Brown, *Personnel and Industrial Psychology* (New York: McGraw-Hill, 1948), 1.

43. Ibid., 2.

44. Ibid., 220.

45. Ellen Leopold, *Under the Radar: Cancer and the Cold War* (New Brunswick, NJ: Rutgers University Press, 2009), 165–166.

46. Logan T. Robertson, "The Role of the Psychologist in Industry," *A.M.A. Archives of Industrial Health* 18, no. 2 (1958): 110.

47. Ibid.

48. Donald Napoli, *Architects of Adjustment: The History of the Psychological Profession in the United States* (Port Washington, NY: Kennikat, 1981), 138. For contemporary accounts, see Joseph Tiffin and Ernest J. McCormick, *Industrial Psychology*, 4th ed. (Englewood Cliffs, NJ: Prentice-Hall, 1958); Keith Davis, *Human Relations in Business* (1957), republished as *Human Relations at Work: The Dynamics of Organizational Behavior*, 3rd ed. (New York: McGraw-Hill, 1967).

49. David M. Potter, *People of Plenty: Economic Abundance and the American Character* (Chicago: University of Chicago Press, 1954), 192.

50. Ibid., 194–195.

51. Ibid., 188. For a useful contextualizing account of *People of Plenty* and the criticism that Potter did not pay enough attention to poverty, see Robert M. Collins, "David M. Potter's *People of Plenty* and the Recycling of Consensus History," *Reviews in American History* 16, no. 2 (1988): 321–335.

52. David Riesman, *Abundance for What?* (New Brunswick, NJ: Transaction, [1964] 1993), 303.

53. "American Life and Times 1900–1950," *Life*, 2 January 1950, 34–35.

54. See Lion Murard, "Atlantic Crossings in the Measurement of Health," in *Medicine, the Market and the Mass Media: Producing Health in the Twentieth Century*, ed. Virginia Berridge and Kelly Loughlin (London: Routledge, 2005), 19.

55. Albert Deutsch, *The Shame of the States* (New York: Harcourt, Brace, 1948).

56. Nathan K. Rickles et al., "Who Goes to a Psychiatrist?," *American Journal of Psychiatry* 106, no. 11 (1950): 845.

57. Although housewives were the largest group (23 percent of the total), the report notes that this is simply "in keeping with the general occupational picture among women" (ibid.).

58. Ibid., 846.

59. Ibid., 848.

60. William I. Greenwald, "Who Goes to a Psychiatrist?: Letter to the Editor," *American Journal of Psychiatry* 107, no. 4 (1950): 306–307.

61. Gerald Gurin, *Americans View Their Mental Health: A Nationwide Interview Survey* (New York: Basic, 1960), xviii–ix.

62. Ibid., 162.

63. Hamilton B. Webb, "The Measurement of Health," *A.M.A. Archives of Industrial Health* 13, no. 2 (1956): 109–111.

64. Harry Levinson, *Men, Management, and Mental Health* (Cambridge: Harvard University Press, 1962), ix.

65. Ibid., xi–xii.

66. Ibid., 11.

67. Ibid., 18.

68. Ibid., 21.

69. Ibid., 167.

70. Clarence P. Oberndorf, "Psychopathology of Work," *Bulletin of the Menninger Clinic* 15, no. 3 (1951): 77–78.

71. Norbert Wiener, "Problems of Organization," *Bulletin of the Menninger Clinic* 17, no. 4 (1953): 138.

72. Alfred J. Marrow, "Experiments in Industrial Management," *Bulletin of the Menninger Clinic* 23, no. 2 (1959): 53.

73. Benjamin Karsh, "Automation's Brave New World," *Nation*, 5 October 1957, 208–210.

74. Elton Rayack, *Professional Power and American Medicine: The Economics of the American Medical Association* (Cleveland: World, 1967), 40.

75. Norman Mailer, "The White Negro," in Norman Mailer, *Advertisements for Myself* (London: Flamingo, 1994), 282.

76. David Riesman, "Character Types and Political Apathy: Some Revisions," 16 May 1948 (Riesman Papers, Harvard University Archives, Cambridge, MA), 11–14.

77. Donald Meyer, *The Positive Thinkers* (Middletown, CT: Wesleyan University Press, [1965] 1988), 178–180.

78. Norman Vincent Peale, *The Power of Positive Thinking* (New York: Simon and Schuster, [1952] 1980), xi.

79. Walker Percy, *The Last Gentleman* (New York: Farrar, Straus and Giroux, 1966), 46.

80. Peale, *The Power of Positive Thinking*, 217.

81. Ibid., 225

82. Ibid., 153.

83. Norman Vincent Peale, *The Tough-Minded Optimist* (New York: Fawcett Columbine, 1961), 129.

84. Quoted in Meyer, The *Positive Thinkers*, 285.

85. Quoted in Arthur Gordon, *One Man's Way: The Story and Message of Norman Vincent Peale* (Englewood Cliffs, NJ: Prentice-Hall, 1972), 248.

86. *Keeping the Nervous Patient on the Job* (St. Louis: Dios Chemical Co., 1944), 4.

87. Ibid., 17.

88. Erica Arthur, "Emasculation at Work: White-Collar Protest Fiction in the 1950s and 1990s" (PhD diss., University of Nottingham, 2004), 37.

89. Crawford H. Greenewalt, *The Uncommon Man: The Individual in the Organization* (New York: McGraw Hill, 1959), 22.

90. Ibid., 26.

91. Ibid., 27; Arthur, "Emasculation at Work," 43.

92. Vance Packard, *The Status Seekers* (New York: McKay, 1959), 8.

93. Ibid., 9.

94. C. Wright Mills, *The Power Elite* (New York: Oxford University Press, 1956).

95. Ibid., 34.

96. Ibid., 38.

97. Arthur, "Emasculation at Work," 45.

98. Peale, The *Tough-Minded Optimist*, 3.

99. Arthur, "Emasculation at Work," 60.

100. Richard Weiss, *The American Myth of Success: From Horatio Alger to Norman Vincent Peale* (Urbana: University of Illinois Press, 1988), 232–233.

101. See Carol V. R. George, *God's Salesman: Norman Vincent Peale and the Power of Positive Thinking* (New York: Oxford University Press, 1993).

102. Ibid., 234.

103. Greenewalt, *The Uncommon Man*, 28.

104. William H. Whyte, *The Organization Man* (New York: Simon and Schuster, [1956] 1960), 22.

105. Dan Wakefield, "From the Dark Towers . . . ,"*Nation*, 5 October 1957, 210–212.

106. Rod Serling, *Patterns: Four Television Plays with the Author's Personal Commentaries* (New York: Simon and Schuster, 1955), 82.

107. See Jack Gould, "*Patterns* Is Hailed as a Notable Triumph," *New York Times*, 17 January 1955.

108. Quoted in Wakefield, "From the Dark Towers . . . ," 212.

109. Ernst Pawel, *From the Dark Tower* (New York: Macmillan, 1957), 24.

110. Ibid., 67.

111. The influence of Dostoevsky's *Notes from Underground* (1864) can be felt in *From the Dark Tower*, as well as Kafka's *The Trial* (1925), which had been available in translation since

the 1930s but which became influential as a proto-existentialist novel in the 1950s. Pawel later wrote a biography of Kafka, *The Nightmare of Reason: A Life of Franz Kafka* (New York: Farrar, Straus, Giroux, 1984).

112. Pawel, *From the Dark Tower*, 59.

113. Ibid., 2.

114. Ibid., 5–6.

115. Ibid., 7, 14.

116. Ibid., 15, 71.

117. Ibid., 242.

118. Ibid..

119. Ibid., 244.

120. Christopher Wilson, *White Collar Fictions: Class and Social Representation in American Literature, 1885–1925* (Athens: University of Georgia Press, 1992), 16.

121. David Riesman, "The Suburban Dislocation," *Annals of the American Academy of Political and Social Science* 314, no. 1 (1957): 123.

122. Harrry Henderson, "The Mass-Produced Suburbs," *Harper's*, November 1953, 25–32, and December 1953, 80–86.

123. Robert C. Wood, *Suburbia: Its People and Their Politics* (New York: Houghton Mifflin, 1959).

124. John Keats, *The Crack in the Picture Window* (Boston: Houghton Mifflin, 1957), xi.

125. William H. Whyte, "How the New Suburbia Socializes," in *The Essential William H. Whyte*, ed. Albert LaFarge (New York: Fordham University Press, 2000), 32.

126. Ibid., 31.

127. Lynn Spigel, *Welcome to the Dreamhouse: Popular Media and Postwar Suburbs* (Durham, NC: Duke University Press, 2001), 3.

128. Riesman, "The Suburban Dislocation," 126.

129. Wood, *Suburbia*, 5.

130. Sloan Wilson, *The Man in the Gray Flannel Suit* (New York: Penguin, [1955] 2002), 69.

CHAPTER 5 — IN THE FAMILY CIRCLE

1. Otis L. Wiese, "Live the Life of McCall's," *McCall's*, May 1954, 27.

2. Christopher Lasch, *Haven in a Heartless World: The Family Besieged* (New York: Basic, 1977), 42.

3. Ibid., 20.

4. John R. Seeley et al., *Crestwood Heights: A Study of the Culture of Suburban Life* (New York: Basic, 1956), 165.

5. Clair Brown, *American Standards of Living, 1918–1988* (Oxford: Blackwell, 1994), 190.

6. Jacqueline Foertsch, *Bracing Accounts: The Literature and Culture of Polio in Postwar America* (Cranbury, NJ: Associated University Presses, 2008), 26–50.

7. Alan E. Nourse, *Ladies' Home Journal Family Medical Guide* (New York: Harper and Row, 1973), 2.

8. Bert Hansen, *Picturing Medical Progress from Pasteur to Polio: A History of Mass Media Images and Popular Attitudes in America* (New Brunswick, NJ: Rutgers University Press, 2009), 10.

9. "These are the tranquillized *Fifties,* / and I am forty" (Robert Lowell, "Memories of West Street and Lepke," in Robert Lowell, *Life Studies* (London: Faber and Faber, [1959] 1985), 99.

10. Consumers' Project (supervised by US Department of Labor), *The Home Medicine Cabinet* (Washington, DC: US Government Printing Office, 1936).

11. Harlan Miller, *There's a Man in the House* (New York: Random House, 1955), 145–146.

12. Ibid., 147.

13. Seeley et al., *Crestwood Heights,* 45.

14. Quoted in *Medicine Avenue: The Story of Medical Advertising in America* (Huntington, NY: Medical Advertising Hall of Fame, 1999), 23.

15. Andrea Tone, *The Age of Anxiety: A History of America's Turbulent Affair with Tranquilizers* (New York: Perseus, 2009), 53–68.

16. Ibid., 115.

17. Bill Davidson, "The Case of the Missing Miracle," *Collier's,* 9 November 1946: 80.

18. Ibid., 83.

19. Dennis Worthen, *Pharmacy in World War II* (Binghamton, NY: Haworth, 2004); David Healy, *The Antidepressant Era* (Cambridge: Harvard University Press, 1999) and *Pharmageddon* (Berkeley: University of California Press, 2012).

20. Ruth Nanda Anshen, "The Family in Transition," in *The Family: Its Function and Destiny,* ed. Ruth Nanda Anshen, rev. ed (New York: Harper's, 1959), ix.

21. Talcott Parsons, "The Social Structure of the Family," in *The Family,* ed. Anshen, 201.

22. Anshen, "The Family in Transition," xiv.

23. Clifford Kirkpatrick, *The Family as Process and Institution* (New York: Ronald, 1955), 573.

24. Deborah Weinstein, "The Pathological Family: A Cultural History of Family Therapy in Post–World War II America," PhD diss., Harvard University, 2002, 2. For a discussion of Theodora Abel and family therapy, see J. LeRoy Gabaldon, "Patterns of an Age: The Psychological Writings of Theodora M. Abel," PhD diss., Fielding Institute, Santa Barbara, CA, 1980. See also Nathan Ackerman, *The Psychodynamics of Family Life: Diagnosis and Treatment of Family Relationships* (New York: Basic, 1958); Murray Bowen, *Family Therapy in Clinical Practice* (New York: Aronson, [1966] 1985).

25. Margaret Mead, *Male and Female: A Study of the Sexes in a Changing World* (New York: William Morrow, 1949), 264.

26. G. P. Murdock, *Social Structure* (New York: Macmillan, 1949), 2.

27. Robert S. Lynd and Helen Merrell Lynd, *Middletown: A Study in Contemporary American Culture* (New York: Harcourt, Brace, 1929) and *Middletown in Transition: A Study in Cultural Conflicts* (New York: Harcourt, Brace, 1937).

28. See Lawrence R. Jacobs, *The Health of Nations: Public Opinion and the Making of American and British Health Policy* (Ithaca, NY: Cornell University Press, 1993), 85–107.

29. Harold Diehl, *Elements of Healthful Living* (New York: McGraw Hill, 1942), 5.

30. Dwight D. Eisenhower, "Health of the American People," 83rd Congress, 2nd Session, 18 January 1954 (Washington: Government Printing Office, 1954), 1, 7.

31. Joint Commission on Mental Illness and Health, *Action for Mental Health: Final Report* (New York: Basic, 1961).

32. Vance Packard and Clifford R. Adams, *How to Pick a Mate: The Guide to a Happy Marriage* (New York: Dutton, 1946), 20.

33. "The American Family in Trouble," *Life*, 26 July 1948, 83.

34. Ibid., 93.

35. Anshen, "The Family in Transition," xvii.

36. J. C. Furnas, *How America Lives* (New York: Henry Holt, 1941), 8.

37. Ibid., 293.

38. Edward Steichen, "Freedom and the Artist," in *Edward Steichen: Selected Texts and Bibliography*, ed. Ronald J. Gedrim (New York: G. K. Hall, 1996), 98.

39. Edward Steichen, *The Family of Man*, thirtieth anniversary ed. (New York: Museum of Modern Art, [1955] 1986), 149, 169.

40. Ibid., 56–59.

41. Eric J. Sandeen, *Picturing an Exhibition: The Family of Man and 1950s America* (Albuquerque: University of New Mexico Press, 1995), 29, 31.

42. Ibid., 74. Sandeen notes that in the 1960s the exhibition was reinterpreted as "an anthology of 1950s middle-class sentimentalism and insensitivity" (75).

43. The quotes are the titles of chapters 5 and 6 in Elaine Tyler May, *Homeward Bound: American Families in the Cold War Era* (New York: Basic, 1988).

44. Earl Lomon Koos, *The Health of Regionville: What the People Thought and Did about It* (New York: Columbia University Press, 1954), 9.

45. Ibid., 138.

46. Ibid., 32.

47. Ibid., 33.

48. Ibid., 34–35.

49. Ibid., 139.

50. Ibid., 144.

51. See, for example, Mary Beth Haralovich, "Sitcoms and Suburbs: Positioning the 1950s Homemaker," *Quarterly Review of Film and Video* 11, no. 1 (1989): 61–83.

52. Seeley et al., *Crestwood Heights*, 45.

53. Amasa B. Ford, *Urban Health in America* (New York: Oxford University Press, 1976), 120–148.

54. Phyllis McGinley, "Suburbia: Of Thee I Sing" in Phyllis McGinley, *A Short Walk from the Station* (New York: Viking, 1951), 11.

55. Ibid., 10.

56. Jo Gill, *Women's Poetry* (Edinburgh: Edinburgh University Press, 2007), 82.

57. Jo Gill, "Anne Sexton's Poetics of the Suburbs," in *Health and the Modern Home*, ed. Mark Jackson (London: Routledge, 2007), 64.

58. Arlene Skolnick, *Embattled Paradise: The American Family in an Age of Uncertainty* (New York: Basic, 1991), 52. For the statistic, see Andrew J. Cherlin, "The Changing American Family and Public Policy," in *The Changing American Family and Public Policy*, ed. Andrew J. Cherlin (Washington: Urban Institute Press, 1988), 5.

59. Skolnick, *Embattled Paradise*, 52.

60. Rebecca Jo Plant, *Mom: The Transformation of Motherhood in Modern America* (Chicago: University of Chicago Press, 2010), 97. See also Sonya Michel, "Danger on the Home Front: Motherhood, Sexuality, and Disabled Veterans in American Postwar Films," *Journal of the History of Sexuality* 3, no. 1 (1992): 113.

61. Helene Deutsch, *The Psychology of Women* (London: Research Press, 1944), 1:220–255.

62. Ferdinand Lundberg and Marynia F. Farnham, *Modern Woman: The Lost Sex* (New York: Harper and Brothers, 1947), 215.

63. Ibid., 16, 10.

64. Lucy Freeman, *Fight against Fears* (New York: Continuum, [1951] 1988).

65. Plant, *Mom*, 98. Writing between the world wars, Harry Stack Sullivan anticipated the antifeminist chorus by suggesting that unhappiness, stress, and neurosis are likely to arise in women who fulfill "the urge to 'be a man'" (*Personal Psychopathology: Early Formulations* [New York: Norton, 1972], 263).

66. Wendy Kline, *Building a Better Race: Gender, Sexuality, and Eugenics from the Turn of the Century to the Baby Boom* (Berkeley: University of California Press, 2001), 152–156.

67. Leonard H. Biskind, *Health and Hygiene for the Modern Woman* (New York: Harper and Brothers, 1957). See also Erich Neumann, *The Great Mother: An Analysis of the Archetype*, trans. Ralph Manheim (New York: Bollingen Foundation, 1955); Theodor Reik, *The Creation of Woman* (New York: George Braziller, 1960).

68. David Riesman, *The Lonely Crowd*, rev. ed. (New Haven: Yale University Press, [1950] 2001), 203.

69. Brandon French, *On the Verge of Revolt: Women in American Films of the Fifties* (New York: Ungar, 1978), xxi.

70. Richard Yates, *Revolutionary Road* (Boston: Little, Brown, 1961).

71. Richard E. Gordon, Katherine K. Gordon, and Max Gunther, *The Split-Level Trap,* (New York: Bernard Geis, 1960), 28.

72. Ibid., 38.

73. Ibid., 42.

74. Ibid., 45–47.

75. Ibid., 48–49.

76. Herbert Gans claimed the opposite: suburban dwellers tried to fit in with their neighbors and did not consume conspicuously (*The Levittowners: Ways of Life and Politics in a New Suburban Community* [New York: Pantheon, 1967]).

77. Plant, *Mom*, 26.

78. T. Swann Harding, "The Consumer and the Medicine Cabinet," *Journal of Home Economics* 22, no. 7 (1930): 561, 565. See also David Cantor, "Cancer, Quackery and the Vernacular Meanings of Hope in 1950s America," *Journal of the History of Medicine and Allied Sciences* 61, no. 3 (2006). 324–368.

79. Nancy Tomes, "'Skeletons in the Medicine Closet': Women and 'Rational Consumption' in the Inter-War American Home," in *Health and the Modern Home*, ed. Jackson, 190.

80. Lynn Spigel, *Welcome to the Dreamhouse: Popular Media and Postwar Suburbs* (Durham, NC: Duke University Press, 2001), 8–9.

81. See, for example, "Congress Must Act on Food Additives," *Ladies Home Journal*, February 1958, 11.

82. Suzanne Douglas, "Positive Thinking," *Ladies' Home Journal*, January 1958, 68.

83. Mary Swartz Rose, "Old and New Emphases in the Teaching of Nutrition," *Journal of Home Economics* 22, no. 1 (1930): 878–884.

84. Mead, *Male and Female*, 247.

85. Daniel Delis Hill, *Advertising to the American Woman 1900–1990* (Columbus: Ohio State University Press, 2002), 86.

86. Holger Frederick Kilander, *Nutrition for Health* (New York: McGraw-Hill, 1951), 22.

87. Ibid., 22–23.

88. Brown, *American Standards of Living*, 199–200.

89. Quoted in Kathleen Brown, "The Maternal Physician: Teaching American Mothers to Put the Baby in the Bathwater," in *Right Living: An Anglo-American Tradition of Self-Help Medicine and Hygiene*, ed. Charles E. Rosenberg (Baltimore: Johns Hopkins University Press, 2003), 100. See Rima D. Apple, "Constructing Mothers: Scientific Motherhood in the Nineteenth and Twentieth Centuries," *Social History of Medicine* 8, no. 2 (1995): 161–178.

90. Brown, "The Maternal Physician," 100.

91. The best historical overview of polio is David M. Oshinsky, *Polio: An American Story* (Oxford: Oxford University Press, 2005). See also Marc Shell, *Polio and Its Aftermath: The Paralysis of Culture* (Cambridge: Harvard University Press, 2005).

92. Apple, "Constructing Mothers," 162.

93. *Infant Care*, 8th ed. (Washington: US Government Printing Office, 1923), 12.

94. For a comparison of *Infant Care* and *Baby and Child Care*, see Nancy Pottishman Weiss, "Mother, the Invention of Necessity: Dr. Benjamin Spock's *Baby and Child Care*," *American Quarterly* 29, no. 5 (1977): 519–546.

95. Thomas Maier, *Dr. Spock: An American Life* (New York: Harcourt. Brace, 1998), 124.

96. Quoted in A. Michael Sulman, "The Humanization of the American Child: Benjamin Spock as a Popularizer of Psychoanalytic Thought," *Journal of the History of the Behavioral Sciences* 9, no. 3 (1973): 258–265.

97. Ibid., 261–263.

98. Spitz's films are available at the History of American Psychology Archive, Akron University. For an early lecture by Spitz on the importance of motherhood, see his "Are Parents Necessary" in *Medicine in a Postwar World* (New York: Columbia University Press, 1948), 37–53.

99. René Spitz, dir., *Psychogenic Disease in Infancy* (1952), www.archive.org/details/PsychogenicD.

100. For a discussion of Harold Skeels's work in the 1930s, see Scot Danforth, *The Incomplete Child: An Intellectual History of Learning Disabilities* (New York: Peter Lang, 2009), 111. After World War II, Skeels worked for the National Institute of Mental Health, where he continued his earlier pediatric research as well as focusing on the impact of mental health on communities.

101. Helene Deutsch, The *Psychology of Women* (London: Research Press, 1946), 2:430.

102. For discussion of these external shaping factors, see Robert R. Sears et al., *Patterns of Child Rearing* (Evanston, IL: Row, Peterson, 1957), 421–446.

103. D. W. Winnicott, *Mother and Child: A Primer of First Relationships* (New York: Basic, 1957), 12.

104. Winnicott argued that by focusing squarely on physical health, pediatrics "at its worst . . . can be said to be the organized exploitation of the betrayal of human nature by instincts" ("Psychoses and Child Care," in D. W. Winnicott, *Through Paediatrics to Psycho-Analysis: Collected Papers, with an introduction by M. Masud R. Khan* [New York: Brunner/ Mazel, 1992], 225).

105. D. W. Winnicott, "Transitional Objects and Transitional Phenomena," *International Journal of Psychoanalysis* 34, no. 2 (1953): 90.

106. Winnicott, *Mother and Child*, 190.

107. Erik Erikson, *Childhood and Society* (London: Vintage, [1950] 1995), 258–259. For a fuller discussion of the "Reflections on the American Identity" chapter in Erikson's book, see

Lawrence J. Friedman, *Identity's Architect: A Biography of Erik H. Erikson* (New York: Scribner, 1999), 178–184.

108. Erikson, *Childhood and Society*, 261.

109. Ibid., 260.

110. Phyllis McGinley, "Girl's-Eye View of Relatives," in Phyllis McGinley, *Times Three* (New York: Viking, 1960), 42.

111. Winnicott, *Mother and Child*, 121.

112. Louis Lyndon, "Uncertain Hero: The Paradox of the American Male," *Woman's Home Companion*, November 1956, 41–43, 107.

113. McGinley, "Girl's-Eye View of Relatives," 42.

114. Deutsch, *The Psychology of Women*, 1:195–196, 158–159.

115. Stephen Cohan, *Masked Men: Masculinity and the Movies in the Fifties* (Bloomington: Indiana University Press, 1997).

116. Robert Lowell, "Eye and Tooth," in Robert Lowell, *For the Union Dead* (New York: Farrar, Straus and Giroux, 1964), 18–19.

117. Cohan, *Masked Men*, 38

118. Lyndon, "Uncertain Hero," 107.

119. Sloan Wilson, *The Man in the Gray Flannel Suit* (New York: Penguin, [1955] 2002), 3.

120. Ibid., 1, 3.

121. William H. Whyte, "How the New Suburbia Socializes," in *The Essential William H. Whyte*, ed. Albert LaFarge (New York: Fordham University Press, 2000), 32.

122. Ibid.

123. Georgie Starbuck Galbraith, "Housebroke," *Ladies' Home Journal*, March 1958, 20.

124. The serious article adjacent to the poem is Dorothy Thompson, "Is Morality 'Normal'?," *Ladies' Home Journal*, March 1958, 11, 20, 169.

125. Whyte, "How the New Suburbia Socializes," 33. This echoes Winnicott's view that, although fathers "can be good mothers for limited periods of time," their primary function is "to protect the mother and baby from whatever tends to interfere with the bond between them" (*Mother and Child*, xi).

126. Quoted in Clarence G. Lasby, *Eisenhower's Heart Attack: How Ike Beat Heart Disease and Held on to the Presidency* (Lawrence: University Press of Kansas, 1997), 71.

127. Berton Roueché, "Ten Feet Tall," *New Yorker*, 10 September 1955, 47. Roueché's article should not be confused with Helen Topping Miller's *A Man Ten Feet Tall* (1957), a medical novel in which Dr. Adam Reagan promises to become a health crusader after seeing his father die due to lack of medical care. Roueché published a series of books on medical detection in the 1950s, including *Eleven Blue Men* (1954) and *The Incurable Wound* (1958).

128. Roueché, "Ten Feet Tall," 48.

129. Ibid., 59.

130. Ibid., 62.

131. Barbara Klinger, *Melodrama and Meaning: History, Culture and the Films of Douglas Sirk* (Bloomington: Indiana University Press, 1994), xii.

132. I have borrowed this tension between being "locked in" and "locked out" from Christopher Orr's reading of Douglas Sirk's narrative technique in "Closure and Containment: Mary Hadley in *Written on the Wind*," *Wide Angle* 4, no. 2 (1980): 28–35.

133. Gordon, Gordon, and Gunther, *The Split-Level Trap*, 33.

134. Wilson, *The Man in the Gray Flannel Suit*, 62.

135. William A. Bellamy, "Malpractice Risks Confronting the Psychiatrist: A Nationwide Fifteen-Year Study of Appellate Court Cases, 1946 to 1961," *American Journal of Psychiatry* 118, no. 9 (1962): 769–780; Donald J. Dawidoff, *The Malpractice of Psychiatrists: Malpractice in Psychoanalysis, Psychotherapy, and Psychiatry* (Springfield, IL: Charles C. Thomas, 1973), 79–85, 96–97.

136. Morton Kramer, *Public Health and Social Problems in the Use of Tranquilizing Drugs* (Washington: Public Health Reports, 1956), 1.

137. Ibid., 22–24. See also Harold Burn, *Drugs, Medicines and Man* (London: Unwin, 1962), 111–122.

138. See Eugenia Kaledin, *Mothers and More: American Women in the 1950s* (Boston: Twayne, 1984), 181.

139. Quoted in Seymour M. Farber and Roger H. L. Wilson, *The Potential of Woman* (New York: McGraw-Hill, 1963), 18.

140. Adrienne Rich, *Of Woman Born: Motherhood as Experience and Institution* (New York: Norton, 1976), 284.

141. Gladys Denny Shultz, "Cruelty in Maternity Wards," *Ladies' Home Journal*, May 1958, 44, 152–153, and December 1958, 58–59, 135–139.

142. Ibid., December 1958, 58.

143. Phillip Knightley et al., *Suffer the Children: The Story of Thalidomide* (New York: Viking, 1979).

144. Ethel Roskies, *Abnormality and Normality: The Mothering of Thalidomide Children* (Ithaca, NY: Cornell University Press, 1972).

145. Kaledin, *Mothers and More*, 175.

146. Barron H. Lerner, *The Breast Cancer Wars: Hope, Fear, and the Pursuit of a Cure in Twentieth-Century America* (Oxford: Oxford University Press, 2001), 76.

147. Edwin M. Schur, *Crimes without Victims: Deviant Behavior and Public Policy* (Englewood Cliffs, NJ: Prentice-Hall, 1965), 11–12.

148. Ibid., 22–23.

149. Joan Didion, *Play It As It Lays* (New York: Farrar, Straus and Giroux, 1970), 62.

150. Mary Calderone, *Abortion in the United States* (New York: Hoeber-Harper, 1958).

151. See Leslie J. Reagan, *When Abortion Was a Crime: Women, Medicine, and Law in the United States, 1867–1973* (Berkeley: University of California Press, 1997), 218–222.

152. Ibid., 201–202.

CHAPTER 6 — OUTSIDE THE CIRCLE

1. Robert E. Gilbert, *The Mortal Presidency: Illness and Anguish in the White House* (New York: Fordham University Press, 1998), 81–82.

2. Craig Allen, *Eisenhower and the Mass Media: Peace, Prosperity, and Prime-Time TV* (Chapel Hill: University of North Carolina Press, 1993), 86–93.

3. Clarence G. Lasby, *Eisenhower's Heart Attack: How Ike Beat Heart Disease and Held on to the Presidency* (Lawrence: University Press of Kansas, 1997).

4. Rose McDermott, *Presidential Leadership, Illness, and Decision Making* (Cambridge: Cambridge University Press, 2008), 198–199.

5. Ibid., 178–179.

6. Ibid., 159, 174. For a discussion of Eisenhower's "coronary crisis" and the increasingly fraught relationship between Eisenhower and Nixon see William Costello, *The Facts About Nixon* (New York: Viking, 1960), 135–152.

7. Another good example is Elia Kazan's 1961 film *Splendor in the Grass*, in which Deanie (Natalie Wood) is driven to a state of psychosis by the conflicting sexual messages of her Kansas town in the late 1920s.

8. John F. Kennedy, "The Soft American," *Sports Illustrated*, 26 December 1960, 15–17.

9. J. Edgar Hoover, *Masters of Deceit* (New York: Henry Holt, 1958), 82.

10. Quoted in Ellen Schrecker, *Many Are the Crimes: McCarthyism in America* (Princeton: Princeton University Press, 1998), 144.

11. Gregory Field, "Flushing Poisons from the Body Politic: The Fluoride Controversy and American Political Culture, 1955–1965," in *The Sixties Revisited: Culture—Society—Politics*, ed. Jurgen Heideking et al. (Heidelberg: Carl Winter, 2001), 469–486.

12. See Michelle M. Nickerson, "The Lunatic Fringe Strikes Back: Conservative Opposition to the Alaska Mental Health Bill of 1956," in *The Politics of Healing: Histories of Alternative Medicine in Twentieth-Century North America*, ed. Robert D. Johnston (New York: Routledge, 2004), 110–123.

13. Arthur Schlesinger Jr., "What McCarthyism Is," *ADA World*, November 1950, 4.

14. Vance Packard, *The Hidden Persuaders* (New York: McKay, 1957), 247. See also David Greenberg, *Nixon's Shadow: The History of an Image* (New York: Norton, 2003), 65–67.

15. Quoted in Greenberg, *Nixon's Shadow*, 62.

16. Jacqueline Foertsch, *Enemies Within: The Cold War and the AIDS Crisis in Literature, Film, and Culture* (Urbana: University of Illinois Press, 2001), 195–196.

17. Ilina Singh, "Bad Boys, Good Mothers, and the 'Miracle' of Ritalin," *Science in Context* 15, no. 4 (2002): 577–603.

18. Erving Goffman, "On Face Work," in Erving Goffman, *Interaction Ritual: Essays on Face-to-Face Behavior* (New York: Anchor, 1967), 31, 45.

19. Carita Huang, "Making Children Normal: Standardizing Children in the United States, 1885–1930," PhD diss., University of Pennsylvania, 2004.

20. Report presented at the Conference of Chief Psychologists in State Mental Health Programs, Bethesda, Maryland, 30–31 August 1952 (Carter Papers, M316, Archives of the History of American Psychology, University of Akron, Akron, OH).

21. John E. Gibson, "How Neurotic Are You?," *Ladies' Home Journal*, March 1958, 47.

22. *Diagnostic and Statistical Manual of Mental Disorders* (Washington: American Psychiatric Association, 1952), vii.

23. Ibid.

24. John C. Spurlock, "From Reassurance to Irrelevance: Adolescent Psychology and Homosexuality in America," *History of Psychology* 5, no. 1 (2002): 38–51.

25. Jennifer Terry, *An American Obsession: Science, Medicine, and Homosexuality in Modern Society* (Chicago: University of Chicago Press, 1999), 324–325; Allan Bérubé, *Coming Out under Fire: The History of Gay Men and Women in World War II* (New York: Free Press, 1990), 14.

26. Spurlock, "From Reassurance to Irrelevance," 39–40. Psychologists disagreed about the age range in which these transitional friendships were most likely to arise, some saying between eight and thirteen years of age and others saying between fourteen and twenty. See Alexander Schneiders, *Personality Development and Adjustment in Adolescence* (Milwaukee: Bruce, 1960).

27. Spurlock, "From Reassurance to Irrelevance," 40. See also Ronald Bayer, *Homosexuality and American Psychiatry: The Politics of Diagnosis* (New York: Basic, 1981).

28. Morris L. Ernst and David Loth, *Sexual Behaviour and the Kinsey Report* (London: Falcon, 1949), 33.

29. Spurlock, "From Reassurance to Irrelevance," 43.

30. Evelyn Hooker, "The Adjustment of the Male Overt Homosexual," *Journal of Projective Techniques* 21, no. 1 (1957): 18–31.

31. *Diagnostic and Statistical Manual of Mental Disorders*, 3rd ed. (Washington: American Psychiatric Association, 1987), 335.

32. Benjamin Spock considered adoption a problem, arguing that adopted children were more prone to neuroses. See *Baby and Child Care*, rev. ed. (London: New English Library, 1969), 520–523. Other evidence at the time suggested that adoption between the ages of three and six was likely to lead to unresolved crises among adopted children. See E. Wayne Carp, *Family Matters: Secrecy and Disclosure in the History of Adoption* (Cambridge: Harvard University Press, 1998), 127–128.

33. In terms of the lowest infant mortality rates in the world, the United States fell from sixth place in 1950 to fourteenth in 1963 and seventeenth in 1977. See Vern L. Bullough and Bonnie Bullough, *Health Care for the Other Americans* (New York: Appleton-Century-Crofts,

1982), 2–3; Gopal K. Singh and Stella M. Yu, "Infant Mortality in the United States: Trends, Differentials, and Projections, 1950 through 2010," *American Journal of Public Health* 85, no. 7 (1995): 957–964.

34. Charles E. Strickland and Andrew M. Ambrose, "The Baby Boom, Prosperity, and the Changing Worlds of Children, 1945–1963," in *American Childhood: A Research Guide and Historical Handbook*, ed. Joseph M. Hawes and N. Ray Hiner (Westport, CT: Greenwood, 1985), 540–541.

35. Benjamin Spock, *Problems for Parents* (London: Bodley Head, 1962), 7.

36. Erik Erikson, *Identity: Youth and Crisis* (New York: Norton, 1968), 96.

37. Ibid., 94.

38. For an earlier discussion of personality growth through childhood and adolescence, see Harry Stack Sullivan's posthumously published *Personal Psychopathology* (New York: Norton, 1972).

39. Erikson, *Insight and Responsibility* (New York: Norton, 1964), 84.

40. Ibid., 87.

41. Spock, *Problems for Parents*, 65.

42. John A. Hutchinson, "The Nuclear Age and the Cold War," in *Dilemmas of Youth: In America Today*, ed. Robert M. MacIver (New York: Harper and Brothers, 1961), 103.

43. Quoted in Dean W. Roberts, "Highlights of the Midcentury Conference on Children and Youth," *American Journal of Public Health* 41, no. 1 (January 1951): 98.

44. Quoted in "War Fear Is Blow to Child Welfare," *New York Times*, 1 December 1950. For changing attitudes toward orphans, see Bernadine Barr, "Spare Children, 1900–1945: Inmates of Orphanages as Subjects of Research in Medicine and the Social Sciences in America," PhD diss., Stanford University, 1992.

45. Quoted in Ann Hulbert, *Raising America: Experts, Parents, and a Century of Advice About Children*, paperback ed. (New York: Vintage, 2004), 192.

46. Inabel B. Lindsay and Caroline F. Ware, "Welfare Agencies and the Needs of Negro Children and Youth," *Journal of Negro Education* 19, no. 3 (1950), 377–378.

47. Carolyn Herbst Lewis argues that "sexual citizenship" was reinforced widely by medical practitioners in the 1950s (*Prescription for Heterosexuality: Sexual Citizenship in the Cold War Era* [Chapel Hill: University of North Carolina Press, 2010]).

48. Jessica Weiss, *To Have and to Hold: Marriage, the Baby Boom and Social Change* (Chicago: University of Chicago Press, 2000), 146–150.

49. Rickie Solinger, *Wake Up Little Susie: Single Pregnancy and Race before Roe v. Wade*, 2nd paperback ed. (New York: Routledge, 2000), 3.

50. Quoted in ibid., 22.

51. Carp, *Family Matters*, 121–125. This view of the risks of divorce continued until at least the mid-1960s. But a 1966 poll suggested that over half of the respondents thought that

it was worse for children to remain with embattled parents than with a single parent after a divorce. See Weiss, *To Have and to Hold*, 187.

52. Paul Starr, *The Social Transformation of American Medicine* (New York: Basic, 1982), 158, 260. For an account of Boston's welfare culture, see Peter C. Holloran, *Boston's Wayward Children: Social Services for Homeless Children, 1830–1930* (Boston: Northeastern University Press, [1989] 1994).

53. Lawrence J. Friedman, *Menninger: The Family and the Clinic* (Lawrence: University Press of Kansas, 1992), 101.

54. Bruno Bettelheim, *Love Is Not Enough* (New York: Free Press, 1950), 16.

55. Ibid., 7.

56. Ibid., 6, 25.

57. Nina Sutton, *Bruno Bettelheim: The Other Side of Madness* (London: Duckworth, 1995), 273–274.

58. Bettelheim, *Love Is Not Enough*, 375.

59. Bruno Bettelheim, *Truants from Life* (Glencoe, IL: Free Press, 1955), 3.

60. Bart Beaty, *Fredric Wertham and the Critique of Mass Culture* (Jackson: University Press of Mississippi, 2005), 7.

61. Fredric Wertham, *Seduction of the Innocent* (New York: Rinehart, 1954), 97.

62. Ibid., 356.

63. Keisha L. Hoerrner, "The Forgotten Battles: Congressional Hearings on Television Violence in the 1950s," *Web Journal of Mass Communications Research* 2, no. 3 (1999), www.scripps.ohiou.edu/wjmcr/vol02/2–3a-B.htm. See also Wilbur Schramm, *Television in the Lives of Our Children* (Stanford: Stanford University Press, 1961).

64. Wertham, *Seduction of the Innocent*, 52.

65. Louis Kaplan, *Mental Health and Human Relations in Education* (New York: Harper and Brothers, 1959), 281–311.

66. See Eva Moskowitz, *In Therapy We Trust* (Baltimore: Johns Hopkins University Press, 2001), 47–60, 66.

67. Joint Committee on Health Problems in Education, *Mental Health in the Classroom: How Would You Help A Child Like This?* (Washington: National Education Association, 1955).

68. Kathleen W. Jones, *Taming the Troublesome Child: American Families, Child Guidance, and the Limits of Psychiatric Authority* (Cambridge: Harvard University Press, 1999).

69. Benjamin Fine, *One Million Delinquents* (Cleveland: World Publishing, 1955), 25–26.

70. Robert Lindner, *Rebel without a Cause: The Hypnoanalysis of a Criminal Psychopath* (New York: Grune and Stratton, 1944), ix.

71. Ibid., 2.

72. Ibid.

73. Robert Lindner, *Must You Conform?* (New York: Rinehart, 1956), 7.

74. Robert Lindner, *Prescription for Rebellion* (London: Victor Gollancz, 1953), 7.

75. J. D. Salinger, *Franny and Zooey* (London: Penguin, [1961] 1964), 26.

76. Lindner, *Must You Conform?*, 15.

77. Ibid., 19.

78. Ibid., 28.

79. Robert Lindner, *The Fifty-Minute Hour* (New York: Bantam, [1955] 1966), vii.

80. Ibid., xiv.

81. Ibid., 3.

82. Ibid., 8.

83. Ibid., 11–12.

84. Ibid., 15–16.

85. Ibid., 37.

86. Ibid., 43–44.

87. Ibid., 27.

88. Frank Riessman, *The Culturally Deprived Child* (New York: Harper and Brothers, 1962), 1. See also Celia S. Heller, *Mexican American Youth: Forgotten Youth at the Crossroads* (New York: Random House, 1966), 64–77.

89. Bettelheim, "The Problem of Generations," in *The Challenge of Youth*, ed. Erik Erikson (New York: Doubleday, 1965), 89–90.

90. David Riesman, introduction to Edgar Z. Friedenberg, *The Vanishing Adolescent* (Boston: Beacon, 1959), 11.

91. Friedenberg, *The Vanishing Adolescent*, 37.

92. Ibid., 34.

93. Ibid., 41–42.

94. Ibid., 202.

95. Ibid., 105.

96. Erikson, "The Problem of Ego Identity," in *Identity and the Life Cycle* (New York: Norton, 1959), 108–77. See also Peter Blos, *On Adolescence: A Psychoanalytic Interpretation* (New York: Free Press, 1962).

97. Paul Goodman, *Growing Up Absurd: Problems of Youth in the Organized Society* (New York: Vintage, 1960), 12.

98. Margaret Parton and Mary Ann MacKaye, "Our Teen-Age Drug Addicts," *Ladies' Home Journal*, March 1958, 174.

99. Ibid., 190.

100. Strickland and Ambrose, "The Baby Boom," 566.

101. Goodman's essay "Being Queer" (1969) was a much more explicit statement of the libidinal drift than *Growing Up Absurd*, in which Goodman valorized childhood sexuality and spontaneity.

102. Thomas Doherty, *Teenagers and Teenpics: The Juvenilization of American Movies in the 1950s* (Philadelphia: Temple University Press, 2002), 63–64.

103. Quoted in K. A. Cuordileone, *Manhood and American Political Culture in the Cold War* (New York: Routledge, 2005), 51.

104. Quoted in ibid., 59.

105. Ibid., 67–69.

106. Robert Anderson, *Tea and Sympathy* (New York: Signet, [1953] 1956), 45.

107. Jackie Byars, *All That Hollywood Allows: Re-reading Gender in 1950s Melodrama* (Chapel Hill: University of North Carolina Press, 1991), 113. See also Robert J. Corber, *Homosexuality in Cold War America: Resistance and the Crisis of Masculinity* (Durham, NC: Duke University Press, 1997).

108. John D'Emilio and Estelle B. Freedman, *Intimate Matters: A History of Sexuality in America* (New York: Harper and Row, 1988), 204.

109. See Philip Pauly, *Biologists and the Promise of American Life: From Meriwether Lewis to Alfred Kinsey* (Princeton: Princeton University Press, 2000), 228–233.

110. Alfred C. Kinsey et al., *Sexual Behavior in the Human Male* (Philadelphia: W. B. Saunders, 1948), 5.

111. Paul Robinson, *The Modernization of Sex: Havelock Ellis, Alfred Kinsey, William Masters, and Virginia Johnson*, with a new preface (Ithaca, NY: Cornell University Press, [1976] 1989), 44.

112. Pauly, *Biologists and the Promise of American Life,* 236.

113. Sol W. Ginsberg, "Atomism of Behavior," in *An Analysis of the Kinsey Reports on Sexual Behavior of the Human Male and Female*, ed. Donald Porter Geddes (New York: New American Library, 1954), 39.

114. Weiss, *To Have and to Hold,* 147.

115. Lewis, *Prescription for Heterosexuality,* 31–35.

116. Terry, *An American Obsession,* 327.

117. Stanley Rachman and John Teasdale, *Aversion Therapy and Behaviour Disorders: An Analysis* (London: Routledge and Kegan Paul, 1969).

118. Quoted in Terence Kissack, "Alfred Kinsey and Homosexuality in the '50s," *Journal of the History of Sexuality* 9, no. 4 (2000): 476–477.

119. Eliza Byard Starr, "Inverts, Perverts, and National Peril: Federal Responses to Homosexuality, 1890–1956," PhD diss., Columbia University, 2002, 188–202, 206–207.

120. Quoted in Neil Miller, *Out of the Past: Gay and Lesbian History from 1869 to the Present* (New York: Vintage, 1995), 261.

121. Henry L. Minton, *Departing from Deviance: A History of Homosexual Rights and Emancipatory Science in America* (Chicago: University of Chicago Press, 2002), 171–173.

122. Herbert E. Huncke, *Guilty of Everything: The Autobiography of Herbert Huncke* (New York: Paragon, 1990), 79.

123. Huncke has been described as Ginsberg's "diabolical angel" (Jonah Raskin, *American Scream: Allen Ginberg's Howl and the Making of the Beat Generation* [Berkeley: University of California Press, 2004], 83).

124. Allen Ginsberg, introduction to Herbert E. Huncke, *The Evening Sun Turned Crimson* (Cherry Valley, NY: Cherry Valley Editions, 1980), 8.

125. Barry Miles, *Ginsberg: A Biography* (New York: Simon and Schuster, 1989), 65–66.

126. Ibid., 96–97.

127. Ibid., 118–25.

128. Allen Ginsberg, *Journals Mid-Fifties 1954–1958*, ed. Gordon Ball (New York: HarperCollins, 1995), 198.

129. Allen Ginsberg, *The Book of Martyrdom and Artifice, First Journals and Poems, 1937–1952*, ed. Juanita Liberman-Plimpton and Bill Morgan (New York: Da Capo, 2006), 359.

130. For a discussion of Naomi Ginsberg's health, see Miles, *Ginsberg*, 21–34, 93–95, 150.

131. Ginsberg, *Journals Mid-Fifties*, 260.

132. Ibid., 335.

133. Tony Trigilio, "'Strange Prophecies Anew': Rethinking the Politics of Matter and Spirit in Ginsberg's 'Kaddish,'" *American Literature* 71, no. 4 (1999): 776.

134. Ibid., 781–782.

135. Allen Ginsberg, *Kaddish and Other Poems 1958–1960* (San Francisco: City Lights, 1961), 17.

136. Allen Ginsberg, *Howl and Other Poems* (San Francisco: City Lights, 1956), 9.

137. Ibid., 15, 11.

138. Carl Goy [Solomon], "Afterthoughts of a Shock Patient," in Allen Ginsberg, *Howl*, 50th anniversary edition, ed. Barry Miles (New York: Harper, 2006), 113–117. For Solomon's writings on psychiatry and surrealism, see Carl Solomon, *Emergency Messages: An Autobiographical Miscellany*, ed. John Tytell (New York: Paragon, 1989).

139. Goodman thought that "Howl" was simply a list of Ginsberg's gripes. See Goodman's 1958 review of *On the Road*, reprinted in *Growing Up Absurd*, 279.

140. Quoted in Trigilio, "'Strange Prophecies Anew,'" 789.

CHAPTER 7 — INSTITUTIONS OF CARE AND OPPRESSION

1. For Eisenhower's healthcare proposals, see Lester A. Sobel, *Health Care: An American Crisis* (New York: Facts on File, 1976), 21–29; Steven Wagner, *Eisenhower Republicanism: Pursuing the Middle Way* (DeKalb: Northern Illinois University Press, 2006), 13–16.

2. Only when cases of polio started to emerge among recently inoculated children did Hobby move to establish a scheme of national distribution of the vaccine, and such was the fallout from her initial reluctance that she resigned in the summer of 1955, only a few months into the vaccination program. See Bert Spector, "The Great Salk Vaccine Mess," *Antioch Review* 38, no. 3 (1980): 291–303.

3. Elton Rayack, *Professional Power and American Medicine: The Economics of the American Medical Association* (Cleveland: World, 1967).

4. Dwight Eisenhower, "Farewell Address to the Nation," 17 January 1961, in *Speeches of the American Presidents*, ed. Janet Podell and Steven Anzovin, 2nd ed. (New York: H. W. Wilson, 2001), 675–678.

5. John F. Kennedy, "Inaugural Address," 20 January 1961, in *Speeches of the American Presidents*, ed. Podell and Anzovin, 687–689.

6. Rose McDermott, *Presidential Leadership, Illness, and Decision Making* (Cambridge: Cambridge University Press, 2008), 118–56.

7. Robert E. Gilbert, *The Mortal Presidency: Illness and Anguish in the White House*, 2nd ed. (New York: Fordham University Press, 1998), 142–175.

8. Ibid., 166.

9. Robert Dallek, *An Unfinished Life: John F. Kennedy, 1917–1963* (Boston: Little, Brown, 2003), 300.

10. Ibid., 471–473.

11. Laurence Leamer, *The Kennedy Women: The Saga of an American Family* (New York: Villard, 1994), 138.

12. Ibid., 227–228, 318–319.

13. Rose Fitzgerald Kennedy, *Times to Remember* (New York: Doubleday, 1974), 286. It is not clear whether Joe Kennedy made a unilateral decision to have the lobotomy performed or whether his wife, Rose, consented. See Ted Schwarz, *Joseph P. Kennedy: The Mogul, the Mob, the Statesman, and the Making of an American Myth* (Hoboken, NJ: Wiley, 2003), 302–305.

14. Ibid., 319–21.

15. Edward Shorter, *The Kennedy Family and the Story of Mental Retardation* (Philadelphia: Temple University Press, 2000), 33–34; Garry Wills, *The Kennedy Imprisonment: A Meditation on Power* (Boston: Little, Brown, 1981), 128.

16. John F. Kennedy, *Kennedy and the Press: The News Conferences*, ed. Harold W. Chase and Allen H. Lerman (New York: Crowell, 1965), 118.

17. Ibid.

18. "Psychiatry: Toward a New Frontier," *Time*, 15 February 1963, 44. *Time* prefaced its report on the president's speech with a reference to Rosemary Kennedy.

19. Joint Commission on Mental Illness and Health, *Action for Mental Health: Final Report* (New York: Basic, 1961), 22.

20. For a discussion of *Action for Mental Health*, see Gerald N. Grob, "The National Institute of Mental Health and Mental Health Policy, 1949–1965," in *Biomedicine in the Twentieth Century: Practices, Policies, and Politics*, ed. Caroline Hannaway (Amsterdam: IOS, 2008), 72–73.

21. See Steven S. Sharfstein, "Whatever Happened to Community Mental Health?," *Psychiatric Services* 51, no. 5 (2000): 616–620.

22. Doris Zames Fleischer and Frieda Zames, *The Disability Rights Movement: From Charity to Confrontation* (Philadelphia: Temple University Press, 2000), 33.

23. One report worried that this health coverage, although well intentioned, simply reinforced white middle-class values. See O. R. Gursslin et al., "Social Class and the Mental Health Movement," in *Mental Health of the Poor*, ed. Frank Riessman et al. (New York: Free Press, 1964), 57–67.

24. See Glen O. Gabbard and Krin Gabbard, *Psychiatry and the Cinema*, 2nd ed. (New York: American Psychiatric Press, 1999), 103. I am indebted to John Horne for this reference to the preview screening of *The Caretakers*.

25. *The Health Care Issues of the 1960s* (New York: Group Health Insurance, 1963), 5.

26. Quoted in Ed Cray, *In Failing Health: The Medical Crisis and the AMA* (Indianapolis: Bobbs-Merrill, 1970), 25.

27. Howard H. Goldman et al., "Deinstitutionalization: The Data Demythologized," *Hospital and Community Psychiatry* 34, no. 2 (1983): 130. The authors argue that despite this shift from inpatient to outpatient, the need to provide institutional care for "chronic and severely disturbed patients" remained high.

28. James W. Trent Jr., *Inventing the Feeble Mind: A History of Mental Retardation in the United States* (Berkeley: University of California Press, 1995), 238.

29. Letter from Karl Menninger to Lillian Smith, 14 March 1944, in *The Selected Correspondence of Karl A. Menninger, 1919–1945*, ed. Howard J. Faulkner and Virginia D. Pruitt (New Haven: Yale University Press, 1988), 400.

30. Michael Harrington, *The Other America* (New York: Macmillan, 1962).

31. Albert Deutsch, *The Mentally Ill in America: A History of Their Care and Treatment from Colonial Times*, 2nd ed. (New York: Columbia University Press, 1949), 518–519.

32. Grob, "The National Institute of Mental Health and Mental Health Policy," 69.

33. Pearl S. Buck, *The Child Who Never Grew* (New York: John Day, 1950), 8.

34. Trent, *Inventing the Feeble Mind*, 230–233.

35. Buck, *The Child Who Never Grew*, 43.

36. Ibid., 46.

37. Ibid.

38. Ibid., 53.

39. Peter Conn, *Pearl S. Buck: A Cultural Biography* (Cambridge: Cambridge University Press, 1996), 111–112.

40. See Stanley Finger and Shawn E. Christ, "Pearl S. Buck and Phenylketonuria (PKU)," *Journal of the History of the Neurosciences* 13, no. 1 (2004), 44–57.

41. Buck, *The Child Who Never Grew*, 56.

42. Maxwell Jones, *Social Psychiatry: A Study of Therapeutic Communities* (London: Tavistock, 1952), 25.

43. Ibid., 156. Frank Leonard praised the British health system, claiming that it was "ten to twenty years ahead" of the US system in terms of humane treatment of mental illness and in limiting involuntary institutionalization (*City Psychiatric* [London: Four Square, 1966], v).

44. Dennie Briggs, *A Life Well Lived: Maxwell Jones—A Memoir* (London: Jessica Kingsley, 2002), 30.

45. Harrington, *The Other America*, 188. For a postwar report on rural health care, see Frederick D. Mott and Milton I. Roemer, *Rural Health and Medical Care* (New York: McGraw-Hill, 1948).

46. See Robert J. Kleiner et al., "Mental Disorder and Status Based on Race," *Psychiatry* 23, no. 3 (1960): 271–274.

47. Robert E. L. Faris and H. Warren Dunham, *Mental Disorders in Urban Areas: An Ecological Study of Schizophrenia and Other Psychoses* (Chicago: University of Chicago Press, 1939).

48. August B. Hollingshead and Fredrick C. Redlich, *Social Class and Mental Illness: A Community Study* (New York: Wiley, 1958); Jerome K. Myers and Bertram H. Roberts, *Family and Class Dynamics in Mental Illness* (New York: Wiley, 1959). These two longitudinal studies were based on statistics drawn from the New Haven, Connecticut, psychiatric census of 1950.

49. Leo Srole and Anita Kassen Fischer, eds., *Mental Health in the Metropolis: The Midtown Manhattan Study*, rev. ed. (New York: Harper, 1975), 9.

50. Ibid., 12.

51. Harrington, *The Other America*, 2.

52. Ibid., 4.

53. E. Franklin Frazier, *The Negro in the United States* (New York: Macmillan, 1949), 636.

54. Abram Kardiner and Lionel Ovesey, *The Mark of Oppression: Explorations in the Personality of the American Negro*, 2nd ed. (Cleveland: Meridian, 1962), 53–54.

55. "The Myth—and the Need," *New York Times*, 17 July 1961.

56. Vern L. Bullough and Bonnie Bullough, *Health Care for the Other Americans* (New York: Appleton-Century-Crofts, 1982), 4.

57. Ibid., 6.

58. Ibid, 8.

59. Samuel K. Roberts Jr., *Infectious Fear: Politics, Disease, and Health Effects of Segregation* (Chapel Hill: University of North Carolina Press, 2009), 5. See also Bullough and Bullough, *Health Care for the Other Americans*, 50, 107.

60. Kardiner and Ovesey, *The Mark of Oppression*, ix.

61. Neil Dayton, *New Facts on Mental Disorders: Study of 89,190 Cases* (Springfield, IL: Thomas, 1940).

62. Benjamin Malzberg, "Mental Disease and 'the Melting Pot,'" *Journal of Nervous and Mental Disease* 72, no. 4 (1930): 379.

63. Benjamin Malzberg, *The Mental Health of the Negro: A Study of First Admissions to Hospitals for Mental Disease in New York State, 1949–1951* (Albany, NY: Research Foundation for Mental Hygiene, 1963), 3–6.

64. Walter A. Adams, "The Negro Patient in Psychiatric Treatment," *American Journal of Orthopsychiatry* 20, no. 2 (1950): 305–310. See also Benjamin Malzberg, "Uses of Alcohol among White and Negro Mental Patients," *Quarterly Journal of Studies on Alcohol* 16, no. 4 (1955): 668–674.

65. Cited by Alvin F. Pouissant, "The Mental Health Status of Black Americans, 1983," in *Handbook of Mental Health and Mental Disorder among Black Americans*, ed. Dorothy S. Ruiz and James P. Comer (New York: Greenwood, 1990), 46.

66. This theme was developed in the United Artists film *Pressure Point* (1962), based on Robert Lindner's case study "Destiny's Tot," in which an African American prison doctor (also played by Poitier) is charged with treating a sociopathic Nazi sympathizer ("Destiny's Tot," in Robert Lindner, *The Fifty-Minute Hour* [New York: Bantam, (1955) 1966], 119–155). For an extended discussion, see Andrea Slane, "The Interracial Treatment Relationship in the Cold War Period: *Pressure Point* in Analysis," in *Celluloid Couches, Cinematic Clients: Psychotherapy in the Movies*, ed. Jerrold R. Brandell (Albany: State University of New York Press, 2004), 47–66.

67. A. B. Sclare, "Cultural Determinants in the Neurotic Negro," in *Mental Health and Segregation*, ed. Martin M. Grossack (New York: Springer, 1963), 173.

68. Janet A. Kennedy, "Problems Posed in the Analysis of Negro Patients," *Psychiatry* 15, no. 3 (1952): 313–327.

69. For a discussion of the wider context of sterilization practices in Virginia, see Pippa Holloway, *Sexuality, Politics, and Social Control in Virginia, 1920–1945* (Chapel Hill: University of North Carolina Press, 2006).

70. See Donald H. Rockwell et al., "The Tuskegee Study of Untreated Syphilis: The Thirtieth Year of Observation," *Archives of Internal Medicine* 114, no. 6 (1964): 792–798. See also James H. Jones, *Bad Blood* (New York: Free Press, 1981); Susan M. Reverby, *Examining Tuskegee: The Infamous Syphilis Study and Its Legacy* (Chapel Hill: University of North Carolina Press, 2009).

71. John Bartlow Martin, "Inside the Asylum," *Saturday Evening Post*, 6 October 1956, 25. Bartlow's focus was the Columbus State Hospital, in Columbus, Ohio.

72. Erving Goffman, *Asylums* (New York: Anchor, 1961), xiii.

73. Ibid., 4–5.

74. For criticism of Goffman's description of total institutions, see Nicos Mouzelis, "On Total Institutions," *Sociology* 5, no. 1 (1971): 113–120.

75. Maxwell Jones, *Social Psychiatry in Practice: The Idea of the Therapeutic Community* (London: Penguin, 1968), 77. See also Maxwell Jones, *Beyond the Therapeutic Community* (New Haven: Yale University Press, 1968), 108–125.

76. Goffman, *Asylums*, 7.

77. Ibid., 18.

78. See R. M. Weinstein, "Goffman's *Asylums* and the Total Institution Model of Mental Hospitals," *Psychiatry* 57, no. 4 (1994): 348–367.

79. Goffman, *Asylums,* 320.

80. Ken Kesey, *One Flew over the Cuckoo's Nest: Text and Criticism*, ed. John Clark Pratt (New York: Penguin, 1973), 341–342.

81. Edward Shorter, *A History of Psychiatry: From the Era of the Asylum to the Age of Prozac* (New York: Wiley, 1997), 275–276.

82. Roger C. Loeb, "Defending the Mental Health Industry," in *Readings on One Flew over the Cuckoo's Nest*, ed. Lawrence Kappel (San Diego: Greenhaven, 2000), 86.

83. J. D. Salinger, *Catcher in the Rye* (London: Penguin, [1949] 1994), 220.

84. Ken Kesey, *Kesey's Garage Sale* (New York: Viking, 1973), 7.

85. Ken Kesey, *One Flew over the Cuckoo's Nest* (New York: Viking, 1962), 218.

86. Ibid., 10.

87. Ibid., 216. Michael E. Staub points out that the anti-authoritarianism demonstrated by McMurphy does not feature at all in *Asylums* (*Madness Is Civilization: When the Diagnosis Was Social, 1948–1980* [Chicago: University of Chicago Press, 2011], 68–69).

88. The United Artists film *The Caretakers* was adapted from Dariel Telfer's 1959 psychosexual novel of the same name.

89. Kesey, *One Flew over the Cuckoo's Nest*, 37, 91.

90. See Erving Goffman, *Frame Analysis: An Essay on the Organization of Experience* (New York: Harper and Row, 1974), 13.

91. Kesey, *One Flew over the Cuckoo's Nest*, 269.

92. Ibid., 68.

93. Catherine Holly (Elizabeth Taylor) is threatened with a lobotomy in the 1959 film *Suddenly, Last Summer* (loosely adapted from Tennessee Williams' one-act play of 1958), linking Catherine's illness to her witnessing prostitution and cannibalism.

94. Erving Goffman, *The Presentation of Self in Everyday Life* (New York: Doubleday, [1956] 1959), 253.

95. For this reading, see Philip Manning, *Erving Goffman and Modern Sociology* (Stanford: Stanford University Press, 1992), 44.

96. Goffman, *Asylums,* 29.

97. Ibid., 14.

98. For a discussion of laughter therapy, see Nicolaus Mills, "Ken Kesey and the Politics of Laughter," *Centennial Review* 16, no. 1 (1972): 82–90.

99. Goffman, *Asylums*, 320.

100. Howard Taubman, "Theater: 'Cuckoo's Nest,'" *New York Times*, 14 November 1963. For reviews of the 1971 stage version, see Kesey, *One Flew over the Cuckoo's Nest*, ed. Pratt, 442–453.

101. Albert F. Wessen, *The Psychiatric Hospital as a Social System* (Springfield, IL: Charles C. Thomas, 1964), 5.

102. Ibid., 18–19.

103. Ibid., 189, 19.

104. Maxwell Jones's permissive techniques at the Belmont Hospital were met with disapproval in the mid-1950s, particularly when the Social Rehabilitation Unit switched from dealing with veterans suffering from war neurosis to people deemed delinquent and psychopathic. See Robert N. Rapoport, *Community as Doctor: New Perspectives on a Therapeutic Community* (London: Tavistock, 1960), 2–3.

105. Howard E. Freeman and Ozzie G. Simmons, *The Mental Patient Comes Home* (New York: John Wiley, 1963), viii–ix, 2.

106. Richard Schickel, "The Frightful Follies of Bedlam," *Life*, 1 December 1967, 12. See also Thomas Szasz, "*The Titicut Follies*: The Forgotten Story of a Case of Psychiatric Censorship," *History of Psychiatry* 18, no. 1 (2007): 123–125; Thomas W. Benson and Carolyn Anderson, *Reality Fictions: The Films of Frederick Wiseman*, 2nd ed. (Carbondale: Southern Illinois University Press, 2002).

107. Mary Frances Robinson and Walter Freeman, *Psychosurgery and the Self* (New York: Grune and Stratton, 1954), 32, 24. Lobotomies declined in frequency in the mid-1950s with the rise of drug treatments.

108. Sylvia Plath, *The Bell Jar* (London: Vintage, [1963] 2006), 1.

109. Allen Ginsberg, *Kaddish and Other Poems 1958–1960* (San Francisco: City Lights, 1961), 35.

110. Ralph Ellison, *Invisible Man* (London: Penguin, [1952] 1965), 193–194. For a discussion of Ellison's psychiatric experience, see J. Bradford Campbell, "The Schizophrenic Solution: Dialectics of Neurosis and Anti-Psychiatric Animus in Ralph Ellison's Invisible Man," *Novel* 43, no. 3 (2010), 443–465; Andrew Fearnley, "Methods to Madness: Race, Knowledge, and American Psychiatry, 1880–2000," PhD diss., University of Cambridge, 2012, 1–3.

111. Martin Cherkasky and Maya Pines, "Tomorrow's Hospitals," *Harper's*, October 1960, 158, 165.

112. For a history of the Milledgeville institution, see Peter G. Cranford, *But for the Grace of God: The Inside Story of the World's Largest Insane Asylum, Milledgeville!* (Augusta, GA: Great Pyramid, 1981).

113. "$14.1 Million Asked for Mental Health," *Atlanta Constitution*, 12 January 1960. "Psychiatry: Out of the Snake Pits," *Time*, 5 April 1963, 82. In 2011 Rosalynn Carter wrote about

her early hospital work and Jack Nelson's exposé of the Milledgeville hospital, and she also reflected on current inadequacies in Georgia's mental healthcare system in "Fixing Ailing System Achievable," *Atlanta Journal-Constitution*, 15 December 2011. For the governor's response to the situation at the hospital, see Harold P. Henderson, *Ernest Vandiver: Governor of Georgia* (Athens: University of Georgia Press, 2000), 101–104.

114. Phil Hardy, *Samuel Fuller* (London: Studio Vista, 1970), 38.

115. Lee Server, *Sam Fuller: Film Is a Battleground* (Jefferson, NC: McFarland, 1994), 88–89.

116. Lisa Dombrowski, *The Films of Samuel Fuller: If You Die, I'll Kill You!* (Middletown, CT: Wesleyan University Press, 2008), 148.

117. Clemmont E. Vontress, "The Negro against Himself," *Journal of Negro Education* 32, no. 3 (1963): 237–242.

118. Jocelyn Landrum-Brown, "Black Mental Health and Racial Oppression," in *Handbook of Mental Health and Mental Disorder among Black Americans*, ed. Ruiz and Comer, 117.

119. Dombrowski, *The Films of Samuel Fuller*, 150.

120. Ibid., 152.

121. Ibid., 154.

122. Kesey, *One Flew over the Cuckoo's Nest*, 3.

123. Sclare, "Cultural Determinants in the Neurotic Negro," 161.

124. Frantz Fanon, *Black Skin, White Masks*, trans. Charles Lam Markmann (New York: Grove, 1982), 111.

125. Goffman, *Asylums*, 60–64.

126. Fanon, *Black Skin, White Masks*, 116.

127. Malzberg, *The Mental Health of the Negro*, 225.

128. Ibid., 223–224.

129. Ibid. See also Norman Q. Brill and Hugh A. Storrow, "Social Class and Psychiatric Treatment," in *Mental Health of the Poor*, ed. Riessman et al., 68–75.

130. Malzberg, *The Mental Health of the Negro*, 227.

131. James Summerville, *Educating Black Doctors: A History of Meharry Medical College* (Tuscaloosa: University of Alabama Press, 1983), 156.

132. For statistics on mental illness among African Americans at mid-century, see Ernest Y. Williams and Claude P. Carmichael, "The Incidence of Mental Disease in the Negro," *Journal of Negro Education* 18, no. 3 (1949): 276–282.

133. Monroe Lerner and Odin W. Anderson, *Health Progress in the United States: 1900–1960* (Chicago: University of Chicago Press, 1963), 121.

134. Gunnar Myrdal, *An American Dilemma: The Negro Problem and American Democracy* (New York: Harper, 1944), 659, 928. See also Richard A. Cuoto, *Ain't Gonna Let Nobody Turn Me Round: The Pursuit of Racial Justice in the Rural South* (Philadelphia: Temple University Press, 1991), 253.

135. Maryland Pennell and Mary Grover, "Urban and Rural Morality from Selected Causes in the North and South," *Public Health Reports* 66, no. 10 (1951): 295–305.

136. Benjamin Pasamanick, "A Survey of Mental Disorder in an Urban Population," in *Mental Health and Segregation*, ed. Grossack, 148–149. See also R. M. Frumkin, "Race and Major Mental Disorders," *Journal of Negro Education* 23, no. 1 (1954): 97–98.

137. The Meharry project is documented in Summerville, *Educating Black Doctors*, 156–157.

138. W. Montague Cobb, "Integration in Medicine: A National Need," *Journal of the National Medical Association* 49, no. 1 (1957): 1–7. See also W. Michael Byrd and Linda A. Clayton, *An American Health Dilemma*, vol. 2, *Race, Medicine and Health Care in the United States* (New York: Routledge, 2002), 249.

139. Max Seham, *Blacks and American Medical Care* (Minneapolis: University of Minnesota Press, 1973), 69–70.

140. Karen Kruse Thomas, "Dr. Jim Crow: The University of North Carolina, the Regional Medical School for Negroes, and the Desegregation of Southern Medical Education, 1945–1960," *Journal of African American History* 88, no. 3 (2003): 223–244; Karen Kruse Thomas, "The Hill-Burton Act and Civil Rights: Expanding Hospital Care for Black Southerners, 1939–1960," *Journal of Southern History* 72, no. 4 (2006): 823–870; Karen Kruse Thomas, *Deluxe Jim Crow: Civil Rights and American Health Policy, 1935–1954* (Athens: University of Georgia Press, 2011).

141. David McBride, *Integrating the City of Medicine: Blacks in Philadelphia Health Care, 1910–1965* (Philadelphia: Temple University Press, 1989), 187; Estelle Massey Riddle, "The Nurse Shortage: A Concern of the Negro Public," *Opportunity* 25 (January 1947): 22–23.

142. Franklin McLean et al., "Progress in Chicago," *Modern Hospital* 79 (August 1952): 68–70.

143. Paul K. Conkin, *Gone with the Ivy: A Biography of Vanderbilt University* (Knoxville: University of Tennessee Press, 1985), 540–545; J. Mack Lofton Jr., *Healing Hands: An Alabama Medical Mosaic* (Tuscaloosa: University of Alabama Press, 1995), 28–29.

144. Dietrich C. Reitzes, *Negroes and Medicine* (Cambridge: Harvard University Press, 1958), xxv–xxvi.

145. Ibid., 8; Charles W. Johnson Sr., *The Spirit of a Place Called Meharry* (Franklin, TN: Hillsboro, 2000), 115; Conkin, *Gone with the Ivy*, 577–580.

146. Anne C. Rose, *Psychology and Selfhood in the Segregated South* (Chapel Hill: University of North Carolina Press, 2009), 70–71; Jeanne Spurlock, "Early and Contemporary Pioneers," in *Black Psychiatrists and American Psychiatry*, ed. Jeanne Spurlock (Washington: American Psychiatric Association, 1999), 3–24.

147. Summerville, *Educating Black Doctors*, 146.

148. "A Proposal for a Program to Increase the Number of Psychologists in the South," the Council of Psychological Resources in the South and the Southern Regional Education Board, 18 August 1955 (Carter Papers, M316, Archives of the History of American Psychology, University of Akron, Akron, OH).

149. Ibid., 3.

150. *Fisk University and Negro Health* (Nashville, TN: Fisk University Department of Publicity, 1937), n.p.

151. Seham, *Blacks and American Medical Care*, 15–16. For an overview of the Hill-Burton Act, see Rosemary Stevens, *In Sickness and in Wealth: American Hospitals in the Twentieth Century* (Baltimore: Johns Hopkins University Press, [1989] 1999), 200–226.

152. Owen Blank et al., "Why White Americans Are Healthier," in *Institutional Racism in America*, ed. Louis L. Knowles and Kenneth Prewitt (Englewood Cliffs, NJ: Prentice-Hall, 1969), 110.

153. Esther Milner, "Some Hypotheses Concerning the Influence of Segregation on Negro Personality Development," *Psychiatry* 16, no. 3 (1953): 291–297.

154. Robert Coles, *The Desegregation of Southern Schools: A Psychiatric Study* (Atlanta: Southern Regional Council, 1963), 5.

155. Byrd and Clayton, *An American Health Dilemma*, 217.

156. Seham, *Blacks and American Medical Care*, 17.

157. Mike Gorman to Mrs. Albert B. Lasker, 19 November 1954, www.docstoc.com/docs/19923727/NATIONAL-MENTAL-HEALTH-COMMITTEE. For Gorman's broader views about inadequate mental health support, see his *Every Other Bed* (Cleveland: World, 1956).

158. P. Preston Reynolds, "Hospitals and Civil Rights, 1945–1963: The Case of *Simpkins v. Moses H. Cones Memorial Hospital*," *Annals of Internal Medicine* 126, no. 11 (1997): 899–900.

159. John A. Kenney Jr., "Medical Rights: The Drive for Medical Equality," *Journal of the National Medical Association* 55, no. 5 (1963): 430–432.

160. Edward H. Beardsley, *A History of Neglect: Health Care for Blacks and Mill Workers in the Twentieth-Century South* (Knoxville: University of Tennessee Press, 1987), 273–274. See also Thomas, "Dr. Jim Crow," 224.

161. Kennedy, *Kennedy and the Press*, 463.

162. Lyndon B. Johnson, "The War on Poverty," in *Speeches of the American Presidents*, ed. Podell and Anzovin, 726.

163. For discussion of the poverty tours, see Beardsley, *A History of Neglect*, 291–297.

164. Nick Kotz, *Let Them Eat Promises: The Politics of Hunger in America* (Englewood Cliffs, NJ: Prentice-Hall, 1969); James Donnelly, "Who Knows, Who Cares," *America*, 1 March 1969, 250–252.

165. For the findings of the Meharry research program under Ralph Hines and a related survey in poor Nashville neighborhoods carried out by George Peabody College in 1966, see Summerville, *Educating Black Doctors*, 157–160.

166. Cray, *In Failing Health*, 20. See also Amasa B. Ford, *Urban Health in America* (New York: Oxford University Press, 1976), 76–94.

167. See Cuoto, *Ain't Gonna Let Nobody Turn Me Round*, 274–275.

168. Paul Goodman, *Growing Up Absurd: Problems of Youth in the Organized Society* (New York: Vintage, 1960), xvi.

CHAPTER 8 — THE HUMAN FACE OF THERAPY

1. Lyndon B. Johnson, "Let Us Continue," 17 November 1963, in *Speeches of the American Presidents*, ed. Janet Podell and Steven Anzovin, 2nd ed. (New York: H. W. Wilson, 2001), 723–724.

2. For a discussion of Johnson's double-edged homage to Kennedy, see Philip Abbott, *Accidental Presidents: Death, Assassination, Resignation, and Democratic Succession* (London: Palgrave Macmillan, 2008), 131–154.

3. Lyndon B. Johnson, "The War on Poverty," 16 March 1964, in *Speeches of the American Presidents*, 728.

4. James T. Patterson, *America's Struggle against Poverty 1900–1980* (Cambridge: Harvard University Press, 1981), 136.

5. Richard M. Nixon, "First Inaugural Address," 20 January 1969, in *Speeches of the American Presidents*, ed. Podell and Anzovin, 769.

6. C. Wright Mills, *The Power Elite* (New York: Oxford University Press, 1956).

7. Lyndon B. Johnson, "The Great Society," 22 May 1964, in *Speeches of the American Presidents*, ed. Podell and Anzovin, 731.

8. Norman Mailer, *The Time of Our Time* (New York: Little, Brown, 1998), 542.

9. Robert F. Rich and William D. White, "Health Care Policy and the United States: Issues of Federalism," in *Health Policy, Federalism, and the American States*, ed. Robert F. Rich and William D. White (Washington: Urban Institute Press, 1996), 19.

10. Lyndon Baines Johnson, *The Vantage Point: Perspectives of the Presidency 1963–1969* (New York: Holt, Rinehart and Winston, 1971), 220, 343. Johnson's perspective was at odds with that of the president of the American Medical Association, Milford O. Rouse, who thought in 1967 that medical care was a privilege, more in line with Nixon's opinion. See Max Seham, *Blacks and American Medical Care* (Minneapolis: University of Minnesota Press, 1973), 2–3.

11. *The Alabama Project on Medicaid* (Birmingham: Alabama Law Institute, University of Alabama, 1997), 2; Eli Ginzberg, *From Health Dollars to Health Services: New York City, 1965–1985* (Totowa, NJ: Rowman and Littlefield, 1986), 8, 20.

12. For Johnson's emphasis on community action and race, see Jill Quadagno, *The Color of Welfare: How Racism Undermined the War on Poverty* (New York: Oxford University Press, 1994).

13. Mailer, *The Time of Our Time*, 542, 544; Herbert Marcuse, "The Individual in the Great Society," in *Towards a Critical Theory of Society*, vol. 2 of *Collected Papers of Herbert Marcuse*, ed. Douglas Kellner (London: Routledge, 2001), 63.

14. Quoted in Jack Valenti, *A Very Human President* (New York: Norton, 1975), 394–395.

15. Philip Rieff, *The Triumph of the Therapeutic* (Chicago: University of Chicago Press, [1966] 1987), 76.

16. Ginzberg, *From Health Dollars to Health Services*, 15.

17. Nixon, "First Inaugural Address," 770.

18. The Mental Health and Mental Retardation Act, 20 October 1966, www.dpw.state .pa.us/ucmprd/groups/wecontent/documents/document/s_001650.pdf.

19. Judith Randal, "The Bright Promise of Neighborhood Health Centers," *Reporter,* 21 March 1968, 15, 16.

20. Ibid., 17. For Howard's contribution to the Taborian Hospital and his career as a civil rights activist (including a year as president of the National Medical Association in the mid-1950s), see David T. Beito and Linda Royster, *Black Maverick: T.R.M. Howard's Fight for Civil Rights and Economic Power* (Urbana: University of Illinois Press, 2009).

21. David T. Beito, "Black Fraternal Hospitals on the Mississippi Delta, 1942–1967," *Journal of Southern History* 65, no. 1 (1999): 109–140.

22. See Seham, *Blacks and American Medical Care*, 90–91.

23. Randal, "The Bright Promise of Neighborhood Health Centers," 18.

24. *The Urban Planner in Health Planning: A Report* (Washington: Department of Health, Education, and Welfare, 1968), 1. For discussion of community projects from a psychiatric perspective, see Leopold Bellak, ed., *Handbook of Community Psychiatry and Community Mental Health* (New York: Grune and Stratton, 1964); Irving N. Berlin, "Transference and Countertransference in Community Psychiatry," *Archives of General Psychiatry* 15, no. 2 (1966), 165–172.

25. Karl Evang et al., *Medical Care and Family Security* (Englewood Cliffs, NJ: Prentice-Hall, 1963), 198–199.

26. T. F. Fox, "Personal Medicine," in *The Health Care Issues of the 1960s* (New York: Group Health Insurance, 1963), 68.

27. "Surgery: The Best Hope of All," *Time,* 3 May 1963, 44–60.

28. Paul S. Rhoads, "The Doctor's Dilemma—Drug Therapy and the Facts of Life," *Archives of Internal Medicine* 107, no. 6 (1961): 810–812.

29. Joseph Turow and Rachel Gans-Boriskin, "From Expert in Action to Existential Angst: A Half Century of Television Doctors," in *Medicine's Moving Pictures*, ed. Leslie J. Reagan et al. (Rochester, NY: University of Rochester Press, 2008), 267–268. Arthur Penn's 1962 film, *The Miracle Worker*, which focused on the educational difficulties of the young Helen Keller (Patty Duke), shared this rehumanizing impulse in the guise of Helen's half-blind tutor, Anne Sullivan (Anne Bancroft).

30. Regina Markell Morantz-Sanchez, *Sympathy and Science: Women Physicians in American Medicine* (New York: Oxford University Press, 1985), 340–342.

31. For an account of occupational health, see Allison Hepler, *Women in Labor: Mothers, Medicine, and Occupational Health in the United States, 1890–1980* (Columbus: Ohio State University Press, 2000). See also Bonnie Noonan, *Women Scientists in Fifties Science Fiction Films* (Jefferson, NC: McFarland, 2005), 48–71.

32. See Ruth H. Howes and Caroline L. Herzenberg, eds, *Their Day in the Sun: Women of the Manhattan Project* (Philadelphia: Temple University Press, 1999).

33. Ellen S. More, *Restoring the Balance: Women Physicians and the Profession of Medicine, 1850–1995* (Cambridge: Harvard University Press, 1999), 186–187.

34. Cited in Julia Kirk Blackwelder, "President Lyndon Johnson and the Gendered World of National Politics," in *Looking Back at LBJ: White House Politics in a New Light*, ed. Mitchell B. Lerner (Lawrence: University Press of Kansas, 2005), 222.

35. Erich Fromm, *The Sane Society*, 360–361.

36. Helen Graham, *The Human Face of Psychology* (Milton Keynes, UK: Open University Press, 1986), 66–67.

37. Sidney Hook, "Science and Mythology in Psychoanalysis," in *Psychoanalysis, Scientific Method, and Philosophy: A Symposium*, ed. Sidney Hook (New York: New York University Press, 1959), 223.

38. William James, "The Will to Believe," in William James, *The Will to Believe and Other Essays in Popular Philosophy* (New York: Dover, [1897] 1956), 21.

39. Quoted in Edward Hoffman, *The Right to Be Human: A Biography of Abraham Maslow* (Wellingborough, UK: Crucible, 1989), 43; Abraham Maslow, *Toward a Psychology of Being*, 2nd ed. (New York: D. Van Nostrand, 1968), 5.

40. Carl Rogers, *Client-Centered Therapy: Its Current Practice, Implications and Theory* (Boston: Houghton Mifflin, 1951), 34.

41. Ibid., x.

42. Ibid., xi.

43. Connections on the theme of anxiety can be made to Rollo May's first book, *The Meaning of Anxiety* (New York: Ronald, 1950) and Ainslie Meares, *The Management of the Anxious Patient* (Philadelphia: W. B. Saunders, 1963).

44. Carl Rogers, *On Becoming a Person: A Therapist's View of Psychotherapy* (Boston: Houghton Mifflin, 1961), 5.

45. Carl Rogers and B. F. Skinner, "Some Issues Concerning the Control of Human Behavior," *Science* 124, no. 3231 (1956): 1057–1065; Carl Rogers, "Education and the Control of Human Behavior," in *Carl Rogers: Dialogues*, ed. Howard Kirschenbaum and Valerie Land Henderson (London: Constable, 1990), 82–152.

46. Rogers, *Client-Centered Therapy*, xi.

47. Ibid., 21, 54.

48. Carl Rogers, "Client-Centered Therapy," in *Carl Rogers: Dialogues*, ed. Kirschenbaum and Henderson, 11.

49. Erving Goffman, "On Face Work," in Erving Goffman, *Interaction Ritual: Essays on Face-to-Face Behavior* (New York: Anchor, 1967), 8.

50. Theodore Isaac Rubin, *Jordi / Lisa and David* (New York: Macmillan, [1962] 1990), 4. See also Jerrold R. Brandell, "Translating Psychotherapy Narratives from Literature onto Film: An Interview with Theodore Isaac Rubin," in *Celluloid Couches, Cinematic Clients:*

Psychotherapy in the Movies, ed. Jerrold R. Brandell (Albany: State University of New York Press, 2004), 217–233.

51. Goffman, "On Face Work," 31.

52. Alan Petigny, The *Permissive Society: America, 1941–1965* (New York: Cambridge University Press, 2009), 77–79.

53. Rogers, *Client-Centered Therapy*, 203.

54. For an overview of third-force psychology, see Linda Sargent Wood, *A More Perfect Union: Holistic Worldviews and the Transformation of American Culture after World War II* (New York: Oxford University Press, 2010), 139–168.

55. Maslow, *Toward a Psychology of Being*, 13.

56. Carl Rogers, "A Therapist's View of Personal Goals," excerpted in *The Carl Rogers Reader*, ed. Howard Kirschenbaum and Valerie Land Henderson (London: Constable, 1990), 436–438.

57. Carl Rogers, "Some Questions and Challenges Facing a Humanistic Psychology," paper presented at the annual meeting of the Association of Humanistic Psychology, Los Angeles, CA, 3 September 1964, 1 (Knapp Papers, M642, Archives of the History of American Psychology, University of Akron, Akron, OH).

58. Ibid., 1–2.

59. Jessie Taft, *Otto Rank* (New York: Julian, 1958), 148.

60. Otto Rank, *Psychology and the Soul: A Study of the Origin, Conceptual Evolution, and Nature of the Soul*, trans. Gregory C. Richter and E. James Lieberman (Baltimore: Johns Hopkins University Press, 1988), 2; Carl Rogers, *Counseling and Psychotherapy: Newer Concepts in Practice* (Boston: Houghton Mifflin, 1942), 28 (see also 85–113). For Rank's influence on Rogers, see E. James Lieberman, *Acts of Will: The Life and Work of Otto Rank* (Amherst: University of Massachusetts Press, 1985), 365, 397.

61. Otto Rank, *Beyond Psychology* (New York: Dover, 1941), 12, 29.

62. Ludwig Binswanger, *Being-in-the-World: Selected Papers of Ludwig Binswanger*, ed. and trans. Jacob Needleman (New York: Basic, 1963), 186.

63. Sigmund Freud, "A Philosophy of Life," in Sigmund Freud, *New Introductory Lectures on Psycho-Analysis*, 3rd ed., trans. W.J.H. Sprott (London: Hogarth, 1946), 202.

64. Binswanger, *Being-in-the-World*, 207–208.

65. Ludwig Binswanger, "The Case of Ellen West," in *Existence: A New Dimension in Psychiatry and Psychology*, ed. Rollo May et al. (New York: Basic, 1958), 329; Binswanger, *Being in the World*, 208–209.

66. Ludwig Binswanger, "The Existential Analysis School of Thought," in *Existence*, ed. May et al., 193.

67. Martin Buber, *I and Thou*, trans. R. G. Smith (Edinburgh: T. and T. Clark, [1937] 1987).

68. Binswanger, "The Case of Ellen West," 315.

69. Frieda Fromm-Reichmann, *Principles of Intensive Psychotherapy* (Chicago: University of Chicago Press, 1960), 30.

70. Binswanger, *Being-in-the-World*, 251.

71. Binswanger, "The Existential Analysis School of Thought," 201.

72. For a discussion of these two cases, see Martin Halliwell, *Romantic Science and the Experience of Self* (Brookfield, VT: Ashgate, 1999), 136–155.

73. Binswanger, "The Existential Analysis School of Thought," 198.

74. Carl Rogers, *A Way of Being* (Boston: Houghton Mifflin, 1980), 165. See also his 1961 article "Ellen West—and Loneliness," in Rogers, *The Carl Rogers Reader*, 157–168.

75. Rogers, *A Way of Being*, 166.

76. Ibid., 174.

77. Ibid., 175.

78. Carl Rogers dialogue with Martin Buber in *Carl Rogers: Dialogues*, ed. Kirschenbaum and Henderson, 43–63.

79. Petigny, *Permissive Society*, 155–157.

80. The two cases (Loretta as a transcript, Gloria in summary) are included in Barry A. Farber et al., *The Psychotherapy of Carl Rogers: Cases and Commentary* (New York: Guilford, 1996), 33–73. Both cases are presented with additional commentary. For the full case of Gloria, see *Operational Theories of Personality*, ed. Arthur Burton (New York: Brunner/Mazel, 1974), 237–254.

81. The results of the collaborative schizophrenia project appeared in 1967, in *The Therapeutic Relationship and Its Impact: A Study of Psychotherapy with Schizophrenics*, which provided evidence suggesting that empathy can help the therapeutic outcome. See Howard Kirschenbaum, *The Life and Work of Carl Rogers* (Ross-on-Wye, UK: PCCS, 2007), 283–297.

82. Rogers, "The Case of Loretta (1958)," in Farber et al., *The Psychotherapy of Carl Rogers*, 34.

83. Ibid., 35.

84. Ibid., 43. For a careful reading of the case study, see Nathaniel J. Raskin, "The Case of Loretta," in Farber et al., *The Psychotherapy of Carl Rogers*, 44–56.

85. For the results of an empathic approach, see Greet Vanaerschot, "Empathy as Releasing Several Micro-Processes in the Client," in *Beyond Carl Rogers*, ed. David Brazier (London: Constable, 1993), 47–71.

86. Brian Thorne, *Carl Rogers* (London: Sage, 1992), 52.

87. Abraham Maslow, *Religions, Values, and Peak-Experiences* (Columbus: Ohio State University Press, 1964).

88. Fred Zimring, "Rogers and Gloria," in Farber et al., *The Psychotherapy of Carl Rogers*, 68.

89. The transcript of the session has 249 additional words in which Gloria reveals her feelings to her father. See Rogers, "The Case of Gloria (1964)," in Farber et al., *The Psychotherapy of Carl Rogers*, 57, 63–64.

90. Richard Noll, *American Madness: The Rise and Fall of Dementia Praecox* (Cambridge: Harvard University Press, 2011), 36–48, 232–275.

91. Lisa Appignanesi, *Mad, Bad and Sad: A History of Women and Mind Doctors from 1800 to the Present* (London: Virago, 2008), 221–229; Janet Colaizzi, *Homicidal Insanity, 1800–1985* (Birmingham: University of Alabama Press, 1989), 109; Sally Cline, *Zelda Fitzgerald: Her Voice in Paradise* (New York: Arcade, 2003), 261–272.

92. Jules D. Holzberg, "Sex Differences in Schizophrenia," *Advances in Sex Research* 1 (October 1963): 241.

93. Ibid., 243.

94. Jonas R. Rappeport and George Lassen, "Dangerousness: Arrest Rate Comparison of Discharged Patients and the General Population," *American Journal of Psychiatry* 121, no. 8 (1965): 776–783; Jonas R. Rappeport and George Lassen, "The Dangerousness of Female Patients: A Comparison of the Arrest Rate of Discharged Psychiatric Patients and the General Population," *American Journal of Psychiatry* 123, no. 4 (1966): 413–419.

95. For discussion of Erich Fromm and Frieda Reichmann's German years, see Lawrence Friedman, *The Lives of Erich Fromm: Love's Prophet* (New York: Columbia University Press, 2013), chapter 1.

96. Fromm-Reichmann, *Principles of Intensive Psychotherapy*, 214.

97. Quoted in Thomas H. McGlashlan and William T. Carpenter, "Identifying Unmet Therapeutic Domains in Schizophrenia Patients: The Early Contributions of Wayne Fenton from Chestnut Lodge," *Schizophrenia Bulletin* 33, no. 5 (2007): 1090.

98. Appignanesi, *Mad, Bad and Sad*, 249–250; Cline, *Zelda Fitzgerald*, 349–362, 400–402.

99. Gail A. Hornstein, *To Redeem One Person Is to Redeem the World: The Life of Frieda Fromm-Reichmann* (New York: Free Press, 2000), 350. Hornstein discusses the mixed reviews of Greenberg's book and the tensions between the different ways of reading it—as case history, disguised autobiography, and fiction (352–355, 371–372).

100. Joanne Greenberg, *I Never Promised You a Rose Garden*, with a new afterword (New York: St Martin's, 2004), 40.

101. Ramírez had been hospitalized since the early 1930s at Stockton State Hosptial, before moving to DeWitt, a former military hospital, in 1948. There he was discovered by a professor of psychology and art, Tarmo Pasto, which led to four solo exhibits between 1951 and 1961 (including "The Art of a Schizophrene" in Oakland and "Art from the Disturbed Mind" at Stanford University, both in 1954), as well as a retrospective at DeWitt after Ramírez's death in 1963. His reputation as an outsider artist has grown since the 1970s and 1980s. See Lynne Cooke et al., *Martín Ramírez: Reframing Confinement* (Madrid: Museo Nacional Centro de Arte Reina Sofía, 2010).

102. Greenberg, *I Never Promised You a Rose Garden*, 14.

103. Ibid., 4–5. The term "midworld" corresponds to Binswanger's description of *Mitwelt* and links to the experience of "co-being" or *Mitsein* (Ludwig Binswanger, "Insanity as

Life-Historical Phenomenon and as Mental Disease: The Case of Ilse," in *Existence*, ed. May et al., 224, 226).

104. Greenberg, *I Never Promised You a Rose Garden*, 106.

105. Hornstein, *To Redeem One Person Is to Redeem the World*, xvii.

106. Ibid., 232.

107. Ibid., 234–235.

108. Greenberg, *I Never Promised You a Rose Garden*, 31.

109. Ibid., 50–51.

110. Ibid., 70.

111. Ibid., 71.

112. Ibid., 116–117, 121.

113. Ibid., 212.

114. Mary Barnes and Joseph Berke, *Mary Barnes: Two Accounts of a Journey through Madness* (London: MacGibbon and Kee, 1971).

115. Binswanger, *Being-in-the-World*, 296; Ludwig Binswanger, *Dream and Existence*, ed. Keith Hoeller (Atlantic Highlands, NJ: Humanities, [1930] 1993), 99.

116. Hornstein, *To Redeem One Person Is to Redeem the World*, 374. For a perceptive reading of Greenberg's text, see Jerrold R. Brandell, "Kids on the Couch: Hollywood's Vision of Child and Adolescent Treatment," in *Celluloid Couches, Cinematic Clients*, ed. Brandell, 22–29.

117. For comparative national suicide statistics in 1955 and 1965, see Erwin Stengel, *Suicide and Attempted Suicide*, rev. ed. (London: Penguin, 1970), 19–22.

118. Appignanesi, *Mad, Bad and Sad*, 340.

119. Jean-Paul Sartre, *Being and Nothingness*, trans. Hazel E. Barnes (London: Methuen, [1943] 1958), 479. For Arbus's view on suicide and her death, see Patricia Bosworth, *Diane Arbus: A Biography* (London: Vintage, [1984] 2005), 220, 309–21.

120. Hal Foster, "Blinded Insights," in Cooke et al., *Martín Ramírez*, 163.

121. Quoted in Eric F. Goldman, *The Tragedy of Lyndon Johnson* (New York: Knopf, 1969), 13.

122. Foster, "Blinded Insights," 163.

123. Robert E. Gilbert, *The Mortal Presidency: Illness and Anguish in the White House* (New York: Fordham University Press, 1998), 193–201.

124. Laura D. Hirshbein, *American Melancholy: Constructions of Depression in the Twentieth Century* (New Brunswick, NJ: Rutgers University Press, 2009), 29.

125. Ibid., 12–13.

126. Laura D. Hirshbein, "Science, Gender, and the Emergence of Depression in American Psychiatry, 1952–1980," *Journal of the History of Medicine and Allied Sciences* 61, no. 2 (2006), 193–194.

127. Ibid., 200–201.

128. Ibid. See also David G. Schuster, *Neurasthenic Nation: America's Search for Health, Happiness, and Comfort, 1869–1920* (New Brunswick, NJ: Rutgers University Press, 2011), 95–110.

129. Quoted in Charlotte Silverman, *The Epidemiology of Depression* (Baltimore: Johns Hopkins University Press, 1968), 136.

130. Hirshbein, *American Melancholy*, 35.

131. For a discussion of overdiagnosis among African Americans, see Diane R. Brown and Verna M. Keith, eds, *In and Out of Our Right Minds: The Mental Health of African American Women* (New York: Columbia University Press, 2003), 39.

132. Data from the National Center for Health Statistics (1970–1989), extrapolated by Jacquelyne J. Jackson, "Suicide Trends of Blacks and Whites by Sex and Age," in *Handbook of Mental Health and Mental Disorder among Black Americans*, ed. Dorothy S. Ruiz and James P. Comer (New York: Greenwood, 1990), 98.

133. A 1954 study concluded that suicide among African Americans fluctuated less with the ups and downs of the business cycle than did suicide among whites. See Andrew F. Henry and James F. Short Jr., *Suicide and Homicide: Some Economic, Sociological and Psychological Aspects of Aggression* (New York: Free Press, 1954), 23–44.

134. "The Meaning of Tragedy in Birmingham," 22 September 1963 (Box 54, Folder 11, Reinhold Niebuhr Papers, Library of Congress Manuscript Room, Washington, DC).

135. James Baldwin, *Another Country* (London: Penguin, 1963), 14.

136. Ibid., 92.

137. For a comparative discussion of modernist urban suicides, see Catherine Morley, *Modern American Literature* (Edinburgh: Edinburgh University Press, 2012), 97–98.

138. Gunnar Myrdal, introduction to Kenneth B. Clark, *Dark Ghetto: Dilemmas of Social Power* (Middletown, CT: Wesleyan University Press, [1965] 1989), xi.

139. Lee Rainwater, *Behind Ghetto Walls: Black Families in a Federal Slum* (Chicago: Aldine, 1970); C. V. Willie et al., eds., *Racism and Mental Health* (Pittsburgh: University of Pittsburgh Press, 1973).

140. Abraham Maslow, "Neurosis as a Failure of Personal Growth," paper presented at the Institute of Man Symposium, Duquesne University, Pittsburgh, PA, 18 November 1966, 9. (Maslow published a version of this lecture as "Neurosis as a Failure of Personal Growth," *Humanitas* 3 [1967]: 153–169).

141. Ibid., 11.

142. Carl Elliott and John Lantos, eds., *The Last Physician: Walker Percy and the Moral Life of Medicine* (Durham, NC: Duke University Press, 1999), 3.

143. Walker Percy, "From Facts to Fiction," in *Signposts in a Strange Land*, ed. Patrick Samway (New York: Farrar, Straus and Giroux, 1991), 188.

144. Bertram Wyatt-Brown, "Inherited Depression, Medicine, and Illness in Walker Percy's Art," in *The Last Physician*, ed. Elliott and Lantos, 114–115.

145. Ibid., 117. For a discussion of Sullivan, see Robert Coles, *Walker Percy: An American Search* (Boston: Little, Brown, 1978), 17–20. For Percy's family background, see Bertram Wyatt-Brown, *The House of Percy: Honor, Melancholy, and Imagination in a Southern Family* (New York: Oxford University Press, 1994).

146. Coles, *Walker Percy*, 176. Percy likened Will Barrett to the epileptic Christ-like figure of Myshkin in Doestovsky's *The Idiot* (1869), combining a medical affliction with an existential commitment to help others (188).

147. Walker Percy, *The Last Gentleman* (New York: Farrar, Straus and Giroux, 1966), 4, 11.

148. Ibid., 12.

149. Ibid., 50.

150. For a suggestion that Will Barrett and Sutter Vaught represent two facets of the novelist's life, see Ross McElwee, "The Act of Seeing with One's Own Eyes," in *The Last Physician*, ed. Elliott and Lantos, 16–37.

CHAPTER 9 — COUNTERCULTURE

1 Herbert Marcuse, *One Dimensional Man: The Ideology of Industrial Society* (London: Sphere, [1964] 1968), 11.

2. Paul A. Robinson, *The Freudian Left: Wilhelm Reich, Geza Roheim, Herbert Marcuse* (New York: Harper and Row, 1969).

3. Abraham Maslow, "The Farther Reaches of Human Nature," *Journal of Transpersonal Psychology* 1, no. 1 (1969): 1.

4. Ibid., 4.

5. Ibid., 6.

6. For British parallels, see Mathew Thomson, *Psychological Subjects: Identity, Culture, and Health in Twentieth-Century Britain* (Oxford: Oxford University Press, 2006), 273–278.

7. Maslow, "The Farther Reaches of Human Nature," 8.

8. Ibid., 8–9.

9. Ibid., 9.

10. I am grateful to Alexander Dunst for our conversations on Herbert Marcuse and Richard Hofstadter, as reflected in Dunst's "Politics of Madness: Crisis as Psychosis in the United States, 1950–2010," PhD diss., University of Nottingham, 2010.

11. Herbert Marcuse, "Beyond One-Dimensional Man," in *Towards a Critical Theory of Society*, vol. 2 of *Collected Papers of Herbert Marcuse*, ed. Douglas Kellner (London: Routledge, 2001), 114.

12. Herbert Marcuse, *Negations: Essays in Critical Theory*, trans. Jeremy J. Shapiro (Boston: Beacon, 1968), 248–249; Alan Watts, "From Time to Eternity," in Alan Watts, *Eastern Wisdom, Modern Life: Collected Talks 1960–1969* (Novato, CA: New World Library, 2006), 109.

13. Marcuse, *Negations*, 251.

14. Buryl Payne, *Getting There without Drugs* (New York: Viking, 1973), ix.

15. Robinson, *The Freudian Left*, 174.

16. Herbert Marcuse, *Eros and Civilization* (London: Ark, [1956] 1987), 241, 243.

17. Ibid., 262. See also the selection of "psychoanalytic interventions" in Herbert Marcuse, *Philosophy, Psychoanalysis and Emancipation*, ed. Douglas Kellner and Clayton Pierce, vol. 5 of *Collected Papers of Herbert Marcuse* (New York: Routledge, 2011), 101–131.

18. Marcuse, *One Dimensional Man*, 9.

19. Ibid., 9–10.

20. Ibid., 196.

21. Ibid., 200–201.

22. Frederick S. Perls, *Gestalt Therapy Verbatim* (Gouldsboro, ME: Gestalt Journal Press, [1969] 1992), 21.

23. Ibid., 22.

24. Ibid., 21. For critical views of Perls, see Joyce Milton, *The Road to Malpsychia: Humanistic Psychology and Our Discontents* (New York: Encounter, 2002); Walter Truett Anderson, *The Upstart Spring: Esalen and the American Awakening* (Reading, MA: Addison-Wesley, 1983).

25. Perls, *Gestalt Therapy Verbatim*, 23.

26. For discussion of Perls at the Esalen Institute, see Martin Shepard, *Fritz: An Intimate Portrait of Fritz Perls and Gestalt Therapy* (New York: Saturday Review Press, 1975), 115–131; Petruska Clarkson and Jennifer Mackewn, *Fritz Perls* (London: Sage, 1993), 24–27.

27. Frederick Perls, "Author's Note" (1969), in Frederick S. Perls et al., *Gestalt Therapy: Excitement and Growth in the Human Personality* (London: Penguin, 1973), vi. See also Perls, *Gestalt Therapy Verbatim*, 57.

28. Perls, *Gestalt Therapy Verbatim*, 29, 22.

29. Ibid., 35.

30. Ibid., 49.

31. Ibid., 48.

32. Anderson, *The Upstart Spring*, 65; Linda Sargent Wood, *A More Perfect Union: Holistic Worldviews and the Transformation of American Culture after World War II* (New York: Oxford University Press, 2010), 5.

33. Anderson, *The Upstart Spring*, 6.

34. Timothy Leary, *Interpersonal Diagnosis of Personality* (New York: Ronald, 1957), 4–5, 8–9, 12.

35. Timothy Leary, *Politics of Ecstasy* (New York: G. P. Putnam's, 1968), 319–320. By 1960 Watts had both a radio show, *Way Beyond the West*, and a television show, *Eastern Wisdom in Modern Life*, both of which were broadcast on the West Coast.

36. Ibid., 92.

37. Ibid., 14. For a contextual discussion, see Robert Greenfield, *Timothy Leary: A Biography* (Orlando, FL: Harcourt, 2006), 341–343.

38. Leary, *Politics of Ecstasy*, 362–363.

39. Timothy Leary, *Changing My Mind, Among Others: Lifetime Writings* (Englewood Cliffs, NJ: Prentice-Hall, 1982), x.

40. Leary, *Politics of Ecstasy*, 365. In the 1970s Leary developed his emphasis on neurology into an eight-phase evolutionary model (*NeuroLogic*, 1973) and then into a twenty-four stage model (*Exo-Psychology*, 1977).

41. Leary, *Politics of Ecstasy*, 371. Leary discussed the ways in which LSD can imprint experience in the early to mid-1960s (*Changing My Mind, Among Others*, 119–130).

42. Leary, *Politics of Ecstasy*, 371.

43. Richard H. King, *Party of Eros: Radical Social Thought and the Realm of Freedom* (New York: Delta, 1973), 158.

44. Norman O. Brown, "Apocalypse: The Place of Mystery in the Life of the Mind," in Norman O. Brown, *Apocalypse and/or Metamorphosis* (Berkeley: University of California Press, 1991), 1, 2.

45. Norman O. Brown, *Love's Body* (New York: Random House, 1966), 222.

46. For an overview of anti-psychiatry, see Digby Tantam, "The Anti-Psychiatry Movement," in *150 Years of British Psychiatry, 1841–1991*, ed. German E. Berrios and Hugh Freeman (London: Gaskell, 1991), 333–347. Discussion of the French and Italian wings of anti-psychiatry lie outside this study: for Gilles Deleuze and Félix Guattari's schizoanalysis, see their *Anti-Oedipus*, trans. Robert Hurley et al. (New York: Continuum, [1972] 2004); for a selection of Basaglia's writings, see *Psychiatry Inside Out: Selected Writings of Franco Basaglia*, ed. Nancy Scheper-Hughes and Anne M. Lovell, trans. Anne M. Lovell and Teresa Shtob (New York: Columbia University Press, 1987).

47. David Cooper, *Psychiatry and Anti-Psychiatry* (London: Paladin, [1967] 1970), 27.

48. David Cooper, introduction to *The Dialectics of Liberation*, ed. David Cooper (London: Penguin, 1968), 7.

49. Marcuse, *Negations*, 253.

50. Ibid., 254.

51. Ibid.

52. Cooper, *Psychiatry and Anti-Psychiatry*, 34.

53. Ibid., 10, 26. The second edition of *Diagnostic and Statistical Manual of Mental Disorders* (*DSM-II*) continued to draw on psychoanalytic concepts to explain personality disorders, but this 1968 edition was arguably as vague as its 1952 predecessor. The second edition underlined the inconsistency of some psychiatric diagnoses and, although it was published at the height of the Vietnam War, skirted around the psychological impact of war. See Basil Jackson, "The Revised Diagnostic and Statistical Manual of the American Psychiatric Association," *American Journal of Psychiatry* 127, no. 1 (1970): 65–73.

54. Thomas J. Scheff, *Being Mentally Ill: A Sociological Theory*, 2nd ed. (New York: Aldine, 1984), 40, 38.

55. Ibid., 159.

56. Ibid., 7.

57. Thomas Szasz, *Insanity: The Idea and Its Consequences* (New York: Wiley, 1987), 12. For a discussion of Szasz within the context of *DSM*, see Rick Mayes and Allan V. Horwitz, "DSM-III and the Revolution in the Classification of Mental Illness," *Journal of the History of the Behavioral Sciences* 41, no. 3 (2005): 249–267.

58. Cooper, *Psychiatry and Anti-Psychiatry*, 10.

59. John Clay, *R. D. Laing: A Divided Self* (London: Hodder and Stoughton, 1996), 117.

60. Szasz believed that patients collude in their invalidism, and he later criticized Laing's patient Mary Barnes for inventing both her condition and her cure (Thomas Szasz, *Schizophrenia: The Sacred Symbol of Psychiatry* [Syracuse, NY: Syracuse University Press, 1976]). For a discussion of Szasz's criticisms of Laing, see Daniel Burston, *The Wing of Madness: The Life and Work of R. D. Laing* (Cambridge: Harvard University Press, 1996), 170–171.

61. Thomas Szasz, "Bootlegging Humanistic Values through Psychiatry" (1962), in Thomas Szasz, *Ideology and Insanity* (Garden City, NY: Doubleday, 1970), 87–97.

62. Bob Mullan, *Mad to be Normal: Conversations with R. D. Laing* (London: Free Association, 1995), 107.

63. Foucault's lectures at the Collège de France in 1973–1974 shared Laing's interest in discipline and surveillance within families. See Mauro Basaure, "Foucault and the 'Anti-Oedipus Movement': Psychoanalysis as Disciplinary Power," *Journal of Psychiatry* 20, no. 3 (2009): 340–359. Laing claims that his work was not heavily influenced by Foucault, except for a section of *The Voice of Experience* (1982) in which he discusses the panopticon as a structure of surveillance. For a critical discussion of Foucault's *Madness and Civilization* in dialogue with anti-psychiatry, see Peter Sedgwick, "Michel Foucault: The Anti-History of Psychiatry," *Psychological Medicine* 11, no. 2 (1981): 235–248.

64. Michel Foucault, *Madness and Civilization: A History of Insanity in the Age of Reason*, trans. Richard Howard (London: Routledge, [1967] 1993), 58.

65. Erving Goffman, "The Insanity of Place," in Erving Goffman, *Relations in Public: Microstudies of the Public Order* (London: Penguin, 1972), 415.

66. Ibid., 422.

67. Ibid., 436.

68. Ibid., 440.

69. Garry Wills, *Nixon Agonistes: The Crisis of the Self-Made Man* (New York: Signet [1970] 1979), 368–376.

70. Herbert Block, *Herblock Special Report* (New York: Norton, 1974), 47, 53.

71. William Costello, *The Facts about Nixon* (New York: Viking, 1960), 290; Jules Whitcover, *The Resurrection of Richard Nixon* (New York: Putnam's, 1970), 23; Arthur J. Schlesinger Jr., "A Skeptical Democrat Looks at President Nixon," *New York Times*, 17 November 1968.

72. Schlesinger, "A Skeptical Democrat Looks at President Nixon."

73. Ibid. Rose McDermott argues that Nixon's "borderline tendency" was one of his psychiatric symptoms that might have affected his foreign policy (*Presidential Leadership, Illness, and Decision Making* [Cambridge: Cambridge University Press, 2008], 159, 187–194).

74. Robert B. Semple, "Sensible Compromise, or a Failure of Leadership?," *New York Times*, 21 September 1969; Robert B. Semple, "Impulsive Nixon Action," *New York Times*, 5 August 1970.

75. Richard M. Nixon, "First Inaugural Address," 20 January 1969, in *Speeches of the American Presidents*, ed. Janet Podell and Steven Anzovin, 2nd ed. (New York: H. W. Wilson, 2001), 769–770; Richard M. Nixon, "Toward an Open World," 18 September 1969, ibid., 770–771.

76. Richard Hofstadter, "The Paranoid Style in American Politics," *Harper's*, May 1964, 77.

77. Media mistrust of Nixon continued into the 1960s, but he faded from the spotlight briefly after losing presidential and gubernatorial elections in 1960 and 1962, and he chose not to run for president in 1964, when Barry Goldwater became the Republican candidate.

78. Hofstadter, "The Paranoid Style in American Politics," 77.

79. Sigmund Freud, "Some Neurotic Mechanisms in Jealousy, Paranoia, and Homosexuality," in *The Standard Edition of the Complete Psychological Works of Sigmund Freud*, trans. and ed. James Strachey (London: Hogarth, 1981), 18:221–232.

80. "Medical Scientists Differ on Safety of Marijuana," *New York Times*, 9 October 1967.

81. Ronald K. Siegel and Louis J. West, *Hallucinations: Behavior, Experience, and Theory* (New York: Wiley, 1975), ix, 81–161. For the 1958 symposium on hallucinations, see Louis J. West, ed., *Hallucinations* (New York: Grune and Stratton, 1962).

82. Payne, *Getting There without Drugs*, xii. Scientists at the State University of New York at Buffalo and the University of Oregon released reports about genetic abnormalities linked to LSD use. See "Study Links LSD to Cell Damage," *New York Times*, 16 May 1967.

83. J. R. Wittenborn et al., eds., *Drugs and Youth: Proceedings of the Rutgers Symposium on Drug Abuse* (Springfield, IL: Charles C. Thomas, 1969); *Youth and Drugs: A Handbook for Parents* (Houston, TX: Parents League of Houston, 1969); and Donald J. Wolk, ed., *Drugs and Youth* (Washington: National Council for Social Studies, 1971).

84. Richard M. Nixon, "President Nixon's Speech to the Congress on Drug Abuse," 17 June 1971, in Richard M. Nixon, *Nixon: The First Year of his Presidency* (Washington: Congressional Quarterly, 1970), 63A–64A.

85. Ibid., 63A.

86. David J. Bentel et al., "Drug Abuse in Combat: The Crisis of Drugs and Addiction among American Troops in Vietnam," in *It's So Good, Don't Even Try It Once: Heroin in Perspective*, ed. David E. Smith and George R. Gay (Englewood Cliffs, NJ: Prentice-Hall, 1972), 60. See John Steinbeck IV, "The Importance of Being Stoned in Vietnam," *Washingtonian*, January 1968, 33–35, 56–60; John Steinbeck IV, *In Touch* (New York: Knopf, 1969), especially 188–193. In an article on Alpha Company, "a microcosm of the Army in evolution," the estimate for

marijuana smoking in Vietnam ranged from 7 percent (by the troop's commander) to 85 percent (by "the senior pothead"), with the troop divided between "juicers" and "smokers"—the groups are described in the text below (John Saar, "You Can't Just Hand Out Orders," *Life*, 23 October 1970. 31–37).

87. George R. Gay et al., "The Haight-Ashbury Free Medical Centre," in *It's So Good, Don't Even Try It Once*, ed. Smith and Gay, 73; "The Binoctal Craze," *US Army Medical Bulletin* 40 (May–June 1969): 40.

88. Steinbeck, "The Importance of Being Stoned in Vietnam," 34–35.

89. David E. Smith and Donald R. Wesson, eds., *Uppers and Downers* (Englewood Cliffs, NJ: Prentice-Hall, 1973), 3; Bentel et al., "Drug Abuse in Combat," 59; "War on Drugs," *Newsweek* (28 June 1971), 32–36.

90. Bentel et al., "Drug Abuse in Combat," 61.

91. Ibid., 63–64.

92. Ibid., 65. The authors discuss the claim that the South Vietnamese government realized in the summer of 1970 that it was could make a profit by allowing US soldiers access to heroin shipped in from Laos, Burma, and Thailand (66).

93. Ibid., 70. Many of the health consequences of the Vietnam War did not become public knowledge until well into the 1970s, and therefore they lie beyond the historical bounds of this study. Reports on physical and psychiatric illness started to emerge during the mid-1970s, together with public sensitivity toward the extensive use of the defoliant Agent Orange between 1965 and 1967. The use was discontinued in spring 1970 (ten months before all herbicides were banned by President Nixon), following studies sponsored by the National Cancer Institute that verified a link between exposure to Agent Orange and birth defects in the children of those who had been exposed. No public investigation into Agent Orange took place until after 1977; after that, there were hearings in Congress over the next two years and an official investigation commissioned by President Carter in 1979.

94. Eldridge Cleaver, *Soul on Ice* (London: Jonathan Cape, 1969), 125, 123.

95. For Cleaver's statement on Leary (including his view that acid does "nothing except [destroy] your own brains and [strengthen] the hands of our enemy"), see Cleaver's taped statement to the underground press and reported in Norman Spinrad, "Leary Busted," *Los Angeles Free Press*, 5 February 1971. See also Greenfield, *Timothy Leary*, 419–420.

96. Kenneth B. Clark, *Dark Ghetto: Dilemmas of Social Power* (Middletown, CT: Wesleyan University Press, 1989), 89–106.

97. Ibid., 104. See Daniel Matlin, *On the Corner: Black Intellectuals and the Urban Crisis* (Cambridge: Harvard University Press, 2013), chapter 1.

98. Cleaver's writing is full of sexualized rhetoric. For example, he positioned James Baldwin as the opposite of black revolutionary power, citing Baldwin's homosexuality as a "racial death wish" (*Soul on Ice*, 102–104).

99. James Summerville, *Educating Black Doctors* (Tuscaloosa: University of Alabama Press, 1983), 184.

100. Ibid., 182–183.

101. William H. Grier and Price M. Cobbs, *Black Rage* (New York: Basic, 1968), xi.

102. Daryl Michael Scott, *Contempt and Pity: Social Policy and the Image of the Damaged Black Psyche, 1880–1996* (Chapel Hill: University of North Carolina Press, 1997), 162–177.

103. See Chester M. Pierce, "The Formation of the Black Psychiatrists of America," in *Racism and Mental Health*, ed. Charles V. Willie et al. (Pittsburgh: University of Pittsburgh Press, 1973), 525–54. Another conference focusing on medicine in the ghetto was held in Portsmouth, New Hampshire, in June 1969, sponsored by the Harvard Medical School, the *Boston Globe*, and the National Center for Health Services Research and Development. Racism was the primary theme, and midway through proceedings a "confrontation" occurred, in which dissatisfied activists mounted an impromptu session demanding the "'truth' concerning the hard realities of money and establishment support for ghetto medicine" (John C. Norman, ed., *Medicine in the Ghetto* [New York: Appleton-Century-Crofts, 1969], 321).

104. Grier and Cobbs, *Black Rage*, 3. For Cobbs's role in the Esalen interracial encounter groups, see Anderson, *The Upstart Spring*, 162–164, 187–188, 196–197.

105. Grier and Cobbs, *Black Rage*, 158–159.

106. Ibid., 161. The case of Miss Y is outlined on 158–160.

107. Ibid., 178–179.

108. Ibid., 179.

109. For a discussion of the racialized crosscurrents of schizophrenia in the 1960s and Cobbs and Grier's claim that some forms of schizophrenia might be a healthy response to institutional racism, see Jonathan M. Metzl, *The Protest Psychosis: How Schizophrenia Became a Black Disease* (Boston: Beacon, 2009), 109–128.

110. Paul Goodman, *New Reformation: Notes of a Neolithic Conservative* (New York: PMPress, [1970] 2010), 31.

111. See Eugene C. Lee and Willis D. Hawley, *The Challenge of California* (Boston: Little, Brown, 1970), 129–140; Lou Cannon, *Governor Reagan: His Rise to Power* (New York: Public Affairs, 2003), 189–194; John Patrick Diggins, *Ronald Reagan: Fate, Freedom, and the Making of History* (New York: Norton, 2007), 135–136.

112. Quoted in Bill Kovach, "Communes Spread as the Young Reject Old Values," *New York Times*, 17 December 1970. West linked the "green rebellion" to "red" and "black" rebellions against government and racism, respectively.

113. Timothy Miller, *The 60s Communes: Hippies and Beyond* (Syracuse, NY: Syracuse University Press, 1999), 68.

114. Ibid., 44, 201.

115. David E. Smith et al., introduction to *The Free Clinic: A Community Approach to Health Care and Drug Abuse*, ed. David E. Smith et al. (Beloit, WI: Stash, 1971), xiv. See also Gregory L. Weiss, *Grassroots Medicine: The Story of America's Free Health Clinics* (Lanham, MD: Rowman and Littlefield, 2006), 28.

116. Richard J. Alexander, "People's Free Clinic," *Texas Medicine* 68, no. 2 (1972): 94–100.

117. Smith et al., introduction to *The Free Clinic*, vi.

118. Ibid., vii.

119. Ibid., viii.

120. David E. Smith and John Luce, *Love Needs Care* (Boston: Little, Brown, 1971), 7, 40.

121. "Proceedings of the First National Free Clinic Council Symposium," in *The Free Clinic*, ed. Smith et al., 6.

122. Alexander, "People's Free Clinic," 95.

123. Smith et al., introduction to *The Free Clinic*, x–xi. For a broader study, see the special issue of *American Journal of Psychiatry* 126, no. 10 (1970), which includes two articles on mental health in urban ghettos.

124. "Proceedings of the First National Free Clinic Council Symposium," 13.

125. Smith and Luce, *Love Needs Care*, 80.

126. David E. Smith and Donald R. Wesson, "Introduction: The Politics of Uppers and Downers," in *Uppers and Downers*, ed. Smith and Wesson, 1.

127. Ibid, 2.

128. Alexander, "People's Free Clinic," 96.

129. Smith and Luce, *Love Needs Care*, 31.

130. Ibid., 34.

131. Ibid., 40.

132. "The Charles Manson Trial (Tate-LaBianca Murder): The Defendants," www.law .umkc.edu/faculty/projects/ftrials/manson/mansondefendants.html.

133. "Proceedings of the First National Free Clinic Council Symposium," 9–10.

134. Timothy Miller, *The Hippies and American Values* (Knoxville: University of Tennessee Press, 1991), 95.

135. Smith and Luce, *Love Needs Care*, 39; George R. Gay, "The Haight-Ashbury Free Medical Clinic," in *It's So Good, Don't Even Try It Once*, ed. Smith and Gay, 73.

136. Jeffrey J. Kripal and Glenn W. Shuck, "Introducing Esalen," in *On the Edge of the Future: Esalen and the Evolution of American Culture*, ed. Jeffrey J. Kripal and Glenn W. Shuck (Bloomington: Indiana University Press, 2005), 5–6.

137. Michael H. Murphy, "Education for Transcendence," *Journal of Transpersonal Psychology* 1, no. 1 (1969): 21–33.

138. Jeffrey J. Kripal, *Esalen: America and the Religion of No Religion* (Chicago: University of Chicago Press, 2007), 3–4, 144.

139. Robert Forte, "The Esalen Institute, Sacred Mushrooms, and the Game of Golf: An Interview with Michael Murphy," in *Timothy Leary: Outside Looking In*, ed. Robert Forte (Rochester, VT: Park Street, 1999), 201, 199.

140. Ibid., 200.

141. Ibid., 201.

142. Quoted in Leo E. Litwak, "A Trip to Esalen," *New York Times*, 31 December 1967.

143. Forte, "The Esalen Institute, Sacred Mushrooms, and the Game of Golf," 199. For a candid account of Esalen's residential program, see Stuart Miller, *Hot Springs: The True Adventures of the First New York Jewish Literary Intellectual in the Human-Potential Movement* (New York: Viking, 1971). For Esalen's wider circle, see Anderson, *The Upstart Spring.*

144. Margaret A. Blair, "Meditation in the San Francisco Bay Area: An Introductory Survey," *Journal of Transpersonal Psychology* 2, no. 1 (1970): 61–70.

145. George Leonard was also a major promoter of Esalen, particularly with the June 1966 special issue of *Look* on California (featuring a photo series about "The Turned-On People" that included images of Murphy and Esalen) and Leonard's 1968 widely read book *Education and Ecstasy*, which was serialized in *Look*. For a discussion of Leonard's promotion of Esalen, see Kripal, *Esalen*, 202–221. For broader discussions of the human potential movement, see Eugene Taylor, *Shadow Culture: Psychology and Spirituality in America* (Washington: Counterpoint, 1999), 235–282.

146. William C. Shutz, *Joy: Expanding Human Awareness* (London: Penguin, 1967), 11, 15.

147. Ibid., 18. Schutz discusses this threefold theory in *FIRO: A Three Dimensional Theory of Interpersonal Behaviour* (New York: Rinehart, 1958).

148. Schutz, *Joy*, 16.

149. Ibid., 11, 189.

150. Josh Greenfield, "Paul Mazursky in Wonderland," *Life*, 4 September 1970, 51–56. See also Mazursky's interview at the Lee Strasberg Theater and Film Institute, included in the 2004 DVD of *Bob & Carol & Ted & Alice.*

151. Dyan Cannon, *Dear Cary: My Life with Cary Grant* (New York: It Books, 2011). Around 1969, Natalie Wood had hopes of playing Deborah Blau in a film version of *I Never Promised You a Rose Garden.*

CONCLUSION

1. Gerald N. Grob, *From Asylum to Community: Mental Health Policy in Modern America* (Princeton: Princeton University Press, 1991), 304.

2. Thomas Kuhn, *The Structure of Scientific Revolutions*, 2nd ed. (Chicago: University of Chicago Press, 1970), 175.

3. Ibid., 181.

4. Carl E. Pitts, "Twelve Years Later: A Reply to Carl Rogers," *Journal of Humanistic Psychology* 13, no. 1 (1973): 75.

5. Ibid., 81.

6. Carl Rogers, "Comment by Carl Rogers," *Journal of Humanistic Psychology* 13, no. 1 (1973): 84.

7. Karl A. Menninger, *The Vital Balance: The Life Process in Mental Health and Illness* (New York: Viking, 1963).

8. Richard M. Nixon, "Annual Message to the Congress on the State of the Union", 22 January 1970, www.presidency.ucsb.edu/ws/index.php?pid=2921

9. Richard M. Nixon, "State of the World Message," 18 February 1970, in Richard M. Nixon, *Richard Nixon: Speeches, Writings, Documents*, ed. Rick Perlstein (Princeton: Princeton University Press, 2008), 194; Richard M. Nixon, "The Present Welfare System," 8 August 1969, ibid.,164; and Richard M. Nixon, "Second State of the Union Message," 22 January 1971, in Richard M. Nixon, *1913: Chronology, Documents, Bibliographical Aids*, ed. Howard F. Bremer (Dobbs Ferry, NY: Oceana, 1975), 129.

10. Richard M. Nixon, "The Rights of Students," 3 June 1969, in *Richard M. Nixon, 1913*, ed. Bremer, 101.

11. Department of Health, Education, and Welfare, "Programs for the Handicapped," 7 December 1970, www.mnddc.org/dd_act/documents/hew_newsletters/12_7_70-PFH-HEW .pdf.

12. For a balanced reading of Nixon's healthcare plans, see Jonathan Engel, *Poor People's Medicine: Medicaid and American Charity since 1965* (Durham, NC: Duke University Press, 2006), 117–122.

13. Judith Groch, *The Right to Create* (Boston: Little, Brown, 1969), 55, 319.

14. John Carothers, *The African Mind in Health and Disease: A Study in Ethnopsychiatry* (New York: Negro Universities Press, 1970); Jean L. Briggs, *Never in Anger: Portrait of an Eskimo Family* (Cambridge: Harvard University Press, 1970).

15. Kenneth Clark, "Behind the Harlem Riots—Two Views," *New York Herald Tribune*, 29 July 1964.

16. Hannah Arendt, *On Violence* (San Diego: Harcourt Brace, 1970); Nathan Leites and Charles Wolf Jr., *Rebellion and Authority: An Analytic Essay on Insurgent Conflicts* (Chicago: Markham, 1970); Joan V. Bondurant, *Conflict: Violence and Nonviolence* (New York: Aldine, 1971).

17. David N. Daniels et al., *Violence and the Struggle for Existence* (Boston: Little, Brown, 1970).

18. Peter G. Bourne, *Men, Stress, and Vietnam* (Boston: Little, Brown, 1970), 114.

19. For a link between schizophrenia and depression, see Sheldon Roth, "The Seemingly Ubiquitous Depression Following Acute Schizophrenic Episodes," *American Journal of Psychiatry* 127, no. 1 (1970): 51–58. For a link between schizophrenia and suicide, see Michael Rotov, "Death by Suicide in the Hospital," *American Journal of Psychotherapy* 2 (April 1970): 216–227.

20. Thomas A. Williams et al., eds., *Recent Advances in the Psychobiology of the Depressive Illnesses* (Washington: National Institute of Mental Health, 1972), 344.

21. Stelazine (a brand of trifluoperazine), manufactured by Smith Kline and French Laboratories in Philadelphia, was advertised in the *American Journal of Psychiatry* throughout

1970; Andrew Scull, "The Mental Health Sector and the Social Sciences in Post–World War II USA. Part 1: Total War and its Aftermath," *History of Psychiatry* 22, no. 1 (2011), 4; Grob, *From Asylum to Community*, 299.

22. For discussions of dependency, see William A. Frosch, "Psychoanalytic Evaluation of Addiction and Habituation," *Journal of the American Psychoanalytic Association* 18, no. 1 (1970): 209–218; R. E. Reinert, "General Observations of Drug Habituation," *Bulletin of the Menninger Clinic* 34, no. 4 (1970): 195–204. For drug use among soldiers on active duty, see Samuel Black et al., "Patterns of Drug Use: A Study of 5,482 Subjects," *American Journal of Psychiatry* 127, 4 (1970): 420–423.

23. Arthur Janov, *The Primal Scream*, first British ed. (London: Abacus, 1973), 62.

24. Ibid., 63, 78.

25. Ibid., 351.

26. Hilde Bruch, "Approaches to Anorexia Nervosa," in *Anorexia and Obesity*, ed. Christopher V. Rowland Jr., (Boston: Little, Brown, 1970), 19. Bruch also published an extended study, *Eating Disorders: Obesity, Anorexia Nervosa, and the Person Within* (New York: Basic, 1973), and a book for general readers, *Golden Cage: The Enigma of Anorexia Nervosa* (Cambridge: Harvard University Press, 1978).

27. Bruch, "Psychotherapy and Eating Disorders," in *Anorexia and Obesity*, ed. Rowland, 348–349, 337.

28. Alice Wolfson, "Health Care May Be Hazardous to Your Health," in *Liberation Now! Writings from the Women's Liberation Movement* (New York: Dell, 1971), 330. See also Sandra Morgen, "Women Physicians and the Twentieth-Century Women's Health Movement in the United States," in *Women Physicians and the Cultures of Medicine*, ed. Ellen S. More et al. (Baltimore: Johns Hopkins University Press, 2009), 162.

29. Ibid., 163–164; Boston Women's Health Book Collective, *Our Bodies, Ourselves*, paperback ed. (New York: Simon and Schuster, 1973).

30. Susan Wells, "Narrative Forms in *Our Bodies, Ourselves*," in *Women Physicians and the Cultures of Medicine*, ed. More et al., 188–189.

31. Boston Women's Health Book Collective, *Our Bodies, Ourselves*, 2.

32. Wells, "Narrative Forms in *Our Bodies, Ourselves*," 201.

33. Boston Women's Health Book Collective, *Our Bodies, Ourselves*, 2. Gloria Steinem shared this concern that women's health issues had been downplayed in the 1940s and 1950s, particularly in relation to her mother's "nervous breakdown," tranquilizer prescription, and hospitalization in the mid-1940s. See Gloria Steinem, "Ruth's Song (Because She Could Not Sing It)," in Gloria Steinem, *Outrageous Acts and Everyday Rebellions* (New York: Signet, 1983), 147–50.

34. Boston Women's Health Book Collective, *Our Bodies, Ourselves*, 3.

35. Shulamith Firestone, *The Dialectic of Sex* (New York: William Morrow, 1970), 36–37, 141–142.

36. Gregory Bateson, *Steps to an Ecology of Mind: Collected Essays in Anthropology, Psychiatry, Evolution, and Epistemology* (Chicago: University of Chicago Press, [1972] 2000), 490.

37. Ibid. See Max Weber, *From Max Weber: Essays in Sociology*, ed. and trans. H. H. Gerth and C. Wright Mills (New York: Oxford University Press, 1958), 323–57.

38. Bateson, *Steps to an Ecology of Mind*, 506.

39. Ibid., 505.

40. Arthur Burton, "Encounter: An Overview," in *Encounter: The Theory and Practice of Encounter Groups*, ed. Arthur Burton (San Francisco: Jossey-Bass, 1969), 2.

41. Noam Chomsky, "A Review of B. F. Skinner's Verbal Behavior," *Language* 35, no. 1 (1959): 26–58.

42. Erving Polster, "Encounter in Community," in *Encounter*, ed. Burton, 151–152.

43. Grob, *From Asylum to Community*, 292.

44. Polster, "Encounter in Community," 138–139. For a cross-cultural study of group therapy, see Carol Wolman, "Group Therapy in Two Languages, English and Navajo," *American Journal of Psychotherapy* 24, no. 4 (1970): 677–85.

45. E. Stanley Godbold Jr., *Jimmy and Rosalynn Carter* (Oxford: Oxford University Press, 2010), 214, 121.

46. Ibid., 215–216.

47. Thomas Szasz, *The Manufacture of Madness: A Comparative Study of the Inquisition and the Mental Health Movement* (New York: Harper and Row, 1970), xv.

48. Ibid., xvi.

49. Ibid., 292. For a more detailed discussion of Szasz's politics, see Michael E. Staub, *Madness Is Civilization: When the Diagnosis Was Social, 1948–1980* (Chicago: University of Chicago Press, 2011), 101–114.

50. Sick societies were frequently depicted in science-fiction stories, where protagonists with disabilities were usually compensated with extraordinary capacities. Examples include John Brunner, *The Whole Man* (1964); Philip K. Dick, *Dr. Bloodmoney* (1965); Anne McCaffrey, *The Ship Who Sang* (1969); and Andre Norton, *The Crystal Gryphon* (1972).

51. For a politicized use of "sick society," see Mark Rudd, "Reply to Uncle Grayson," *Up Against the Wall* 3, no. 1 (1968), 1–2. Rudd, the leader of the Students for a Democratic Society at Columbia University, was addressing the university's president.

52. Saul Bellow, *Mr. Sammler's Planet* (London: Penguin, [1970] 2007), 259.

Index

About the Author

Martin Halliwell is a professor of American studies at the University of Leicester, in the United Kingdom. His published work spans American cultural and intellectual history, the history of medicine and psychology, modern and contemporary American literature, American film after 1945, and avant-garde and popular culture. He is the author of eight monographs and two edited volumes, including *The Constant Dialogue: Reinhold Niebuhr and American Intellectual Culture* (2005), *American Thought and Culture in the 21st Century* (2008) and *William James and the Transatlantic Conversation* (2014). He was the eighteenth chair of the British Association for American Studies (2010–2013). He is the current chair of the English Association, and is a Fellow of the Royal Society of Arts.

CPSIA information can be obtained at www.ICGtesting.com
Printed in the USA
BVOW09s1143161014

370999BV00004B/11/P

"Martin Halliwell offers fresh and inventive insights into the postwar period, showing mastery over an amazing range of material to demonstrate how fully the therapeutic triumphed in American culture." — STEPHEN WHITFIELD, Max Richter Professor of American Civilization, Brandeis University

"Following varied terms of health and illness, mind and body, through successive changes in the healing arts, Halliwell shows the postwar 'triumph of the therapeutic' in a wholly new light." —HOWARD BRICK, Louis Evans Professor of U.S. History, University of Michigan

Therapeutic Revolutions examines the evolving relationship between American medicine, psychiatry, and culture from World War II to the dawn of the 1970s. In this richly layered intellectual history, Martin Halliwell ranges from national politics, public reports, and healthcare debates to the ways in which film, literature, and the mass media provided cultural channels for shaping and challenging preconceptions about health and illness.

Beginning with a discussion of the profound impact of World War II and the Cold War on mental health, Halliwell moves from the influence of work, family, and growing up in the Eisenhower years to the critique of institutional practice and the search for alternative therapeutic communities during the 1960s. Blending a discussion of such influential postwar thinkers as Erich Fromm, William Menninger, Erving Goffman, Erik Erikson, and Herbert Marcuse with perceptive readings of a range of cultural texts that illuminate mental health issues—among them *Spellbound, Shock Corridor, Revolutionary Road,* and *I Never Promised You a Rose Garden*—this compelling study argues that the postwar therapeutic revolutions closely interlink contrasting discourses of authority and liberation.

MARTIN HALLIWELL is a professor of American studies and deputy pro-vice-chancellor for Internationalization at the University of Leicester, U.K. He was the 18th chair of the British Association for American Studies (2010-13). He is a fellow of the Royal Society of Arts, and the author of eight monographs and two edited volumes, most recently *William James and the Transatlantic Conversation.*

Cover photograph: Publicity still from *The Incredible Shrinking Man* (Jack Arnold, Universal, 1957)

Cover design by David Drummond

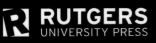

RUTGERS
UNIVERSITY PRESS

Visit our website at rutgerspress.rutgers.edu

ISBN 978-0-8135-6065-6

90000

9 780813 560656